Mary,
Thank you for your outstanding chapter. — Jake

Pediatric Outpatient Procedures

J. B. Lippincott Company

Philadelphia
New York   London
Hagerstown

Jacob A. Lohr, MD

Formerly:
McLemore Birdsong Professor
   and Vice Chairman
Director, Ambulatory Services
Chief, General Pediatrics Division
Department of Pediatrics
University of Virginia
Children's Medical Center
Charlottesville, Virginia

Currently:
Professor and Associate Chairman for
   Ambulatory Programs
Chief, Community Pediatrics Division
Department of Pediatrics
University of North Carolina
   School of Medicine
Chapel Hill, North Carolina

With 26 additional contributors

Pediatric Outpatient Procedures

Illustrations by

William C. Ober, MD

Clinical Assistant Professor
Department of Family Medicine
University of Virginia
Health Sciences Center
Charlottesville, Virginia

and

Claire W. Garrison, RN, BFA

Crozet, Virginia

Production Manager: Janet Greenwood
Production: Ruttle, Shaw & Wetherill
Compositor: Ruttle, Shaw & Wetherill
Printer/Binder: Halliday Lithograph

To my father, Dr. Dermot Lohr,
a trusted family physician in his community

and

To my mother, Blanche Grimes Lohr,
a saintly lady

1   3   5   6   4   2

Library of Congress Cataloging-in-Publication Data

Pediatric outpatient procedures / [edited by] Jacob A. Lohr, with 26
    additional contributors; illustrations by William C. Ober and
    Claire W. Garrison.
        p.   cm.
    Includes bibliographical references.
    Includes index.
    ISBN 0-397-50897-2
    1. Ambulatory care for children.   I. Lohr, Jacob A.
    [DNLM: 1. Ambulatory Care—in infancy & childhood.   2. Ambulatory
Care—methods.   3. Outpatient Clinics, Hospital.   WS 200 P37135]
RJ47.P38   1991
618.92—dc20
DNLM/DLC
for Library of Congress   90-13405
                                                                     CIP

The authors and publisher have exerted every effort to insure that drug selection and
dosage set forth in this text are in accord with current recommendations and practice at
the time of publication. However, in view of ongoing research, changes in government
regulations, and the constant flow of information relating to drug therapy and drug
reactions, the reader is urged to check the package insert for each drug for any change in
indications and dosage and for added warnings and precautions. This is particularly
important when the recommended agent is a new or infrequently employed drug.

Contributors

Peter A. Blasco, M.D.
Center for Children with Chronic Illness and Disability
University of Minnesota
Minneapolis, MN

Karen A. Bringelsen, M.D.
Assistant Professor
Director, Comprehensive Hemophilia Program
Department of Pediatrics
University of Virginia
Children's Medical Center
Charlottesville, VA

Bruce T. Carter, M.D.
Clinical Associate Professor
Departments of Ophthalmology and Pediatrics
University of Virginia
Health Sciences Center
Charlottesville, VA

Richard A. Christoph, M.D.
Assistant Professor
Director, Pediatric Emergency Services
University of Virginia
Children's Medical Center
Charlottesville, VA

Mary W. Clark, M.D.
Associate Professor of Surgery
Division of Orthopedics
Milton S. Hershey Medical Center
Hershey, PA

Leigh G. Donowitz, M.D.
Associate Professor
Department of Pediatrics
University of Virginia
Children's Medical Center
Charlottesville, VA

Kenneth E. Greer, M.D.
Professor
Department of Dermatology
University of Virginia
Health Sciences Center
Charlottesville, VA

Gregory F. Hayden
Professor
Department of Pediatrics
University of Virginia
Children's Medical Center
Charlottesville, VA

Peter W. Heymann, M.D.
Associate Professor
Chief, Pediatric Allergy and Pulmonary Medicine Division
Department of Pediatrics
University of Virginia
Children's Medical Center
Charlottesville, VA

Stuart S. Howards, M.D.
Professor
Department of Urology
Chief, Pediatric Urology Division
University of Virginia
Health Sciences Center
Charlottesville, VA

Richard W. Kesler, M.D.
Medical Alumni Professor and Vice Chairman
Department of Pediatrics
University of Virginia
Children's Medical Center
Charlottesville, VA

Paul R. Lambert, M.D.
Professor
Director, Otology and Neurotology
Department of Otolaryngology, Head and Neck Surgery
University of Virginia
Health Sciences Center
Charlottesville, VA

Elizabeth L. Lawton, R.N., P.N.P.
Clinical Pediatric Nurse Practitioner
Ambulatory Pediatrics
Department of Pediatrics
University of Virginia
Children's Medical Center
Charlottesville, VA

Jacob A. Lohr, M.D.
Professor and Associate Chairman for Ambulatory Programs
Chief, Community Pediatrics Division
Department of Pediatrics
University of North Carolina School of Medicine
Chapel Hill, NC

Marie Lynd, M.D.
Elmwood Pediatric Group
Rochester, NY

Andrew B. Martof, D.D.S.
Associate Professor
Department of Dentistry
University of Virginia
Health Sciences Center
Charlottesville, VA

Eugene D. McGahren, M.D.
Fellow, Pediatric Surgery
Children's Hospital Medical Center
Seattle, WA

Joan McIlhenny
Assistant Professor
Co-Director, Pediatric Radiology Division
Department of Radiology
University of Virginia
Health Sciences Center
Charlottesville, VA

Deborah D. Murphy, R.N.
Clinician A, Allergy Division
Ambulatory Pediatrics
Department of Pediatrics
University of Virginia
Children's Medical Center
Charlottesville, VA

Elaine S. Pomeranz, M.D.
Acting Director
Pediatric Emergency Services
University of Michigan
Ann Arbor, MI

Michael F. Rein, M.D.
Professor
Department of Internal Medicine
University of Virginia
Health Sciences Center
Charlottesville, VA

Bradley M. Rodgers, M.D.

Professor
Chief, Pediatric Surgery Division
Department of Surgery
University of Virginia
Health Sciences Center
Charlottesville, VA

Alan D. Rogol, M.D., Ph.D.

Professor of Pediatrics and Pharmacology
Chief, Endocrinology and Metabolism Division
University of Virginia
Children's Medical Center
Charlottesville, VA

Frank T. Saulsbury, M.D.

Associate Professor
Department of Pediatrics
University of Virginia
Children's Medical Center
Charlottesville, VA

Robert F. Selden, M.D.

Associate Professor
Director, Cystic Fibrosis Center
Department of Pediatrics
University of Virginia
Children's Medical Center
Charlottesville, VA

Deborah E. Smith, M.D.

Assistant Professor
Head, Section of Adolescent Medicine
Department of Pediatrics
University of Virginia
Children's Medical Center
Charlottesville, VA

James L. Sutphen, M.D.

Associate Professor
Chief, Pediatric Gastroenterology Division
Department of Pediatrics
University of Virginia
Children's Medical Center
Charlottesville, VA

Preface

The goal of this book is to provide well-illustrated guidelines for the performance of medical procedures for children seen as outpatients. The book is written for students of nursing and medicine, residents in training in pediatrics, family medicine, or emergency medicine, and nurses and physicians who provide care for children in outpatient facilities.

This textbook provides a framework within which pediatric outpatient procedural methods can be learned, refined, and taught. It is not the intent of this textbook to replace the "See one, do one, teach one" method, because written guidelines cannot supplant the learning experiences garnered from watching the skilled hands of a teacher carry out a procedure, from practicing the technique oneself, or from accepting the responsibility of accurately teaching the method to a learner.

The guidelines for each procedure, with a few exceptions, are described within the same format: 1) Purpose, 2) Selection of Patients, 3) Equipment and Supplies, 4) Description of Procedure, 5) Side Effects and Complications, and 6) Interpretation. It is hoped that familiarity with this simple format will make the guidelines for any of the individual procedures "user friendly."

A limited number of references are included in the chapters. The contributors were asked to provide only references for newer or controversial procedures and key references with which the readers may not be familiar.

I thank the editors of J. B. Lippincott Company for asking me to edit this text and Robert Dershowitz for his encouragement in undertaking the challenge. I appreciate the extended efforts of those who wrote the chapters; their experience and expertise are clearly reflected in the chapters' guidelines and illustrations. I am indebted to my associate, Elizabeth Lawton, whose viewpoints as an experienced clinic head nurse and nurse practitioner influenced the descriptions of procedures in virtually every chapter. I praise my friends, William Ober and Claire Garrison, who painstakingly created the drawings. Dr. Ober's prior experience as a family practitioner and Ms. Garrison's previous career as a pediatric nurse provided knowledge from which drawings of remarkable detail and accuracy arose. I note the contribution of Thomas Cutitta, who provided most of the photography. I acknowledge the editorial assistance of Austin Spruill, who as a pediatric resident, and Martha McGavic, who as a medical student, reviewed the completed chapters and offered many valuable comments. I am grateful to my secretary, Lisa Morris, whose contributions as typist, proofreader, editorial assistant, and organizer were essential.

Jacob A. Lohr, MD

Contents

Chapter 1

Body Measurements

Alan D. Rogol

Elizabeth L. Lawton

A. Growth Measurements

1. Purpose: The continued growth of a child is a tangible outward sign that in general the child's health is good. How a child compares with his peers can be derived from comparison of that child with the normal group represented on a standard growth chart. More importantly, the longitudinal measurements on an individual are a dynamic statement of the general condition of that specific child.

Tanner[1] has proposed that children should be measured accurately to identify individuals or groups of individuals within a community who require special care, to identify an illness that influences growth, or to define an ill child's response to therapy. Measurement also can be used as an index of the health and nutrition of a population or subpopulation. A more complete discussion of this subject is found in an excellent textbook by Rallison.[2]

Cross-sectional data are derived from the measurements of many children at various ages and are generally used to derive the "standard" growth charts. However, individual children do not necessarily grow according to standard curves, and longitudinal growth charts derived from growth points of the same child over time more accurately describe the growth pattern of an individual.

2. Selection of Patients:

a. Indications: Infants and children should have length and weight measurements recorded at all well visits. Occasionally, measurements at the time of acute illnesses will be useful. Certainly, the chronically ill or inappropriately developed patient should have measurements obtained at every visit.

b. Contraindications and Precautions: If a child is to be measured, it is important to measure him accurately to ensure an appropriate interpretation of the growth curve. There are no contraindications to obtaining growth measurements except in patients whose unstable condition would be jeopardized by the procedures.

3. Equipment and Supplies (See Appendix for equipment and supplies manufacturers and suppliers. Appendix is keyed to italicized words in the equipment and supplies lists):

a. Length/height

(1) *Neonates and infants*

· Physical growth *curve* appropriate for age and sex

· Commercially available *measuring device* with a fixed head board and a movable foot board (See Figure 1-1)

(2) *Children over approximately 2 years of age*

· Physical growth *curve* appropriate for age and sex

· Nonstretchable measuring tape permanently mounted to a wall or door

· Right-angle board or other device such as a large plastic right-angle triangle (See Figure 1-2)

b. Height velocity

· Height velocity *curve* for appropriate sex

· Same equipment as for height measurements (See above)

c. Weight

(1) *Neonates and infants*

· Physical growth *curve* appropriate for age and sex

· Scale *paper*

· Basket or pan *scale* (manual with beam and nonde-tachable weights or electronic). Regular maintenance is required to assure consistency of weight measurements. Accuracy should be to one tenth of a kilogram.

(2) *Children*

· Physical growth *curve* appropriate for age and sex

· Platform *scale* (manual with beam and nondetachable weights or electronic). Regular maintenance is required to ensure consistency of weight measurements. Accuracy should be to one tenth of a kilogram.

d. Head circumference

· Nonstretchable measuring *tape*, preferably one designed specifically for measuring head circumferences (See Figure 1-3)

e. Chest circumference

· Nonstretchable measuring *tape* (See Figure 1-4)

f. Body proportions

· Nonstretchable measuring *tape* (See Figures 1-5 and 1-6)

g. Skeletal maturation

· Standards from Atlas of Greulich and Pyle[3]

· Chart from Tanner and colleagues[1]

h. Adult height prediction

· Chart from Tanner and colleagues[1]

· Table from Bayly and Pinneau in Greulich and Pyle[3]

· Same equipment as for height measurement (See above)

i. Dental maturation

· Chart from Sinclair[4]

4. Description of Procedures:

a. Length/height

(1) Neonates infants

Small inaccuracies of length measurement can easily affect percentiles of length on growth curves. Unfortu-

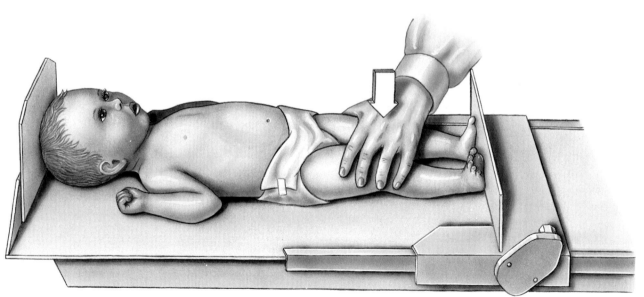

Figure 1-1.
Growth measurements—Length of an infant. Technique.

nately, several frequently used techniques yield inconsistent measurements. Placing a pen or pencil mark at points representing the top of the head and the bottom of the feet on the disposable paper covering the examination table pad and then measuring between the points can lead to erroneous measurements, because the paper often slips while the reference points are being made. Inaccuracies also result from plotting a recumbent length measurement on a growth curve derived from standing height measurements or plotting standing height measurement on a growth curve derived from recumbent length measurements. Lastly, height measurements made with the adjustable height bar on a platform scale may be misleading, because the bars often do not rest on a horizontal plane.

- Position the neonate or infant with his head against the head board of the measuring device and with the eye–ear plane perpendicular to the base of the measuring device (Figure 1-1). Have a parent or an assistant maintain the patient in this position.
- Hold the patient's knees flat and move the foot board until the feet are against it in a vertical position (Figure 1-1). In infants, take advantage of the archer's (tonic neck) reflex to have one leg straight against the measuring surface. Some recommend that both legs be fully extended before the measurement is taken. Less than full extension of the lower extremities, trunk, and neck will affect the accuracy of the procedure.
- Make the measurement from a fixed tape measure that rests along the edge of the device or with a tape measure held between the position of the head and foot boards.
- Record the measurement on the patient's visit form and on the physical growth curve.

(2) Children and adolescents

Standing height is measured for children older than 2 years of age, although supine length charts often include children up to 36 months of age. Diurnal variations of up to 0.7 cm in height may occur, with maximum height on arising. Under ideal circumstances, serial height measurements would all be obtained at the same time of day.

- Remove the child's shoes.
- Have the child stand against the vertical plane (wall or door) to which the measuring tape is attached. The heels, buttocks, shoulders, and back of the head should be touching the door or wall (Figure 1-2). The eye–ear plane should be perpendicular to the door or wall. The feet, including the heels, should be flat on the floor.
- Lower the right-angle device until it touches the top of the head.
- Read the height from the measuring tape where the lower edge of the right-angle device rests.
- Record the measurement on the patient's visit form and on the physical growth curve.

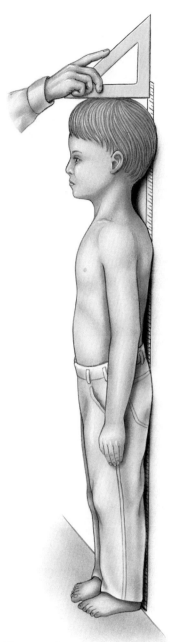

Figure 1-2.
Growth measurements—Height of a child or adolescent. Technique.

b. Height velocity
- Plot on a height velocity curve the serial height measurements obtained according to the above description.

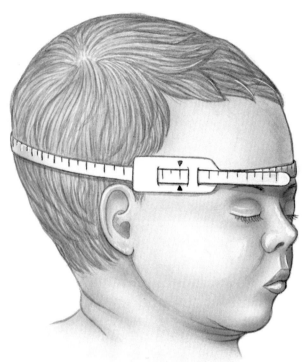

Figure 1-3.
Growth measurements—Head circumference. Technique.

c. Weight

Weight inaccuracies result from scales that are not properly balanced or maintained. The most useful weights are obtained with the patient completely undressed. The importance of respecting a child's or adolescent's modesty may require weighing the patient at least partially clothed. It is particularly important in comparing serial weights that the patient be weighed under the same conditions, including being dressed in a similar manner and ideally being weighed on the same scale. The weight should always be obtained with the patient as motionless as possible and not touching anything other than the pan or platform of the scale. It is equally important that no one is touching the patient during the procedure. The uncooperative infant or child who refuses to be weighed in the conventional manner may be indirectly weighed by having a parent hold the child in her arms, obtaining the weight of both parent and child, and subtracting the weight of the parent from the total weight. This method is not ideal but sometimes is the only alternative.

(1) Neonates and infants
  • Place a piece of scale paper or a diaper in the basket or pan scale to insure cleanliness and to avoid the discomfort of the baby being placed on the cold metal of the scale.

  • Balance the scale to zero weight.
  • Place the patient in the basket or pan scale and adjust the beam weights until the beam is balanced and the patient's weight is indicated. On an electronic scale, adjustment of beam weights is not necessary and the patient's weight is digitally indicated.
  • Record the weight on the patient's visit form and on the physical growth curve.

d. Head circumference
  • Place the nonstretchable tape or head circumference measuring device around the head so that the tape rests just above the eyebrows and ears and over the occipital protuberance, providing the largest occipital–frontal circumference (Figure 1-3). Occasionally, a particular hairstyle or the presence of a shunt, a bandage, or swelling resulting from trauma may preclude an accurate measurement.
  • Gentle restraint of the infant's hands by the parent may be necessary to prevent the infant from interfering with the procedure.

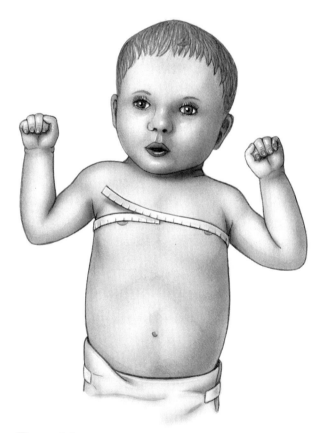

Figure 1-4.
Growth measurements—Chest circumference. Technique.

· Release the tape or device and obtain a second measurement. If the two measurements do not coincide, obtain additional measurements until consistent results are found.

· Record the measurement on the patient's visit form and on the physical growth curve.

e. Chest circumference

· Place the nonstretchable tape around the chest so that the tape rests at the level of the nipples (Figure 1-4).

· Take the measurement at the point of full expiration.

· Record the measurement on the patient's visit form.

f. Body proportions

Arm Span

· Use the nonstretchable measuring tape to measure on a horizontal plane from the center of the back to the tip of the longest finger. Hold the patient's arm at shoulder height in the mid-plane of his body (Figure 1-5).

· Determine the arm span by multiplying the measurement by 2 and record it on the patient's visit form.

Upper-to-Lower Segment Ratio

· Use the nonstretchable tape to measure the distance from the upper edge of the symphysis pubis to the soles of the feet to determine the lower segment length (Figure 1-6). Subtract this measurement from the height measurement (See page 2) to obtain the upper segment length.

· Calculate the ratio of the upper-to-lower length using the formula

U/L = upper segment length/lower segment length

· Record the ratio on the patient's visit form.

g. Skeletal maturation

· Obtain radiographs of appropriate bony structures.

· Identify the growth centers of the radiographed bones and compare their development with standards established by Greulich and Pyle (hand, wrist, or knee)[3] or by Tanner and colleagues (hand and wrist).[1]

· Record the bone or maturational age and compare it with the chronologic age.

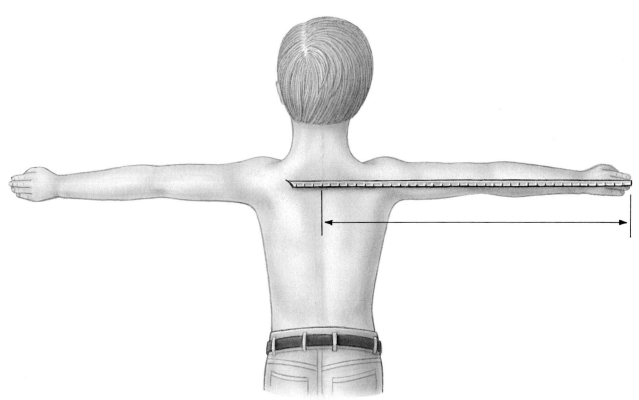

Figure 1-5.
Growth measurements—Body proportions (arm span). Technique.

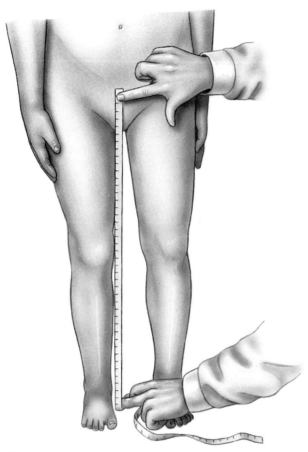

Figure 1-6.
Growth measurements—Body proportions (upper-to-lower segment ratio). Technique.

   h. Adult height prediction
     • Record present height.
     • Record present bone age.
     • Use tables in reference 1 or 3 to predict adult height.
   i. Dental maturation
     • Determine the number and location of the erupted primary (deciduous or "milk") and/or secondary (permanent) teeth and compare with standard dental maturation charts.[5]
     • As an alternative, obtain dental radiographs and compare them with additional standard dental maturation charts.[5]
5. Side Effects and Complications: None
6. Interpretation: Accurate, up-to-date growth charts are an essential tool for assessing a child's growth pattern. They are not only a sensitive indicator of a deviation from normal, but also an objective and easily understood visual representation of normal growth to share with a child's parents.

The height and weight curves are ordinarily interpreted together. An abnormality of one may exist independently of the other, but commonly abnormalities of height and weight are interrelated. Any apparent abnormality on the growth curves requires remeasurements before an interpretation is made. Examples of well-recognized normal variations of growth curves and deviations from normal are illustrated in Figure 1-7A–H:

   A. Normal decrease in weight percentiles and assumption of a new curve early in life.
   B. Genetic short stature
   C. Malnutrition
   D. Exogenous obesity
   E. Hypothyroidism
   F. Growth hormone deficiency
   G. Cushing's syndrome
   H. Congenital virilizing adrenal hyperplasia

The serially plotted head circumference of the infant is particularly important during the first year of life, when brain growth is most rapid and when abnormalities of brain or skull development are usually manifest. The head circumference curve often generally approximates the length and weight curves of the infant, but may normally assume a curve that rests percentiles away from either of the other curves. Regardless of the location of the head circumference curve, current measurements should not deviate significantly from that infant's previously established curve. Deviations are particularly concerning if they deviate beyond the upper and lower percentiles of the normal range of head growth.

Chest circumference measurements uncommonly provide a useful indicator of abnormal growth. In the newborn period the measurement should be somewhat less than the head circumference. By 1 year of age the chest circumference exceeds the head circumference. Visually apparent abnormalities of bony development of the chest may be reflected in actual measurements. An abnormally large chest circumference may be an early manifestation of obesity.

An arm span is related to the height and the stage of development.[6] The upper-to-lower segment ratio is also determined by developmental age, as the axial and appendicular skeletons grow at different rates at various stages of development. Diagnoses of many chondrodystrophies can be entertained in patients who have abnormal skeletal proportions.

Figure 1-7.
Growth measurements—Interpretation of height and weight curves. A, Normal decrease in weight percentiles and assumption of a new normal curve early in life. **B**, Genetic short stature. **C**, Malnutrition. **D**, Exogenous obesity.

(figure continued on page 8)

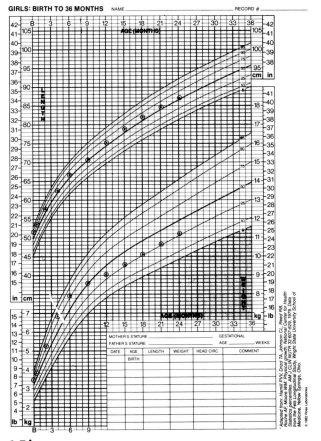

1-7A

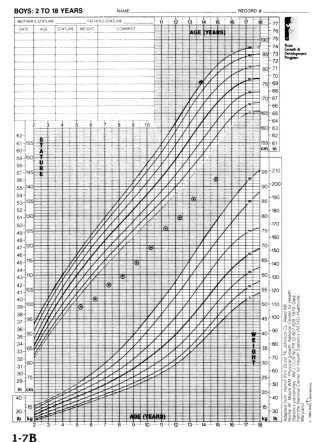

1-7B

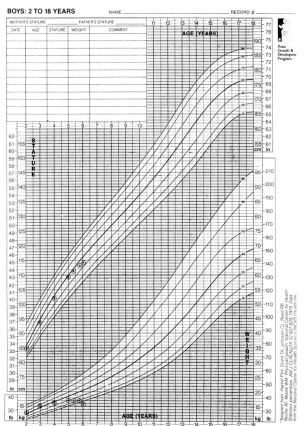

1-7C

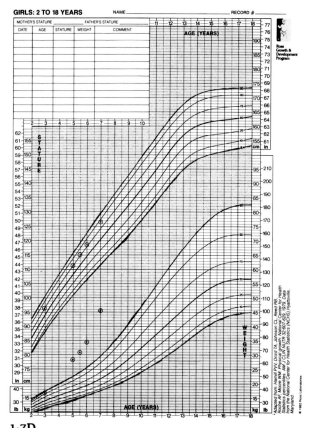

1-7D

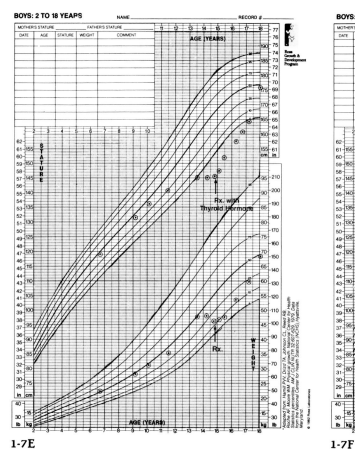

1-7E

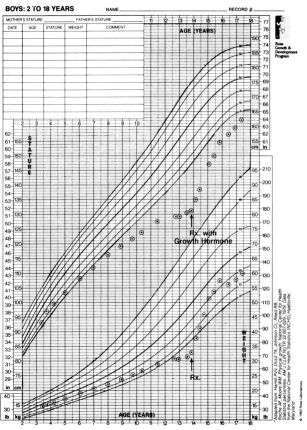

1-7F

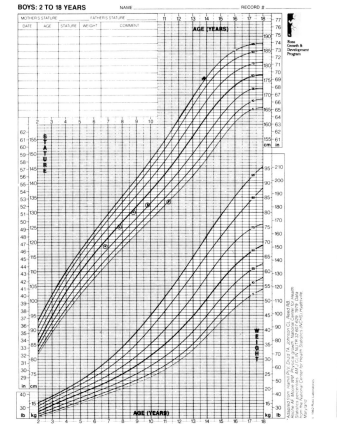

1-7G

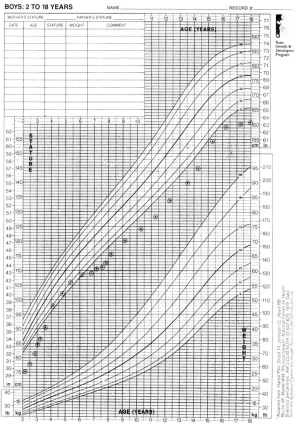

1-7H

Figure 1-7. (continued)
E, Hypothyroidism. **F**, Growth hormone deficiency. **G**, Cushing's syndrome. **H**, Congenital virilizing adrenal hyperplasia.

Radiographs obtained to determine skeletal maturation or bone age are compared with those of "average" children of various ages or by specific objective scoring criteria as established by Greulich and Pyle[3] or Tanner and colleagues.[1] This concept is the same as that of height age in that it represents that degree of skeletal maturation that an average child of that chronologic age should have attained. Dental maturation ("dental age") also may be determined in a similar manner by comparing the child's erupted teeth with standard charts.[5] There is, however, greater variance in the dental development than in the skeletal development.

Adult height can be predicted by comparing the child's present bone age and height with standard charts.[1,3] These predictions are not extremely accurate, as the child's adult height will be the result of many factors such as state of nutrition, general health, heights of the parents, age of onset of puberty, and the duration of the pubertal growth spurt.

References

1. Tanner JM, Whitehouse RH, Marshall WA, et al. Assessment of skeletal maturity and prediction of adult height. London: Academic Press, 1975.
2. Rallison ML. Growth disorders in infants, children and adolescents. New York: John Wiley and Sons, 1986, 144–75.
3. Greulich WW, Pyle SE. Radiographic atlas of skeletal development of the hand and wrist. 2nd ed. Stanford: Stanford University Press, 1959.
4. Sinclair D. Human growth after birth. Oxford: Oxford University Press, 1978, 98–116.
5. Garn SM, Rohman CG, Silverman FN. Radiographic standards for postnatal ossification and tooth calcification. Med Radiogr Photogr 1967; 43:45–66.
6. Wilkins LW. Methods of endocrine study and diagnoses, clinical and development studies in diagnosis and treatment of endocrine disorders in childhood and adolescence. 3rd ed. Springfield: Charles C. Thomas, 1965, 28–43.

Chapter 2

Vital Signs Measurements

Elizabeth L. Lawton

Jacob A. Lohr

A. Pulse Measurements

1. Purpose: The purpose of assessing the pulse is to determine cardiac rate and rhythm.

2. Selection of Patients:

a. Indications: The pulse should be assessed at all patient encounters.

b. Contraindications and Precautions: None

3. Equipment and Supplies (See Appendix for equipment and supplies manufacturers and suppliers. Appendix is keyed to italicized words in the equipment and supplies lists):

- Stethoscope
- Watch or clock

4. Description of Procedure:

The pulse ordinarily is assessed by either palpation or auscultation. In the seriously or critically ill patient, a more technical method may be used (See Blood Pressure Measurements—Oscillometric method, page 17).

- Count the pulse over a 30-second period and then multiply the resultant number by 2 to establish a rate per minute. In determining pulse rhythm you may have to palpate or auscultate for a full minute. Certainly if pulse irregularity is noted, monitor the pulse for at least a minute.
- Note and record variations in pulse quality or amplitude.

Palpation Method

- You can palpate the pulse and determine rate, rhythm, and amplitude at a femoral, radial, brachial, or carotid artery or over the apex of the cardiac precordium. Palpate a peripheral pulse with one, two, or three fingers. Do not use your thumb, because you may sense the thumb's pulse and mistake it for the patient's pulse. Palpate the cardiac apex with the palm of your hand. In infants, palpate the pulse at a femoral artery, which lies

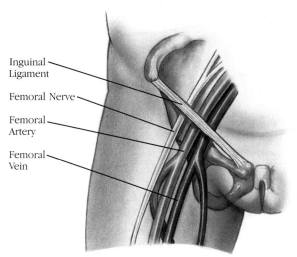

Inguinal Ligament
Femoral Nerve
Femoral Artery
Femoral Vein

Figure 2-1.
Pulse measurements—Palpation method. Anatomic location of femoral artery.

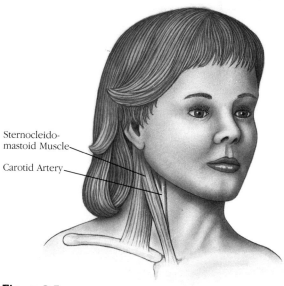

Sternocleido-
mastoid Muscle
Carotid Artery

Figure 2-3.
Pulse measurements—Palpation method. Anatomic location of carotid artery.

relatively superficially and somewhat medially just below the level of the inguinal ligament between the femoral nerve and the femoral vein (Figure 2-1) or palpate the cardiac apex. The infant should be supine and not crying. Beyond infancy, palpate the pulse at the radial artery, which lies just proximal to the wrist crease, lateral to the flexor carpi radialis tendon, and in a line with the space between the index and middle fingers (Figure 2-2). Under routine circumstances the carotid artery pulse is not used to determine a pulse rate, because of the potential to partially or totally occlude it. The pulse of the carotid artery, which can be palpated along the medial border of either sternocleidomastoid muscle (Fig-

ure 2-3), is assessed in the acute management of critically ill children.

Auscultation Method
· The pulse rate and quality can be evaluated by auscultation with a stethoscope over the cardiac precordium, preferably over the apex.

5. Side Effects and Complications: None
6. Interpretation: Normal pulse rates for age are noted in Table 2-1.

The normal pulse ordinarily has a regular rhythm. Activity (exercise) or stress (systemic disease, fever, hot or cold en-

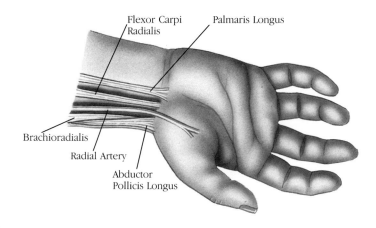

Flexor Carpi Radialis
Palmaris Longus
Brachioradialis
Radial Artery
Abductor Pollicis Longus

Figure 2-2.
Pulse measurements—Palpation method. Anatomic location of radial artery.

Table 2-1. Normal Pulse Rates for Age

Age	Normal Resting Pulse Rates (per minute)
Birth	100–170
Neonates	120–160
1 Year	80–140
2 Years	80–130
3 Years	80–120
4 Years	80–120
6 Years	75–115
8 Years	70–110
10 Years	70–110
Adolescence	70–90

vironment, fright, crying, etc.) will usually increase the pulse rate. For example, fever can increase the pulse rate by 8 to 10 beats per minute for each degree of fever. The respiratory cycle may influence the pulse rate and rhythm by increasing the rate during inspiration and decreasing it during expiration.

B. Respiration Measurements

1. Purpose: The purpose of assessing respirations is to determine respiratory rate and rhythm, depth of respirations, and signs of respiratory distress.

2. Selection of Patients:

a. Indications: Respirations should be assessed at all patient encounters.

b. Contraindications and Precautions: None

3. Equipment and Supplies (See Appendix for equipment and supplies manufacturers and suppliers. Appendix is keyed to italicized words in the equipment and supplies lists):

- Clock or watch
- Stethoscope

4. Description of Procedure:

Respirations can be assessed by observation, palpation, or auscultation. Regardless of the method, the patient should be as comfortable as possible during the procedure.

- Determine the respiratory rate and rhythm by observation or palpation of the associated thoracic excursions in older children or of abdominal movements in infants and small children. You also can determine rate and rhythm by auscultation over the lung fields.
- Measure the rate over a 30- to 60-second period and record as number of respirations per minute.
- Observe the rhythm over the same period and record as "regular" or "irregular (with or without periods of apnea)."
- Also observe the depth of respirations and record as "normal," "deep," or "shallow."

- Finally, note and record any degree of difficulty or distress and whether it is associated with inspiration or expiration.

5. Side Effects and Complications: None

6. Interpretation: The normal respiratory rates grouped by age are shown in Table 2-2. The rate may be increased by exercise or stress (hot or cold environment, fright, crying, etc.) or by many disease states, including those associated with fever, acidosis, hypoxia, or shock. The rate may be decreased by central nervous system disease, especially that associated with increased intracranial pressure, by alkalosis, or by sedatives or other drugs and toxins.

Depth of respiration can be affected by hypoxia, acidosis, alkalosis, central nervous system disease, and respiratory disease.

Respiratory difficulty may accompany exercise or stress and many disease states, including respiratory and cardiac disorders. Inspiratory distress is usually seen with upper airway obstruction, and expiratory distress is more often associated with lower airway obstruction.

C. Temperature Measurements

1. Purpose: The purpose of assessing the temperature is to determine as accurately as possible the body core temperature.

2. Selection of Patients:

a. Indications: The temperature should certainly be assessed for all patients with suspected illness. We assess temperature at all patient encounters.

b. Contraindications and Precautions: There are no contraindications and precautions except as noted under the specific methods described.

3. Equipment and Supplies (See Appendix for equipment and supplies manufacturers and suppliers. Appendix is keyed to italicized words in the equipment and supplies lists):

- *Thermometers* (Fahrenheit or Centigrade scale)
  —Mercury (glass) with covers
  —Electronic with probe covers
  —Ear thermometer with probe covers
  —Forehead strips
  —Enclosed in a pacifier

Table 2-2. Normal Respiratory Rates for Age

Age	Normal Respiratory Rates (per minute)
Birth	30–50
Neonates	40–60
1 Year	30–40
6 Years or older	16–20

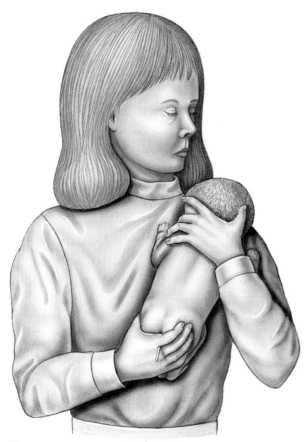

Figure 2-4.
Temperature measurements—Rectal temperature.
Positioning of infant in the mother's arms and holding of thermometer in place.

· *Lubricant*
· 2 × 2 gauze *pads*
· Watch or clock

4. Description of Procedures:

Rectal Temperature Measurement

This is the most accurate of the standard methods for assessing temperature. It is the procedure of choice in the patient under 4 years of age, in the uncooperative or unconscious patient, or in the patient with seizures. The procedure is contraindicated in the patient with neutropenia, because of the possibility of introducing colonic organisms into the bloodstream during the procedure. The procedure can be painful or even hazardous in the patient with rectal disease or vulvovaginitis.

· Depending on age and level of cooperation, have the patient held in the parent's arms (Figure 2-4) or recumbent on the examination table (Figure 2-5). Some suggest that you not carry out the procedure with a patient lying on her back, because the thermometer could be inserted at an angle that could lead to breaking the thermometer or perforating the rectum. Others are of the opinion that in infants virtually any comfortable position is satisfactory. You may need to have the extremities and trunk restrained. In the case of the unusually uncooperative patient, do not proceed with the procedure until the patient is calmed or restrained.

· Explain the procedure to the patient old enough to understand.

Mercury Thermometer

· Check the reading on the thermometer to be sure the mercury has been "shaken down" to below a normal reading. During reading, hold the distal ("non-bulb") end of the thermometer between the thumb and index fingers and rotate it slowly until the meniscus of the mercury is clearly visible. If a thermometer cover is being used, the cover may need to be slipped down toward the "bulb" end of the thermometer so that the mercury level can be readily seen.

· Remove the patient's diaper or underwear, keeping in mind her modesty.

· Lubricate the bulb (silver end) with lubricating jelly.

· Separate the buttocks and insert the thermometer bulb 2 to 5 cm into the rectum.

· Keep the thermometer in place by holding it with your fingers and squeezing the buttocks together (See Figures 2-4 and 2-5).

· Keep the thermometer inserted for 3 to 4 minutes.

· Remove the thermometer from the patient's rectum, remove the plastic cover from the thermometer, wipe off any lubricant from the thermometer, determine the temperature reading, and record the reading in the patient's record.

· Wipe any excess lubricant from the patient's buttocks and replace the diaper or underwear.

Electronic Thermometer

· The method is the same as for the glass thermometer except you insert the electronic thermometer probe, encased in a plastic cover, into the rectum. The temperature reading is displayed on a screen as soon as the maximum temperature is registered, usually within a minute.

Oral Temperature Measurement

Although less accurate than the rectal temperature, the oral method is generally the procedure of choice in the routine patient 4 years of age or older. The patient should be cooperative and alert and should have had nothing to eat or drink for at least 15 minutes before the procedure. Occasionally,

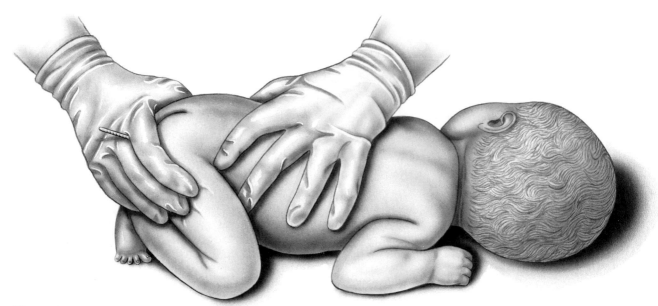

Figure 2-5.
Temperature measurements—Rectal temperatures. Positioning of patient on the
examination table and holding of thermometer in place.

the procedure cannot be used in patients with oral lesions
because of associated discomfort. Mouth breathing, either
voluntary or associated with nasal congestion, may falsely
lower the temperature reading.

- Explain the procedure to the patient.
- Place the bulb tip of the glass thermometer or the tip
of the probe of the electronic thermometer under the
tongue in the right or left posterior sublingual area
(Figure 2-6).
- Ask the patient to keep her mouth closed and to
breathe through her nose so that the reading is not
falsely low.
- Hold the thermometer in place or ask the patient to
do so.
- Keep the thermometer in place for up to 10 minutes
or until the thermometer reading is displayed on the
electronic thermometer.
- Note the temperature and record it.

Axillary Temperature Measurement

This method is known to be less accurate than rectal or oral
methods and is not used unless the more accurate methods
are contraindicated in a particular patient. An electronic thermometer is not recommended, because it is known to be
inaccurate in assessing axillary temperatures.

- Explain the procedure to the child.
- From the front of the patient place the glass thermo-

meter tip deep in the axilla with the long axis of the
instrument parallel to the roof of the axilla (Figure 2-7).
- Hold the child's arm against the chest cage so that the
bulb of the thermometer or tip of the probe is completely covered.
- Keep the thermometer in place for at least 10 minutes
and the probe in place until a reading is displayed.
- Remove the thermometer or probe, note the temperature, and record the temperature in the patient's record.

Ear Thermometer Method
(Infrared Tympanic Thermometry)

This method can be used in patients of any age. The procedure is noninvasive, painless, instantaneous, and provides an
accurate assessment of core temperature. However, the instruments are expensive. The probe senses the infrared energy emitted by the tympanic membrane and ear canal, dig-
itilizes the signal, and transmits it to the microprocessor. The
presence of ear wax apparently does not affect the instrument's accuracy. Inflammation of the tympanic membrane,
however, will falsely elevate the reading.

- Explain the procedure to the child.
- Gently place the covered probe at the external auditory meatus.
- The tympanic membrane temperature will be displayed on the screen within seconds.

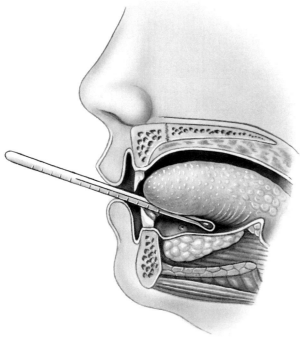

Figure 2-6.
Temperature measurements—Oral temperatures. Proper placement of the thermometer under the tongue.

· Remove the probe from the ear canal and discard the disposable cover.
· Note and record the temperature.

Other Methods
Liquid crystal forehead strips and pacifier thermometers are available.

These methods are attractive because of ease of use, patient acceptance, and limited cost. They have been shown to be inaccurate, however, and we do not recommend their use.
5. Side Effects and Complications: There are no significant problems associated with temperature measurements except as noted under the specific methods.
6. Interpretation: A rectal temperature greater than 38.0°C is considered a fever (See Fever Management Procedures, page 30). Ordinarily, oral temperatures are about 1° lower than corresponding rectal temperatures, and axillary temperatures are about 1° lower than corresponding oral temperatures.

D. Blood Pressure Measurements
1. Purpose: The purpose of the procedure is to provide an accurate assessment of arterial blood pressures.

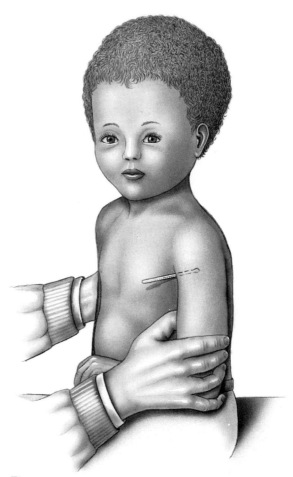

Figure 2-7.
Temperature measurements—Axillary temperatures. Proper placement of the thermometer in the axilla.

2. Selection of Patients:
a. Indications: The procedure is indicated in all ill patients and is indicated routinely in all patients 2 years of age or older.
b. Contraindications and Precautions: The presence of an arterial shunt or an intravenous line in an extremity is a contraindication to obtaining a blood pressure measurement in that extremity.
3. Equipment and Supplies (See Appendix for equipment and supplies manufacturers and suppliers. Appendix is keyed to italicized words in the equipment and supplies list):
· *Sphygmomanometer* with appropriate size upper arm and thigh cuffs. Upper arm cuffs come in standard sizes ranging in width from 3 to 20 cm. Thigh cuffs come in standard sizes, ranging in width from 16 to 24 cm.

- Stethoscope
- Elastic *bandage*
- Doppler ultrasound *instrument*
- Ultrasound *lubricant*
- Oscillometric vital signs *monitor*

4. Description of Procedures:

Auscultation Method

This method is the most commonly used procedure for the indirect measurement of systolic and diastolic pressures. It is noninvasive, simple, accurate, and inexpensive.

- Explain or demonstrate the procedure to the child.
- Have the patient in a sitting or supine position.
- Loosen or remove the child's clothing from the extremity (usually the arm) from which pressures will be obtained.
- Attach to the extremity a cuff that is at least one half the length of the upper arm (or thigh). Some recommend using a cuff that is no longer than two thirds the length of the upper arm (or thigh). We advocate using the largest cuff that can be placed between the antecubital fossa and the axilla (or between the popliteal fossa and the inguinal area.) The rubber bag in the cuff must encircle the extremity being used.
- Palpate the pulse of the brachial artery, which lies above the antecubital fossa along the lower medial border of the biceps brachii (Figure 2-8) (for upper extremity measurements) or of the popliteal artery, which lies in the center of the popliteal fossa (Figure 2-9), posterior tibial artery, which lies posterior to the medial malleolus (See Figure 20-25, page 273), or dorsalis pedis artery, which lies in the medial dorsal surface of the foot (See Figure 20-23, page 272) (for lower extremity measurements).
- Close the air valve and inflate the cuff to approximately 50 mm Hg above the expected systolic pressure.
- Place the diaphragm or bell of the stethoscope lightly over the artery.
- While listening carefully for vascular sounds, slowly release the air valve so that the cuff pressure decreases by approximately 2 to 3 mm Hg per second on the mercury column.
- The first vascular sound is heard when the pressure in the occluded vessel exceeds the pressure of the cuff. The pressure reading at this point represents the systolic pressure. Mentally note this reading as you proceed.
- Continue to slowly lower the pressure while listening. The point at which the vascular sounds disappear is commonly accepted as the diastolic pressure. The point at which the sounds begin to decrease in intensity, however, is thought to more precisely represent the true diastolic pressure.

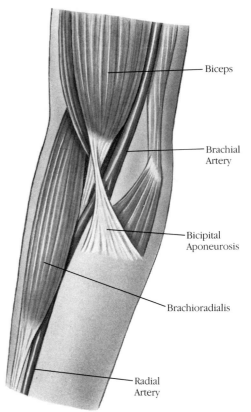

Biceps

Brachial Artery

Bicipital Aponeurosis

Brachioradialis

Radial Artery

Figure 2-8.
Blood pressure measurements—Palpation method.
Anatomic location of the brachial artery.

- Repeat the procedure until reproducible measurements of both systolic and diastolic pressures are obtained.
- Remove the cuff and record the systolic and diastolic pressures in the patient's chart.

Flush Method

This method is used in infants in whom an auscultatory measurement is not possible. It estimates the mean arterial pressure rather than the systolic or diastolic pressure.

- The patient should be in a relaxed supine position.
- Apply the cuff to the forearm or to the calf.
- Elevate the extremity as high as possible (at least above the level of the heart) and tightly wrap the portion of the extremity distal to the cuff. Start at the fingers or toes and wrap toward the cuff edge (Figure 2-10).
- Inflate the cuff to 150 to 200 mm Hg and remove the wrap. The hand or foot should be white.
- In good lighting (preferably sunlight) and with the

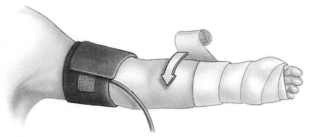

Figure 2-10.
Blood pressure measurements—Flush method. Technique.

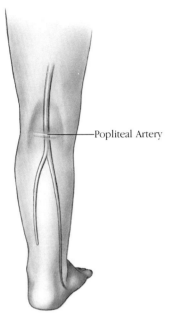

Figure 2-9.
Blood pressure measurements—Auscultation method.
Anatomic location of the popliteal artery.

Popliteal Artery

extremity at the same level as the heart, slowly lower the cuff pressure by opening the sphygmomanometer bulb valve. The pressure should drop no faster than 5 mm Hg every 2 to 3 seconds. While the pressure drops, observe the skin of the extremity distal to the cuff for return of blood flow, which is evidenced by the abrupt appearance of pink coloration starting at the lower cuff edge and spreading distally.
· Note the cuff pressure at which the pink coloration appeared and record as a mean arterial pressure (noting that it was obtained "by flush method").
· Repeat the procedure to obtain a reproducible result.

Palpation Method

This method is used when the auscultatory and flush methods are not feasible. It provides an assessment of systolic pressure only.
· Explain the procedure to the child if she is old enough to understand.
· Have the patient in a sitting or supine position.
· Place on the upper arm the largest cuff that will fit between the antecubital fossa and the axilla (See Auscultation Method, page 16).
· Close the air escape valve on the sphygmomanometer bulb and inflate the cuff until the pulse of the brachial artery (See Figure 2-8) is no longer palpable.

· Keep the palpating finger(s) over the artery and slowly release the pressure from the cuff by opening the bulb valve. The pressure should drop no faster than 5 mm Hg per second until the pulse is palpable.
· Record the pressure at which the pulse is first palpable. Repeat the procedure to be certain that a reproducible measurement has been obtained. Record the reading as a systolic pressure (noting that it was obtained "by palpation"), realizing that this reading will be 5 to 10 mm Hg lower than a systolic measurement using the auscultatory method.

Doppler Ultrasound Method

This method is indicated for infants and small children who must have an accurate determination of systolic blood pressure and who are difficult to assess with the auscultatory method. It is particularly useful in the critically ill or anesthetized patient.
· Explain the procedure to the child or a parent.
· Place the cuff as you would for the auscultatory method (See Auscultation Method).
· Coat the Doppler transducer with lubricant and place it beneath the cuff over the selected artery (brachial or popliteal) (See Figures 2-8 and 2-10, pages 16 and 17). Use the flow signal of the Doppler to locate the artery.
· Inflate the cuff to above the expected systolic pressure and slowly release the pressure while listening for the "tapping" sound that signals the systolic pressure.
· A "whooshing" sound may be noted in conjunction with the pulsing sound and represents the vessel wall signal. As the pressure is reduced, the vessel wall signal will change to a muffled sound, allowing you to estimate the diastolic pressure. Note the pressure reading and record as the "estimated diastolic pressure."

Oscillometric Method

This method is indicated for patients of any age who require an accurate measurement of blood pressures. It is especially

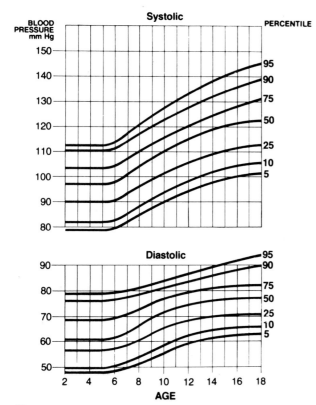

Figure 2-11.
Percentiles of blood pressure measurement for females (right arm, seated).

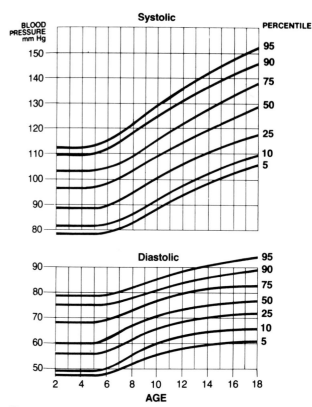

Figure 2-12.
Percentiles of blood pressure measurement for males (right arm, seated).

useful in the critically ill patient. It is a noninvasive procedure and provides automatic readings of systolic, diastolic, and mean pressures as well as pulse rate.

· Explain the procedure to the child or parents.
· Select an appropriate size cuff (See Auscultation Method, page 16).
· Connect the uninflated cuff to the hose.
· Place the cuff around the patient's extremity observing the mark on the inside of the cuff, which is placed over the selected artery. The cuff should be snug but not tight enough to impede venous return between determinations. The extremity should be placed at the same level as the heart.
· Push in the "Power On" switch.
· Press "Start" and await determinations of systolic, diastolic, mean arterial pressure, and pulse.
· Note the determinations and record them on the patient's record.
· Press the "Power Off" switch and remove the cuff from the patient.

5. Side Effects and Complications: There are no significant side effects or complications in an otherwise healthy child, other than the discomfort associated with a highly pressurized cuff. Patients with bleeding disorders may develop petechiae or ecchymoses distal to an inflated cuff.

6. Interpretation: Blood pressure measurements are affected by a wide variety of factors. Blood pressures vary with age. At birth systolic pressures are 60 to 90 mm Hg and diastolic pressures are 20 to 60. The pressures increase by 2 to 3 mm Hg per year until adult levels of around 120 mm Hg systolic and 80 mm Hg diastolic are reached. Pulse pressures (systolic pressure minus diastolic pressure) will normally vary between 20 and 50 mm Hg.

Blood pressures are also affected by gender (Figures 2-11 and 2-12).

The importance of cuff size has been noted. The statement that "The most common cause of 'hypertension' is a cuff that is too small" remains true.

Systolic pressures in the leg are equal to those in the arm in infants less than 1 year of age. In older infants and children, the leg pressure is 10 to 30 mm Hg higher than that in the arm.

Activity, stress, and the degree of cooperation can affect accuracy. Blood pressures also vary with the respiratory cycle, as does the pulse rate. Systolic and/or diastolic pressures are affected by a variety of cardiac, renal, central nervous system, metabolic, and other disorders and by certain drugs and toxins.

Chapter 3

Immunization, Medication, and Tuberculin Skin Test Administration Procedures

Elizabeth L. Lawton

Gregory F. Hayden

The administration of immunizations, medications, and tuberculin skin tests is an essential aspect of comprehensive child care. The specific procedures for administration vary according to the route of delivery (oral, subcutaneous, intramuscular, intravenous, rectal, topical, or intradermal) and will be discussed separately, but the following general guidelines apply to most routes of administration.

Explanation and Support

A brief description of the vaccine, medication, or skin test (why it is being given, the route of administration, expected effects, associated side effects, and treatment for anticipated side effects, if applicable) should be given to the child and parent to decrease apprehension and concern. It is often helpful to use a supportive approach based on the child's age, level of understanding, and developmental level.

Informed Consent

The child and/or her parent (or legal guardian) should be provided with detailed written and verbal information concerning any immunization(s) to be administered. The benefits and risks of the vaccine(s) should be explained. A signed consent form should be obtained and placed in the medical record to document that parents have been made aware of the possibility of a serious vaccine reaction. When appropriate, the same exchange of information (and documentation) should occur before medication administration.

Documentation

For immunizations, record in a permanent office log or file, and in the patient's permanent medical record, the date and type of vaccine administered, the manufacturer's name, the lot number, the signature and title of the person administering the vaccine, and the address of the facility where the vaccine was administered. The vaccine expiration date, the site, and the route of administration can also be recorded.

Storage

Proper storage of immunizations, medications, and skin tests is essential to maximize the benefits from their administration. Specific recommendations for handling and storage should be carefully followed. Refrigerators and freezers should contain thermometers to verify the appropriate storage temperature, which is checked on a regular basis.

Mixing

Immunizations and medications are available in a variety of formulations requiring varying levels of reconstitution. Recommendations for accurate preparation should be carefully followed for each vaccine and medication. An immunization or medication should be prepared for patient administration methodically in a quiet area free of distractions.

Dosing and Patient Identity

Proper identification of the patient by name is imperative before the procedure. Carefully check and recheck drug name, dosage to be given, and patient information before dosing. The dosage of most medications will be calculated on an individual basis for each pediatric patient, using her weight in kilograms. Most vaccines and tuberculin skin tests are given in standard doses according to an established schedule, which should be made available in advance to the patient, parents, or guardians.

Infectious Disease Precautions

Careful handwashing with soap and water before and after the procedure is essential to minimize the risk of transmission of infectious agents to or from the patient. Use a separate disposable needle and syringe for each immunization or medication. Discard all used materials in a puncture-proof contaminated materials container for proper disposal.

Restraint

Some form of positioning and restraint is often needed to administer immunizations, medications, and tuberculin skin tests safely to the pediatric patient. A nonfamily member, preferably a member of the health care team, should immobilize the child's arms and legs, assist in the procedure, and then help to comfort the child.

Proper Route

The preferred route of administration for medications often depends on the age and cooperation of the child and the condition for which the medication is being prescribed. The dosage and efficacy of some drugs may differ when given by alternative routes. Recommended routes of administration for currently available vaccines are shown in Table 3-1.

A. Administration of Oral Immunizations and Medications

1. Purpose: The purpose of this procedure is to provide oral immunizations and medications to patients. Orally administered medications include syrups, elixirs, suspensions, drops, tablets, capsules, and sprinkles. Most include flavoring or coloring agents. The only commonly used oral vaccine, live attenuated oral polio virus vaccine, comes as a sorbitol-flavored liquid in a unit dose.

2. Selection of Patients: For indications, contraindications, and precautions, consult the current edition of the Red Book, medication package insert, and other specific references as appropriate.

3. Equipment and Supplies (See Appendix for equipment and supplies manufacturers and suppliers. Appendix is keyed to italicized words in the equipment and supplies lists):

- Nipple
- Calibrated dropper
- Accurate measuring spoon/cup
- *Syringe* (See Figure 20-7, page 262) without attached needle
- Water or unsweetened fruit juice to follow medication as desired
- Absorbent wipes/tissue
- Spoons to crush tablets, if necessary
- Soft foods such as pudding or applesauce, if mixing sprinkles
- Ice, if a problem with taste is anticipated

4. Description of Procedure:

- Explain to the parents and to an older child the side effects and potential risks associated with the selected oral immunization or medication.
- Obtain informed consent for immunizations.
- Wash your hands.
- Prepare the immunization or medication according to the guidelines included in the accompanying package insert. Measure the medication using a calibrated device. Medication doses often are calculated on the basis of patient weight or size. A unit dose need not be measured if the entire amount is to be given as a single dose.
- Recheck the immunization or medication label, dose, and amount to be given.
- Pills and tablets may be crushed to powder between

Table 3-1. Vaccines Available in the United States, by Type and Recommended Routes of Administration

Vaccine	Type	Route
BCG (Bacillus of Calmette and Guérin)	Live bacteria	Intradermal or subcutaneous
Cholera	Inactivated bacteria	Subcutaneous or intradermal*
DTP (D = Diphtheria) (T = Tetanus) (P = Pertussis)	Toxoids and inactivated bacteria	Intramuscular
HB (Hepatitis B)	Inactive viral antigen	Intramuscular
Haemophilus influenzae b Polysaccharide (HibPV) or Conjugate (HibCV)	Bacterial polysaccharide or Polysaccharide conjugated to protein	Subcutaneous or intramuscular† Intramuscular
Influenza	Inactivated virus or viral components	Intramuscular
IPV (Inactivated Poliovirus Vaccine)	Inactivated viruses of all 3 serotypes	Subcutaneous
Measles	Live virus	Subcutaneous
Meningococcal	Bacterial polysaccharides of serotypes A/C/Y/W-135	Subcutaneous
MMR (M = Measles) (M = Mumps) (R = Rubella)	Live viruses	Subcutaneous
Mumps	Live virus	Subcutaneous
OPV (Oral Poliovirus Vaccine)	Live viruses of all 3 serotypes	Oral
Plague	Inactivated bacteria	Intramuscular
Pneumococcal	Bacterial polysaccharides of 23 pneumococcal types	Intramuscular or subcutaneous
Rabies	Inactivated virus	Subcutaneous or intradermal‡
Rubella	Live virus	Subcutaneous
Tetanus	Inactivated toxin (toxoid)	Intramuscular§
Td or DT¶ (T = Tetanus) (D or d = Diphtheria)	Inactivated toxins (toxoids)	Intramuscular§
Typhoid	Live-attenuated bacteria or inactivated bacteria	Oral Subcutaneous‖
Yellow fever	Live virus	Subcutaneous

* The intradermal dose is lower.
† Route depends on the manufacturer; consult package insert for recommendation for specific product used.
‡ Intradermal dose is lower and used only for preexposure vaccination.
§ Preparations with adjuvants should be given intramuscularly.
¶ DT = tetanus and diphtheria toxoids for use in children ages <7 years. Td = tetanus and diphtheria toxoids for use in persons aged ≥7 years. Td contains the same amount of tetanus toxoid as DTP or DT but a reduced dose of diphtheria toxoid.
‖ Boosters may be given intradermally unless acetone-killed and dried vaccine is used.
Printed with permission by Morbidity and Mortality Weekly Report 1989;38(13):207.

two spoons and then mixed with flavoring Do not crush enteric-coated tablets. Capsules may be greased with a small amount of butter or margarine to facilitate swallowing Chewable tablets may be chewed.

· Crushed pills and tablets or liquid medications may be mixed with a small amount of food or drink to disguise the taste if necessary. Ice may be used to decrease taste sensation by having an older child suck on ice chips before medication administration. Make sure the entire dose of medication is taken and that the medication and food or drink are compatible. Do not mix immunizations or medications with formula or milk, because the infant may subsequently reject this food source.

· Open capsules containing sprinkles just before administration and mix the contents into a spoonful of cold soft food that does not need chewing. Do not attempt to subdivide the contents of a sprinkle capsule, because of the possibility of a dosing error.

· When there is a choice, offer the patient the most palatable form of the medication. Offer the older child choices where appropriate and acceptable (liquid or pills, given with juice or water, etc.). A variety of measuring devices are available for the administration of liquid medications.

· Position the infant and younger child in a semireclining position with adequate head support (Figure 3-1). Position the older child sitting upright. Restrain the patient by gentle immobilization of the hands and feet, depending on the child's age, level of understanding, and cooperation.

· Administer the immunization or medication after explaining the procedure to the patient and/or parent.

· Place the immunization or medication onto the back of the tongue and give slowly to facilitate swallowing.

· Follow the immunization or medication with water or unsweetened fruit juice, if necessary, making sure the entire amount has been swallowed.

· Discard used equipment and supplies in an appropriate trash container.

5. Side Effects and Complications: The administration of oral immunizations and medications may cause gagging, choking, vomiting, or aspiration if the child is not properly positioned or the medication or vaccine is given too rapidly. The uncooperative child may spit the medication out if it is not placed on the back of the tongue and a swallow is not elicited. Refer to standard references (including the current edition of the Red Book and package inserts) and other specific references for additional information.

B. Administration of Subcutaneous (SQ) Immunizations and Medications

1. Purpose: The purpose of this procedure is to provide subcutaneous immunization and medication to patients.

2. Selection of Patients: For indications, contraindications, and precautions consult the Red Book, medication package insert, and other specific references as appropriate.

3. Equipment and Supplies (See Appendix for equipment and supplies manufacturers and suppliers. Appendix is keyed to italicized words in the equipment and supplies lists):

· One milliliter (Tuberculin) *syringe* with a 22- to 26-gauge ⅝- to ¾-inch long) *needle* (Figure 3-2)

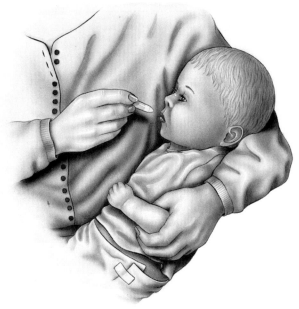

Figure 3-1.
Administration of oral immunizations and medications.
Positioning of patient.

· Isopropyl *alcohol* (70%)
· 2 × 2 gauze *pads*
· Sterile adhesive bandage *strip*

4. Description of Procedure:

· Explain to the patient and parent the reason for the immunization or medication.

· Obtain informed consent for immunization.

· Wash your hands.

· Prepare the immunization or medication according to the guidelines included in the package insert. Check the label and calculate the dosage, if necessary.

· Clean the rubber top of the vial with alcohol. Unwrap the syringe, attach the needle, and uncap the needle, remembering to keep the needle sterile.

· Pull back the syringe plunger, filling the syringe with air.

· Holding the vial upside down with one hand, insert the needle into the vial's rubber top with the other hand, and inject the air into the vial.

· Pull back the plunger, filling the syringe with medication to the correct dosage mark.

· Remove the needle and attached syringe from the vial, and holding the syringe upright, tap the syringe gently so that the air bubbles will rise to the top.

· Readjust the dose at eye level, expelling excess air, and carefully recap the needle.

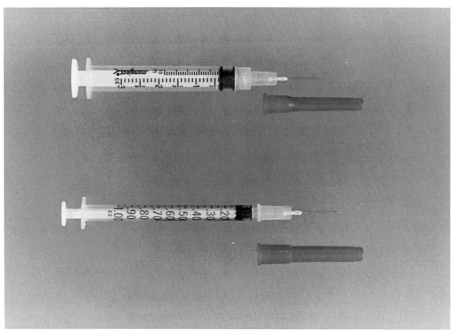

Figure 3-2.
Administration of subcutaneous and intramuscular immunizations and medications, intravenous medications, and intradermal tuberculin skin tests.
Equipment and supplies: 1. One-milliliter (tuberculin) syringe with 25-gauge, ⅝-inch needle; 2. Three-millimeter syringe with 25-gauge, ⅝-inch needle.

• Locate a proper injection site, usually the posterior aspect of the upper arm (Figure 3-3) or the outer aspect of the upper thigh.
• Position the patient in a comfortable sitting or recumbent position allowing access to the chosen injection site.
• Restrain the child's arms, hands, and legs if required. Get assistance if necessary and allow the parent to provide support.
• Clean the injection site with alcohol, and wipe the site with gauze.
• With the thumb and index finger, grasp (gently pinch) the skin around the injection site, raising the skin to ½ inch. Offer a brief explanation regarding expected pain. Tell the child that there will be a quick "ouch."
• Insert the needle with a dartlike motion into the skin at a 45-degree angle (Figure 3-3). Release the raised skin and retract the plunger to check for blood aspiration. If none appears, inject the medication slowly. If blood is aspirated, withdraw the needle and syringe without injecting the immunization or medication. Change the needle and slightly alter the injection site.
• Following injection, withdraw the needle and syringe,

and wipe the injection site with gauze if oozing or bleeding occurs.
• Apply a sterile adhesive bandage strip, if desired.
• Discard the uncapped needle and syringe in an appropriate contaminated materials container.
• Comfort the child with praise and offer the child a nonfood reward.
5. Side Effects and Complications: Discomfort or pain and slight bleeding at the injection site may occur. Refer to the Red Book, package insert, or other standard references for additional information.

C. Administration of Intramuscular (IM) Immunizations and Medications
1. Purpose: The purpose of this procedure is to administer intramuscular immunizations and medications.
2. Selection of Patients: For indications, contraindications and precautions, consult the Red Book, medication package insert, and other specific references as appropriate.
3. Equipment and Supplies (See Appendix for equipment and supplies manufacturers and suppliers. Appendix is keyed to italicized words in the equipment and supplies lists):

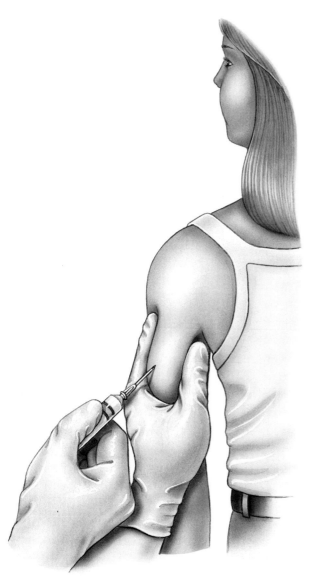

Figure 3-3.
Administration of subcutaneous immunizations and medications. Proper injection site (posterior aspect of the upper arm) and technique.

· Three-millimeter *syringe* and *needle* with needle gauge (usually 25 for infants and 20 to 22 for children) dependent on medication viscosity and needle length (⅝ inch to 1 inch) sufficient to reach the selected muscle mass (See Figure 3-2, page 24).
· Isopropyl *alcohol* (70%)
· 2 × 2 gauze *pads*
· Sterile adhesive bandage *strip*

4. Description of Procedure:
· Explain to the child and parents the reason for the intramuscular immunization or medication.
· Obtain informed consent from the parent or guardian.
· Wash your hands.
· Prepare the immunization or medication according to the guidelines included in the package insert.
· Check the label and calculate the dose.
· Clean the rubber top of the vial with alcohol.
· Unwrap the syringe and attach the needle, remembering to keep the needle sterile.
· Pull back the plunger, filling the syringe with air.
· Holding the vial upside down with one hand, insert the needle into the vial's rubber top with the other hand and inject the air into the vial.
· Pull back the plunger, filling the syringe with medication to the correct dosage mark.
· Remove the needle and syringe from the vial, holding the needle upright.
· Tap the syringe gently to remove air bubbles, readjust the dosage at eye level, and carefully recap the needle.
· Locate a proper injection site, depending on the child's age and the bulk of the muscle mass.
· In the infant or small child the anterolateral aspect of the upper thigh (vastus lateralis muscle) is preferred (Figure 3-4). This site is located approximately one third the distance downward from the hip to the knee, bordered by the mid-anterior thigh in front and the mid-lateral thigh on the side.
· In the older child or adolescent the outer aspect of the upper arm (deltoid muscle) (Figure 3-5) is preferred. This site is bordered above by the lower edge of the acromion, below by a line on the same plane as the roof of the axilla and laterally by the lines one third (anterior border) and two thirds (posterior border) of the way around the arm, starting at the anterior axillary line. In the younger child the size of deltoid muscle mass must be considered.
· Although the posterior gluteal area was commonly used for intramuscular injections in previous years, this site has several disadvantages: 1) The gluteal muscles are incompletely developed in small children, making the site unacceptable in this group of patients. 2) The sciatic nerve or the superior gluteal artery may be injured with misdirected injections. 3) Rabies vaccine and hepatitis B vaccine may be ineffective if injected into fat tissues of the buttocks. Except in small children, the upper outer quadrant of the buttocks (gluteus medius muscle; Figure 3-6) may be used when large volumes or multiple injections are necessary (e.g., immunoglobulin for hepatitis A prophylaxis or penicillin). The portion of the gluteus medius that is safe for injections lies

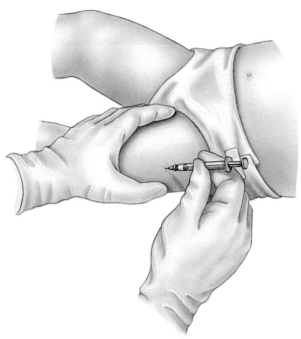

Figure 3-4.
Administration of intramuscular immunizations and medications. Proper injection site (anterolateral thigh [vastus lateralis muscle]) and technique for an infant or small child.

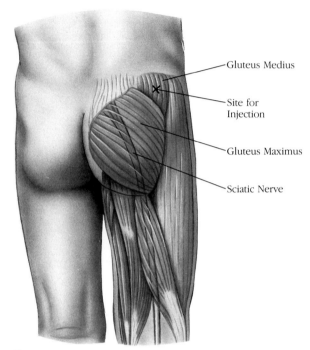

Figure 3-6.
Administration of intramuscular medications. Proper injection site (upper outer quadrant of the buttocks [gluteus medius muscle]) for large volume or multiple injections.

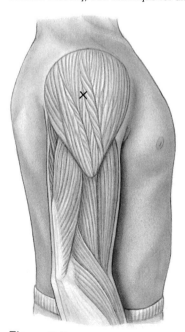

Figure 3-5.
Administration of intramuscular immunizations and medications. Proper injection site (outer aspect of upper arm [deltoid muscle]) for an older child or adolescent.

superior and lateral to a diagonal line drawn from the greater trochanter of the femur to the posterior superior iliac spine.

· Position the patient in a comfortable position (supine for vastus lateralis; standing, sitting, or recumbent for deltoid; and prone for gluteus medius injections), allowing access to the chosen injection site. The selected site should be fully exposed.

· Restrain the child's arms, hands, and legs if required. Get assistance if necessary. Allow the parents to comfort the child.

· Clean the injection site with alcohol. Wipe the site with gauze. Tell the child that there will be a quick "ouch."

· Insert the needle with a dartlike motion into the selected muscle mass at a 90-degree angle to the skin (see Figure 3-5).

· Retract the plunger to check for blood return. If none appears, slowly inject all immunization or medication. If blood is aspirated, withdraw the needle and syringe without injecting the immunization or medication. Change the needle and slightly alter the injection site.

• Withdraw the needle and syringe and wipe the injection site with gauze if oozing or bleeding occurs.
• Gently massage the site to promote absorption.
• Discard the uncapped needle and syringe in an appropriate contaminated materials container.
• Comfort the child with praise and offer a small non-food reward.
• Apply a sterile adhesive bandage strip, if desired.

5. Side Effects and Complications: Pain and bleeding may occur at the injection site. Limping may follow thigh injections. Rare complications may include infection, sterile abscess, cyst formation, local atrophy, scarring, or nerve impairment. Refer to the Red Book, package insert, and other standard references for additional information.

D. Administration of Intravenous (IV) Medications

1. Purpose: The purpose of this procedure is to provide intravenous medication to patients.

2. Selection of Patients: For indications, contraindications, and precautions consult the Red Book, package insert, and other specific references as appropriate.

3. Equipment and Supplies (See Appendix for equipment and supplies manufacturers and suppliers. Appendix is keyed to italicized words in the equipment and supplies lists):

• *Syringe* and *needle* with sizes dependent on medication volumes to be administered (See Figure 3-2)
• Isopropyl *alcohol* (70%)
• Functioning intravenous line with volume control chamber (See Infusion Procedures, page 275)

4. Description of Procedure:

• Explain the reason for the intravenous medication to the child and parent.
• Obtain informed consent.
• Wash your hands.
• Prepare the medication according to specific guidelines included in the package insert.
• Determine whether the medication is compatible with the intravenous fluid being administered.
• Position the patient in a comfortable sitting or recumbent position that allows access to the intravenous site.
• Restrain the child's arms, legs, and hands, if necessary.
• Reassure an older child that the needle will not be stuck into her skin (as it was when the intravenous line was started), but only into her intravenous tubing ("The shot is for your IV and not for you."). Warn her that the medication may burn or sting.
Z Make sure the intravenous line is not infiltrated, that there is no irritation at the intravenous insertion site, and that the tube connections are intact.
• Wipe the stopper on the volume control chamber with alcohol and inject the medication into the chamber,

checking dilution with the amount of existing fluid.
• Adjust the rate of administration (drops per minute).
• Label the volume control chamber with the name of the medication, the drops per minute, and your signature.
• If necessary, closely observe the patient while the drug is infusing.
• Note and chart any worrisome reactions occurring during the infusion and provide treatment as needed.
• Check and readjust the drip rate as necessary.
• After the medication has totally infused, flush the tubing with intravenous fluid, and readjust the flow to the prescribed infusion rate.
• Recheck the intravenous site and surrounding tissue for evidence of infiltration.
• Remove the medication label from the volume control chamber and record in the medical chart.

5. Side Effects and Complications: Crying, movement, or position often affects intravenous fluid flow. Infiltration and subsequent extravasation of medication and intravenous fluids occur as a result of improper needle or catheter placement. Venous spasm and hematoma may also occur as a complication. Thrombophlebitis, infection, and embolism may occur in rare instances.

E. Administration of Rectal Medications

1. Purpose: The purpose of this procedure is to administer rectal suppositories (for the administration of enemas, see Gastrointestinal Procedures, page 126).

2. Selection of Patients: For indications, contraindications, and precautions consult specific references, including the medication package inserts.

3. Equipment and Supplies (See Appendix for equipment and supplies manufacturers and suppliers. Appendix is keyed to italicized words in the equipment and supplies lists):

• Warm water to facilitate insertion of refrigerated suppository
• Nonsterile *gloves*
• Access to bathroom/toilet

4. Description of Procedure:

• Explain to the child and parents the reason for the rectal medication.
• Prepare the medication to be administered according to the guidelines included in the package insert.
• Check dosage and label.
• Do not divide suppositories.
• Remove the suppository covering and moisten the pointed end with warm water.
• Use disposable rubber gloves or plastic bags or wrap to protect your fingers.
• Position the child with the rectum exposed, maintaining her modesty.

- Have the child lie on the left side with one knee or both knees bent to the chest (See Figure 12-1, page 127).
- Restrain the hands, arms, and legs, as necessary.
- Gently insert the pointed end of the suppository into the rectum, past the anal sphincter. Hold a finger at the rectal opening for a few seconds to prevent expulsion of the suppository or hold the buttocks gently together.
- Wash your hands.
- Record the procedure in the patient's permanent medical chart.

5. Side Effects and Complications: Refer to standard references and the package insert for information regarding specific suppositories.

F. Administration of Topical Medications

1. Purpose: The purpose of this procedure is to provide application of topical medications to patients.

2. Selection of Patients: For indications, contraindications, and precautions consult specific references, including the medication package insert.

3. Equipment and Supplies (See Appendix for equipment and supplies manufacturers and suppliers. Appendix is keyed to italicized words in the equipment and supplies lists):
- *Gloves*
- Tongue *blades*

4. Description of Procedure:
- Explain the reason for application of topical medications to the patient and parents.
- Position the child so that skin areas that need medication are accessible. Maintain the patient's modesty.
- Restrain the hands, arms, and legs as necessary.
- Make sure the skin site is clean.
- Remove any remaining topical creams or ointments that have been previously applied.
- Apply a small amount of topical medication onto the gloved hand or the tongue depressor.
- Apply smoothly, using downward strokes to the skin area to be treated. Carefully cover the entire treatment area. Use medication sparingly.
- Remove your gloves and wash your hands.
- Discard the used supplies in an appropriate contaminated materials container.
- Chart the procedure in the patient's permanent medical chart. Note and chart any adverse effects (i.e., stinging, burning, increased skin irritation, itching, erythema, etc.).

5. Side Effects and Complications: Patients may become allergic to a medication's active ingredients, its vehicle, or its preservatives. Systemic absorption of topical medication is enhanced with occlusive dressings, prolonged treatment, denuded skin, and large body surface applications. Plastic occlusive dressings may enhance the development of skin atrophy, infection, and striae. Refer to standard references and package insert for additional information regarding specific medications.

G. Administration of Tuberculin Skin Tests

1. Purpose: The purpose of this procedure is to screen patients for exposure to tuberculosis.

2. Selection of Patients:

a. Indications: Most pediatric patients are screened at regular intervals or on suspected exposure. Annual tuberculin skin testing has been recommended for high-risk children from areas with an increased incidence of tuberculosis.

b. Contraindications and Precautions: Because of the potential for severe local reactions, tuberculin testing with purified protein derivative (PPD) should not be done routinely for those known to have previously positive tuberculin reactions. Reactivity to tuberculin testing may be suppressed or altered for those who have had recent immunization with certain live virus vaccines, who have concurrent viral infections, or who are taking immunosuppressive medication. Prior immunization with bacille Calmette-Guérin (BCG) may sensitize an individual for a varying length of time.

3. Equipment and Supplies (See Appendix for equipment and supplies manufacturers and suppliers. Appendix is keyed to italicized words in the equipment and supplies lists):
- Tine *test* and *PPD,* for Mantoux test
- Isopropyl *alcohol* (70%)
- 2 × 2 gauze *pads*
- Plastic tuberculin *syringe* with ⅝- to ¾-inch 25- to 26-gauge *needle*, with short bevel (See Figure 3-2)

Forms available: Tuberculin screening tests are available as multiple-puncture tines coated with old tuberculin or dried PPD and packaged in a disposable preloaded unit dose in boxes of 25. All multiple-puncture tests are equivalent to five tuberculin units (TU) of PPD Mantoux. For intradermal testing (Mantoux test), PPD in standard strength (5 TU per 0.1 ml) is packaged in 1-ml or 5-ml vials. Also available but rarely used in general practice are strengths of one TU per 0.1 ml (used primarily in those individuals suspected of being previously sensitized) and 250 TU per 0.1 ml (used exclusively in those individuals considered at risk who fail to react to a 5-TU injection). Both the 1-TU and the 250-TU strengths are supplied in 1-ml vials. All strengths are ready to use.

Storage: Tine applicators should be stored at room temperature (15° to 30°C). PPD for intradermal testing (Mantoux test) should be stored at between 2° and 8°C and protected from light when being used. After opening, a vial of PPD is stable for 1 month; it should be discarded after that period.

4. Description of Procedure:
- Ascertain exposure to tuberculosis and the history of any previous tuberculin testing.

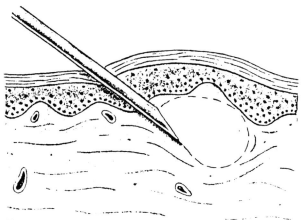

Figure 3-8.
Administration of tuberculin skin tests—Intradermal test.
Technique.

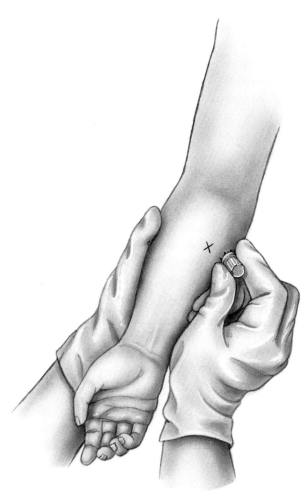

Figure 3-7.
Administration of tuberculin skin tests—Tine test.
Technique.

• Explain to the patient and parent the reason for skin testing and the method of application to be used.
• Assemble the equipment and supplies.
• Wash your hands.
• If administering the Mantoux test, draw up 0.1 ml of appropriate strength solution into a tuberculin syringe. Do not draw up the solution more than 1 hour before administration.
• Position the patient so that the flexor surface of the forearm is accessible.
• Restrain the arm as necessary. For the tine test, apply the impregnated tine disk firmly to the skin surface with even pressure for at least 1 second before removing the disk (Figure 3-7). The puncture sites should be visible. For the Mantoux test, inject 0.1 ml of tuberculin antigen superficially into the top skin layers (intradermally) with the needle bevel up to produce a white bleb (6 to 10 mm in diameter; Figure 3-8). The bleb will disappear in a few minutes.
• Mark the test area with a pen to enable checking the area for induration at 48 to 72 hours.
• Discuss the interpretation of the skin test. Specifically, describe the difference between inflammation ("redness") and induration ("an elevation of skin that can be felt with the fingertip").

5. Side Effects and Complications: Local reactions including pain, pruritis, ulceration, and necrosis may occur in patients who have been previously sensitized.

6. Interpretation: The skin tests should be carefully examined at 48 and 72 hours after administration. Any degree of palpable induration indicates a reaction that a health care provider should measure in millimeters with a ruler held transversely to the long axis of the forearm. You may give the patient or parent a comparison card, usually supplied with the packaged tine tests, to take home and send back after the test reading; but warn the patient or parent that if any degree of induration exists, the reaction should be medically evaluated. A positive or equivocal tine test should be confirmed with a standard Mantoux PPD 5-TU test. Induration of 10 mm or more is a positive reaction to a Mantoux test. A positive Mantoux test signifies exposure and infection, not necessarily disease. Diagnostic tests such as chest radiograph and sputum examination, however, may be indicated, depending on reaction to previous Mantoux tests and the patient's history of possible exposure. Induration less than 10 mm calls for further evaluation dependent on clinical judgment and suspected exposure. All positive TB reactions need to be reported to appropriate public health authorities. Refer to the Red Book for additional guidelines.

Chapter 4

Fever Management Procedures

Elaine S. Pomeranz

Jacob A. Lohr

Fever Reduction

Fever is an increase in the setpoint of the hypothalamic thermostat. In contrast, hyperpyrexia occurs when the hypothalamic setpoint is normal but the usual mechanisms used to dissipate heat are overwhelmed and body temperature increases out of control (e.g., malignant hyperthermia).

Fever is a common chief complaint in pediatric practice. Its importance is magnified by its great concern to parents. Studies have shown that many parents, regardless of education and socioeconomic class, believe that untreated fever has the potential to cause brain damage or death. Consequently, extraordinary measures such as alcohol baths and ice water enemas have been tried in an effort to control fever. Misconceptions regarding fever management are not limited to parents. Surveys of house officers indicate that unproven methods such as sponge bathing and alternating doses of aspirin and acetaminophen are often recommended.[1]

1. Purpose: The management of fever is controversial. Research has shown that fever is a response to infection that has been preserved evolutionarily and phylogenetically, implying that it is adaptive.[2] In fact, some organisms have been shown to cease replication at temperatures easily attained by febrile children.[3] It also has been shown that fevers are self-limited and will plateau at less than 41° to 42°C if untreated.[4] For these reasons, some would advocate not treating fever in otherwise healthy children. However, most physicians treat fever to make children more comfortable. Some authors suggest that the discomfort range for fever begins at approximately 39.5°C.[5,6]

2. Selection of Patients:

a. Indications: We define a fever as a rectal temperature of greater than 38.0°C (100.4°F) or an oral temperature of 37.0°C (98.6°F). An occasional healthy child, however, may normally have a temperature that exceeds this level as part of a diurnal variation. Studies of normal circadian rhythm show an increase of up to 0.8°C over the course of the day, with the peak being reached at around 6:00 P.M. In children younger than 18 months, the range may be even greater, with a diurnal difference of up to 1.4°C.

In most cases, treatment of fever is optional. The clearest indication for treating a fever of greater than 38.0°C rectal or 37.0°C oral is the case of a child less than 6 years old with a history of febrile seizures, although it has not been proven that fever management actually prevents the seizures.

Administration of an antipyretic with the diphtheria-pertussis-tetanus vaccination appears to minimize fever in the ensuing 24-hour period.

It has been suggested that fever itself may contribute to the mortality associated with sepsis[7] and that antipyretic treatment should therefore be added to antibiotic treatment of a septic child.

Most physicians would treat rectal temperatures above 39.5°C to reduce discomfort.

b. Contraindications and Precautions: The most important caveat in treatment of fever is that symptomatic treatment alone is not appropriate in an infant younger than 2 months of age in whom fever may be the only sign of serious illness, in an immunocompromised patient, or in any child who appears ill (lethargy, dehydration, significant anorexia, etc.).

A child of any age who is immunocompromised because of chronic illness or immunosuppressive medications should not have fever assessed or treated rectally because there is a risk of introducing bacteria from the gastrointestinal tract into the bloodstream.

We suggest that in general the child with a fever that is persistent beyond 72 hours' duration should be evaluated.

Chickenpox or influenza infections are considered contraindications for treating fever with aspirin because of the association of this drug with Reye's syndrome in children with these illnesses.

Factitious fevers may occur with overbundling or outside activity in hot weather. In this case, skin temperature is much closer to rectal temperature than if a genuine fever exists. Waiting approximately 30 minutes after removing clothes may be necessary before checking the temperature again.

3. Equipment and Supplies (See Appendix for equipment and supplies manufacturers and suppliers. Appendix is keyed to italicized words in the equipment and supplies lists):

- Thermometer
  - Electronic (digital) *thermometer*
  - Mercury *thermometer*
- Petroleum *jelly*
- Acetaminophen in several preparations:
  - Infant drops (80 mg per 0.8 mL)
  - Elixir or syrup (160 mg per 5 mL)
  - Tablets (80 mg, 325 mg)

  - Suppositories (120 mg, 325 mg, 650 mg), refrigerated
- 5-mL *syringes*

4. Description of Procedure:

a. *Measurement of temperature*
- Your first step in fever management is accurate assessment. Remember that oral temperatures are approximately 1°C lower than rectal temperatures in a child who is not hyperventilating. Hyperventilation lowers oral temperature even further. Axillary temperatures have been shown to be inaccurate unless measured over a period of at least 11 minutes.[8] Palpation is not a reliable method for parents or health professionals to detect fever,[9,10] nor are liquid crystal strips.[11]
- Rule out overbundling and allow a 30-minute cool-down period if necessary.
- Digital thermometers take the least amount of time to use and their accuracy of maximum temperature measurement is enhanced by the fact that they signal when the temperature plateaus.
- Mercury thermometers are useful to have available for parent education, but take approximately 3 minutes to use rectally and need to be held under the tongue for 10 minutes for accurate oral temperature measurement.[12]
  - Rectal temperatures are usually measured in the infant or young child (unless they are immunocompromised); thermometers should be inserted to a maximum depth of approximately 5 cm (less in infants) (See Vital Sign Measurements, Temperature Measurements, page 12).
  - When checking oral temperature in older children, ascertain that they have not recently had a hot or cold beverage and remind them not to mouth breathe.

b. *Treatment of fever*
- Effective treatment of fever is directed at lowering the hypothalamic setpoint, and this can only be achieved pharmacologically. Cold baths are uncomfortable and actually increase heat generation by producing shivering, and therefore are counterproductive. Remember that the main reason for treating fever is comfort, so the treatment should not cause more discomfort than the fever itself. Ice water enemas, cited as "cruel and unusual punishment,"[13] should never be used.
- Aspirin and acetaminophen were until recently the only antipyretics approved for use in children in the United States. Because of concern regarding the association of aspirin and Reye's syndrome, acetaminophen is probably the safest drug for the treatment of the febrile child, although it should be noted that it has the disadvantage of lacking anti-inflammatory properties. In other countries, nonsteroidals such as ibuprofen have been

used for their combined antipyretic and anti-inflammatory activity, and ibuprofen is available now for these purposes for children in the United States.

· The practice of alternating aspirin and acetaminophen has not been shown to be effective; and when the two are combined, the possibility of increased toxicity has been raised.[14]

· Alcohol baths should not be used, because inhalation of alcohol fumes during sponging has been associated with hypoglycemia and coma.[15]

Although sponging with tepid water is not detrimental, it has not been shown to add to the efficacy of acetaminophen alone unless it is continued for more than 30 minutes.[16]

· Acetaminophen suppositories can be used instead of oral preparations and are recommended for the febrile child who is also vomiting (See Administration of Rectal Medications, page 27). Most require refrigeration prior to use.

· The recommended dosage for acetaminophen either orally or rectally is 10 to 15 mg/kg every 4 hours. Because it is difficult to be precise with suppositories, a table of suggested suppository doses is provided (Table 4-1).

c. *Education of parents*

· Education of parents regarding antipyretic use is probably the most crucial aspect of fever management.

· Parents often have misconceptions about the danger of fever and need to be reassured that it will not increase the severity of the illness or cause brain damage if untreated.

· Inform parents about normal diurnal variation in body temperature and what constitutes fever. Your discussion should include determining what type of thermometer they have and which scale (centigrade or fahrenheit) they use and instructing them in the thermometer's use.

· Many parents are concerned about febrile seizures. It may reassure them that 3% of children aged 6 months to 6 years have febrile seizures, and that the seizures are almost always benign.

· Discourage overbundling.

· Remind parents that although fevers do not require treatment except for comfort, dehydration can be a concern in young children particularly, and increased fluid intake is important.

· Discourage parents from awakening a child from sleep to treat fever unless the child has a history of febrile seizures.

· Emphasize that fever, even in the absence of other signs or symptoms, requires medical evaluation if it occurs in the infant younger than 2 months of age.

· Studies show that parents frequently underdose with acetaminophen. Therefore, it is important to review with the parents the appropriate preparation, dosing, and administration of acetaminophen. A 5-mL syringe is helpful in demonstrating these actions and can be given to the parents to take home.

· Remind the parents that they can purchase acetaminophen suppositories and that the suppositories have a shelf life of at least 2 years when refrigerated.

5. Side Effects and Complications: Treatment of fever probably has negligible side effects or complications if serious illness is ruled out or treated appropriately. However, one should recall that some research suggests that fever is helpful in fighting infection and that treating fever therefore may not always be beneficial.

Aspirin has been associated with gastric irritation and anemia, especially if used chronically. It has also been associated with Reye's syndrome, as mentioned earlier.

Acetaminophen appears to be safe when used in the correct dose, but causes severe morbidity and mortality if abused. Therefore, use the same caution and respect as you do for any other medication.

Table 4-1. Acetaminophen Suppository Dose Per Age of Child

Age	Acetaminophen Dose (mg)	Suppository Dose (portion of selected suppository size)
2–3 months	40	~⅓ of 120 mg
4–11 months	80	~⅔ of 120 mg
12–24 months	120	All of 120 mg
2–3 years	160	~½ of 325 mg
4–5 years	240	~¾ of 325 mg
6–8 years	325	All of 325 mg
9–10 years	400	~⅔ of 650 mg
11–12 years	480	~¾ of 650 mg
>12 years	650	All of 650 mg

References

1. Weiss J, Herskwitz L. House officer management of the febrile child. Clin Pediatr 1983; 22:766–9.
2. Keusch GT. Fever: To be or not to be. NY State J Med 1976; 76:1998–2001.
3. Vaughn LK, Veale WL, Cooper KE. Antipyresis: Its effects on mortality of bacterially infected rabbits. Brain Res Bull 1980; 5:69.
4. DeBois EF. Why are fever temperatures over 106°F so rare? Am J Med Sci 1949; 217:361.
5. Schmitt BD. Fever phobia: Misconceptions of parents about fevers. Am J Dis Child 1980; 134:176–81.
6. Casey R, McMahan F, McCormick MC, Pasqueriello PS Jr, Zavod W, King FH Jr. Fever therapy: An educational intervention for parents. Pediatrics 1984; 73:600–5.
7. Cockett ATK, Goodwin WE. Hypothermia as a therapeutic adjunct

in management of bactermia shock after urological surgery. J Urol 1961; 85:358–64.

8. Nichols GA, Ruskin MM, Glor BAK, Kelly WH. Oral, axillary, and rectal temperature determinations and relationships. Nurs Res 1966; 15:307–10.

9. Banco L, Veltri D. Ability of mothers to subjectively assess the presence of fever in their children. Am J Dis Child 1984; 138:976–8.

10. Bergeson PS, Steinfeld HJ. How dependable is palpation as a screening method for fever? Clin Pediatr 1974; 13:350–1.

11. Reisinger KS, Kao J, Grant DM. Inaccuracy of the clinitemp skin thermometer. Pediatrics 1979; 64:4–6.

12. Nichols GA. Measurements of oral temperature in children. J Pediatr 1968; 72:253–6.

13. Yaffe SJ. Management of fever in infants and children. In: Fever. Lipton JM, ed. New York: Raven Press, 1980.

14. Bickers RG, Roberts RJ. Combined aspirin/acetaminophen toxicity. J Pediatr 1979; 94:1001–3.

15. Moss MH. Alcohol induced hypoglycemia and coma caused by alcohol sponging. Pediatrics 1970; 46:445–7.

16. Steele RW, Tanaka PT, Lava RP, Bass JW. Evaluation of sponging and of oral antipyretic therapy to reduce fever. J Pediatr 1970; 77:824–9.

Chapter 5

Infection Control Procedures

Leigh G. Donowitz

In an ideal world, physicians caring for children with infection would provide for them waiting, examination, and treatment space separate from the areas used to care for uninfected and thus susceptible children. This luxury of space and facilities is generally not available and even in situations where it is, the infectious disease often is not diagnosed until after the child has waited and been examined.

The goal of this chapter is to 1) outline routine isolation methods, 2) recommend specific isolation methods for selected infectious diseases commonly seen in the outpatient setting, 3) recommend specific precautions to be used in the routine care of the immunocompromised and thus highly susceptible patient, and 4) suggest routine cleaning, disinfection, and handwashing methods.

Table 5-1 is a list of isolation methods developed by the Centers for Disease Control and modified for outpatient use.

Table 5-2 is a list of common pediatric outpatient infections and/or specific organisms with the recommended isolation category and specific recommendations on the infective material, incubation period, and special necessary precautions. The listed diseases and organisms are common pediatric diagnoses and pathogens where specific recommendations have been made. Other common pediatric infections such as upper respiratory infections, pharyngitis, otitis media, flu syndromes, and sinusitis are not listed in this table and do not have recommended isolation procedures. Careful handwashing and routine room cleaning between patients would be all that is required in such instances.

Screening of all personnel for rubella, mumps, varicella, and tuberculosis should be a routine practice. Immunization of susceptible personnel against rubella and mumps should be mandated. Hepatitis B vaccine should be provided for all employees handling blood and body secretions. Influenza vaccines should be provided each year for all health care personnel. The varicella vaccine may be recommended in the near future for all susceptible health care personnel.

Table 5-1. Categories of Isolation

Type of Isolation/Precaution	Private Examination Room	Gown	Gloves	Mask	Negative-Pressure Ventilation
Strict	Yes	Yes	Yes	Yes	Yes
Contact	Yes	Indicated if soiling is likely	Indicated for touching infective material	Indicated for those who come close to patient	No
Respiratory	Yes	No	No	Indicated for those who come close to patient	No
Acid-fast bacilli	Yes	No	No	Only when patient is coughing and does not reliably cover mouth	Yes
Enteric	Indicated if patient hygiene is poor. May share room with patient infected with same organism.	Indicated if soiling is likely	Indicated for touching infective material	No	No
Drainage/secretion	No	Indicated if soiling is likely	Indicated for touching infective material	No	No
Blood/body fluid	Indicated if patient hygiene is poor. May share room with patient infected with same organism.	Indicated if soiling is likely	Indicated for touching infective material	No	No

Table 5-2. Common Pediatric Infectious Diseases and Recommended Isolation Procedures

Disease	Infective Material	Incubation Period	Isolation Category	Comments*
Acquired immune deficiency syndrome (AIDS)	Blood, semen, and possibly other body secretions	Unknown	Blood/body fluid	Avoid needlestick injury; the presence of opportunistic infections may require additional isolation precautions.
Bronchiolitis/croup; cause unknown	Respiratory secretions	Variable, depending on cause	Contact	Respiratory syncytial virus, parainfluenza viruses, adenoviruses, and influenza viruses have been associated with this syndrome.
Chickenpox (varicella)	Respiratory secretions and lesion secretions	8–21 days; varicella-zoster immune globulen (VZIG) may prolong incubation up to 28 days.	Strict	
Conjunctivitis (pink eye) Bacterial	Purulent exudate			
Chlamydia		24–72 hours	Drainage/secretion	Isolate for 48 hours of specific treatment.
		5–12 days or longer	Drainage/secretion	
Gonococcal		1–5 days	Contact	Isolate for 24 hours of specific treatment.
Viral and cause unknown		12 hours to 3 days	Drainage/secretion	A private room may be indicated if patient hygiene is poor.
Diarrhea—infective cause suspected	Feces	Depends on cause	Enteric	
Campylobacter	Feces	1–10 days	Enteric	
C. difficile	Feces	Unknown	Enteric	
E. coli	Feces	12–72 hours	Enteric	
Diphtheria Cutaneous	Lesion secretions	2–5 days, occasionally longer	Contact	Isolate until 2 cultures from skin lesions are negative, taken at least 24 hours apart after cessation of antibiotics.
Pharyngeal	Respiratory secretions		Strict	Maintain isolation until 2 cultures from both nose and throat are negative, taken 24 hours apart after cessation of antibiotics.
Encephalitis, cause unknown but infectious agent suspected	Feces	Variable, depending on causative agent	Enteric	Precautions for enteroviruses are generally indicated until a definitive diagnosis can be made.

Disease	Source of infection	Incubation period	Type of precaution	Isolation instructions
Enterobiasis (pinworms)	None			
Epiglottitis, due to *Haemophilus influenzae*	Respiratory	Probably less than 10 days	Respiratory	Isolate for 24 hours of specific treatment.
Erythema Infectiosum, "Fifth disease"	Respiratory secretions	4–14 days, usually 12–14 days	Respiratory	Isolate for 7 days after onset.
Gastroenteritis				
Campylobacter species	Feces	1–7 days or longer	Enteric	
Clostridium difficile	Feces	Unknown	Enteric	
Crytosporidium species	Feces	Not precisely known; probably 10 days	Enteric	
E. coli (pathogenic)	Feces	2–6 hours	Enteric	
Giardia lamblia	Feces	5–25 days or longer	Enteric	
Norwalk agent	Feces	24–48 hours	Enteric	
Rotavirus	Feces	Approximately 48 hours	Enteric	
Salmonella species	Feces	6–72 hours	Enteric	
Shigella species	Feces	1–7 days	Enteric	
Unknown cause	Feces	Vary with specific agent	Enteric	
Vibrio parahaemolyticus	Feces	5–29 hours	Enteric	
Viral	Feces	Vary with specific agent	Enteric	
Yersinia enterocolitica	Feces	1–3 weeks	Enteric	
German measles (Rubella)	Respiratory secretions	14–21 days, usually 16–18 days	Contact	Isolate for 7 days after onset of rash. Infants with congenital rubella require isolation for first year unless culture negative after 3 months of age.
Giardiasis	Feces	2–7 days	Enteric	
Gonococcal infections	Purulent exudate		Contact	Isolate for 24 hours of specific treatment.
Haemophilus influenzae infections	Respiratory secretions	Probably less than 10 days	Respiratory	Isolate for 24 hours of specific therapy.
Hand, foot, and mouth disease	Feces	Usually 3–5 days	Enteric	Isolate for 7 days after onset.
Hepatitis A (infectious)	Feces	15–50 days, usually 25–30 days	Enteric	A private room is required for a patient who is not toilet trained, has diarrhea, or has poor personal hygiene.
Hepatitis B (serum)	Blood and body fluids	50–180 days	Blood/body fluid	Infants born to HbsAg–positive mothers should be placed on Blood and Body Fluid Precautions.

continued on page 38

Table 5-2. Common Pediatric Infectious Diseases and Recommended Isolation Procedures (*Continued*)

Disease	Infective Material	Incubation Period	Isolation Category	Comments*
Herpangina	Feces	3–6 days	Enteric	Isolate for 7 days after onset.
Herpes simplex Mucocutaneous, recurrent	Lesion secretions	2–12 days	Drainage/secretion	Exposed lesions should be covered for day-care and school-age children infected as newborn infants or sexually abused with recurrences of genital HSV. Exclusion from day care or school is not indicated for oral lesions.
Impetigo	Lesion secretions	Approximately 10 days	Contact or Drainage/Secretion, depending on the extent of the infection.	Isolate for 24 hours of specific therapy.
Infectious mononucleosis	Respiratory secretions may be		None	
Influenza	Respiratory secretions	1–3 days	Contact	Viral shedding usually ceases within 7 days but may be longer in children. During epidemics, patients with influenza may be cohorted.
Lice (Pediculosis)	Infested area	Approximately 8–10 days after eggs hatch	Contact	Isolate for 24 hours after specific therapy. Mask not necessary.
Measles (Rubeola)	Respiratory secretions	6–21 days, usually 8–12 days	Respiratory	Persons who are susceptible to measles ideally should stay out of room. Persons who are not susceptible do not need to wear a mask. Isolate for minimum of 4 days after rash onset.
Meningitis				
Aseptic (nonbacterial or viral)	Feces	Vary with specific infectious agent	Enteric	
Fungal			None	
Haemophilus influenzae	Respiratory secretions	Probably 2–4 days	Respiratory	Isolate for 24 hours of specific therapy.
Listeria monocytogenes			None	
Neisseria meningitidis	Respiratory secretions	1–10 days, usually 2–4 days	Respiratory	Isolate for 24 hours of specific therapy. Prompt evaluation and follow-up of exposed persons is necessary.
Pneumococcal			None	
Tuberculosis			None	If pulmonary tuberculosis present, AFB precautions are necessary.
Other diagnosed bacterial			None	

Infection	Source of Infectious Material	Incubation Period	Precautions	Comments
Meningococcemia (meningococcal species)	Respiratory secretions		Respiratory	Isolate for 24 hours of specific therapy. Prompt evaluation and follow-up of exposed persons is necessary.
Mumps	Respiratory secretions	12–25 days, usually 16–18 days	Respiratory	Isolate for 9 days after onset. Persons who are not susceptible do not need to wear a mask.
Pediculosis (head, body, and pubic louse)	Infested area	Approximately 8–10 days after eggs hatch	Contact	Isolate for 24 hours of specific therapy. Mask not necessary.
Pertussis (whooping cough)	Respiratory secretions	7–21 days, usually 7–10 days	Respiratory	Isolate for 7 days of specific therapy: If not treated, isolate for 3 weeks after onset of paroxysms. Prompt evaluation and follow-up of exposed persons is necessary.
Pinworm infection (Enterobiasis)			None	
Pneumonia Bacterial not listed elsewhere			None	Respiratory secretions may be infective.
Chlamydia cause unknown	Respiratory secretions		Drainage/secretion	Precautions indicated for most likely cause.
Fungal			None	
Haemophilus influenzae	Respiratory secretions		Respiratory	Isolate for 24 hours of specific therapy.
Legionella		Probably less than 10 days	None	Respiratory secretions may be infective.
Meningococcal	Respiratory secretions		Respiratory	Isolate for 24 hours of specific therapy. Prompt evaluation and follow-up of exposed persons is necessary.
Multiply resistant bacterial	Respiratory secretions and possibly feces		Contact	Includes gram-negative bacilli resistant to all tested aminoglycosides, S. aureus resistant to methicillin, Pneumococcus resistant to penicillin, and H. influenzae resistant to ampicillin and chloramphenicol. In outbreaks, cohorting of infected and colonized patients may be indicated.
Mycoplasma	Respiratory secretions		None	Respiratory secretions may be infective.
Pneumococcal			None	Respiratory secretions may be infective.
S. aureus	Respiratory secretions		Contact	Isolate for 48 hours of effective therapy.
Streptococcus, group A	Respiratory secretions		Contact	Isolate for 24 hours of effective therapy.
Viral	Respiratory secretions		Contact	

continued on page 40

Table 5-2. Common Pediatric Infectious Diseases and Recommended Isolation Procedures (Continued)

Disease	Infective Material	Incubation Period	Isolation Category	Comments*
Respiratory Syncytial Virus (RSV)	Respiratory secretions	5–10 days	Contact	During epidemics, infected patients may be cohorted in the same room.
Ringworm			None	
Roseola infantum (exanthen subitum, Sixth disease)			None	
Rubella (German measles)	Respiratory secretions	14–21 days, usually 16–18 days	Contact	Isolate for 7 days after onset of rash. Infants with congenital rubella require isolation for first year unless culture negative after 3 months of age.
Scabies	Infested areas	2–6 weeks in persons without previous exposure; 1–4 days after repeat exposure.	Contact	Isolate for 24 hours after effective therapy. Masks are not needed.
Staphylococcal infections		Variable; usually 1–10 days for bullous impetigo and scalded skin syndrome.		
Skin, wound, or burn infections				Major = not contained in a dressing. Minor = adequately contained in a dressing.
Major	Pus		Contact	
Minor	Pus		Drainage/secretion	
Enterocolitis	Feces		Enteric	
Pneumonia or draining lung	Respiratory secretions		Contact	Isolate for 48 hours of effective therapy.
Scalded skin syndrome	Lesion drainage		Contact	
Toxic shock syndrome			Drainage/secretion	No evidence of person-to-person transmission has been documented.
Streptococcal infections group A		Usually 1–3 days		
Impetigo	Lesion secretions		Contact or drainage/ secretion, depending on the extent of the infection.	

Disease	Infective material	Incubation	Type of precautions	Comments
Pharyngitis	Respiratory secretions		Drainage/secretion	Isolate for 24 hours of effective therapy.
Pneumonia	Respiratory secretions		Contact	Isolate for 24 hours of effective therapy.
Scarlet fever	Respiratory secretions		Drainage/secretion	Isolate for 24 hours of effective therapy.
Syphilis Congenital	Lesion secretions and blood	10–90 days	Drainage/secretion Blood/body fluid	Isolate for 24 hours of effective therapy. Gloves must be worn when handling infant, as open lesions are highly infective.
Tapeworm Taeniasis Cysticercosis Other			None	
Tinea (ringworm)		2–10 weeks	None	
Tuberculosis Extrapulmonary, draining lesion	Pus		Drainage/secretion	A private room is important for children.
Pulmonary (positive sputum or cavity)	Respiratory secretions		AFB	Isolate 2–3 weeks after effective therapy initiated and sputum smears show reduction in number of TB organisms and cough decreasing.
Primary			None	
Skin test positive with no evidence of active disease			None	
Atypical (mycobacteria other than tuberculosis)			None	Must be receiving chemotherapy.

* Isolate for duration of illness unless specific directions given.

For patients coming to the office when phone contact before their arrival suggests a particular infection that is highly transmissible (e.g., chickenpox, meningococcus, measles), it would be important to directly admit that patient to an examination room and avoid waiting rooms and other crowded patient care areas. Immediately on entry into the health care system, these patients also can have a mask placed that would help reduce transmission to health care providers and other patients.

There is a group of patients in any general practice that will require special precautions because they lack immunity to routine pathogens. Specifically, patients with neutropenia of less than 1000 total white blood cells per cubic milliliter; transplantation patients; patients maintained on immunosuppressive or cytotoxic agents, including corticosteroids; newborns (especially premature newborns); and patients with congenital or acquired immunodeficiencies all should be included in this group of patients requiring special care to avoid exposure to infectious agents. If possible, these patients should be scheduled for the first appointment of the day to avoid their waiting in a potentially infectious environment. They should be admitted directly to a clean examination room. No infected employees, however minor the infection, should care for these patients. Careful handwashing before their routine examination, testing, and therapy should be required. Scrupulous technique should be maintained with all equipment used with these patients. They should have no routine rectal temperatures performed. All invasive procedures (blood drawing, intravenous insertion, etc.) should be preceded by a 5-minute iodophor disinfection of the proposed insertion site.

The following recommendations are general guidelines to be used for all patients:

1. An infant or child on isolation should not share toys with other children.
2. Isolation rooms assigned to patients with contagious airborne infections should be kept at negative pressure in relation to the anteroom or hallway. Negative pressure can be obtained by supplying less air to the area than is removed by the ventilation system. An inexpensive exhaust fan (12-inch diameter with speed of 1550 revolutions per minute) in the window of a private room can be used to create negative pressure for Strict, Respiratory, or Acid-Fast Bacilli isolation. Ideally, one examination room in each office is equipped in this fashion.

3. Gowns, gloves, and masks should be worn as indicated by the type of isolation category. Gowns should be worn only once, and discarded. Disposable single-use gloves are recommended; the wearing of gloves is not a substitute for handwashing. Masks should only be worn once; tied to cover the nose and mouth; and changed whenever moist.
4. Infected specimens should be securely sealed, bagged, and appropriately marked with an isolation sticker indicating the type of isolation required.
5. All needles should be disposed of by placing in special needle boxes and should always be treated as contaminated. Needles should never be recapped.
6. Linen from an isolation room should be handled as little as possible. It should be placed in a laundry bag, then double-bagged and placed in an appropriate area for pickup.
7. No special precautions are necessary for dishes unless they are visibly contaminated with infective material. The water temperature and dishwasher detergent used is sufficient to decontaminate dishes.
8. Routine and terminal cleaning of the isolation room is the same as used in other examination rooms, except housekeeping personnel should follow isolation precautions during routine and terminal cleaning. Furniture and floor should be cleaned with a disinfectant-detergent.
9. If an isolated patient must be transported to another area, use gown, gloves, and mask as indicated by the isolation category. The patient should wear a clean gown and dressings. A clean sheet should be placed over the stretcher or wheelchair and wrapped around the patient, leaving the face exposed if the patient is on Strict, Contact, Respiratory, or Acid-Fast Bacilli isolation. It is preferable to place a clean mask on the patient if indicated. The transporter should wear a mask when this cannot be done.
10. Handwashing before and after each patient contact is the single most important means of preventing the spread of infection. The use of an antimicrobial preparation should be considered for handwashing, especially after the care of a patient on isolation.
11. If a child is a patient at high risk for being infected with a human immunodeficiency virus (hemophiliac, homosexual, drug abuser) or is born to a high-risk mother, blood and body fluid precautions should be exercised when drawing blood from such a patient.

Chapter 6

Developmental Screening

Peter A. Blasco

The purpose of developmental screening is both to identify the child who may be developmentally delayed and to confirm normal developmental progress. The advantage in the first instance is the early identification of and early intervention for specific disabling conditions (Table 6-1). Of equal value is the opportunity to reassure parents that a child is progressing as expected. Such reassurance then becomes a basis for anticipatory guidance about upcoming developmental events. The pediatrician benefits, too, from an ongoing education in the developmental sequences of normal children that will facilitate the recognition of developmental retardation.

What features would the pediatric practitioner like to see in a developmental screen test? First of all, one wants accuracy; that is, a test that really does distinguish the normal from the delayed child. Secondly, one wants something that is both easy and relatively quick to administer and interpret. Thirdly, it ought to be fun to do and, in the best of all circumstances, it would be educational.

Traditionally, pediatricians have employed several methods for developmental screening: clinical judgment, parental history, developmental questionnaires, formal developmental screening tests, and informal screening assessments. Only the last, informal screening assessment, fulfills the desired requirements. Clinical judgment or acumen, for most of us, is an exceedingly poor method for screening development. It needs to be supplemented with something more objective. Relying solely on parental history can be misleading if you have an unreliable or inexperienced parent. The third option, the use of formal questionnaires filled out ahead of time, is dependent on parental experience and literacy. Perhaps what questionnaires offer most is to educate parents and, more importantly, to prime them to be thinking about developmental issues before they enter the physician's office. This value is realized only if the practitioner is prepared to follow

Table 6-1. Developmental Disabilities

Mental retardation
Cerebral palsy
Communication disorders (including autism)
Learning disabilities
Minimal brain dysfunction/attention deficit disorder
Blindness (visual impairment)
Deafness (hearing impairment)

up with something of substance in the office. Formal developmental screening tests, such as the Denver Developmental Screening Test (DDST), developed by William Frankenburg, and the Developmental Screening Inventory (DSI), originally developed by Arnold Gesell, are widely publicized and used. In the pediatrician's office, however, they are rarely used as they were designed and intended: most pediatricians have had little or no training in the method of administering these tests, few have a full compliment of test materials, and both are time consuming. Their reliability is not as good as generally believed, although the DSI is consistently better than the DDST.

The last option and the preferred method of screening is the informal approach. Practically speaking, most pediatricians are already using this approach. It allows for elements of all the above options, but also allows for shortcuts to save time. The key to good informal screening is a sound familiarity with the principles of developmental assessment, especially the separation of intellectual and motor entities. Employing these principles allows the practitioner to better understand and interpret any screening test or full assessment that relates to intelligence, behavior, or motor competence in children. Another concept to keep in mind is that external factors such as motivation, quality of experience, physical well-being, and others do not themselves constitute innate intellectual or motor potential. They are, however, critical to achievement; that is, the expression of one's innate abilities. These factors are not directly measured by the developmental screening process, but they may need to be accounted for in interpreting results.

In thinking about the entire pediatric physical, neurologic, and developmental examination, the developmental portion consists almost exclusively of items that can be observed with the parent doing the interacting or that fall into a framework of play rather than intrusive examination. It makes good sense to approach the overall examination with the developmental aspects first, hopefully allowing one to gain valuable information and also some rapport with the patient based on a pleasant interaction. Portions of the physical and neurologic examinations that require hands-on manipulation, often

threatening to the young child, may be slipped into the developmental exam (joint range of motion, muscle tone, palpation of the spine, coordination on reach, etc.) without damaging one's rapport in the least. A successful developmental examination almost always puts the patient (and parent) at ease and often improves the quality of the rest of the physical and neurologic examinations.

Informal Developmental Screening

There are three *independent* statements that the examiner should strive to make about each child at the conclusion of the developmental evaluation (whether a full assessment or simple screening). These are:

1. A clear statement as to the child's motor competence;
2. A clear, quantitative statement as to the child's intellectual level; and
3. A general impression of the child's behavior.

Most developmental tests recognize four distinct streams of development that are examined separately. One must appreciate what information each of these areas provides about mental and motor competence. The four streams, as described by Gesell,[1,2] are motor milestones (including gross and fine motor), language milestones (expressive and receptive), problem-solving milestones (sometimes referred to as fine motor or adaptive abilities), and psychosocial (or affective) milestones (Table 6-2). Each of these areas will be defined in more detail. As a simple and important starting point, remember that motor milestones are excellent indicators of motor competence but correlate poorly with intellectual development. Language and problem-solving skills provide the best early insights into a child's intellectual potential, and their evolution is very much independent of motor competence. They may be obscured, however, by motor disability and therefore may be more difficult to demonstrate. Psychosocial abilities are critical to understanding the whole child and to making a meaningful statement about behavior. They may or may not lend additional information to the assessment of intellectual and motor competence.

A final principle of developmental assessment has to do with arithmetic. The easiest and most useful way to think about a child's developmental progress is in terms of a single median age at which specific milestones are met rather than in terms of a "range of normal" for every milestone. In other words, a table with milestones matched up to a median age of accomplishment is generally more meaningful than bar graphs giving a span of ages for each milestone. This is not to say that a range of normal does not exist. It certainly does. The point is to concentrate one's effort on identifying a single age level (or a very narrow age range) for the child being tested, thus allowing comparison with the "average child" of

Table 6-2. Streams of Development

Language
    Expressive
    Receptive
Motor
    Fine
    Gross
Problem-solving
    (visual-motor)
Psychosocial
    (affective)

Table 6-3. Gross Motor Development

Prone:	Head up	1 month
	Chest up	2 months
	Up on elbows	3 months
	Up on hands	4 months
Roll:	Front to back	3–5 months
	Back to front	
Sit with support		5 months
Sit without support		7 months
Come to sit		8 months
Pull to stand		8–9 months
Cruise		9–10 months
Walk with 2 hands held		10 months
Walk with 1 hand held		11 months
Walk alone		12 months
Run (stiff-legged)		15 months
Walk up stairs (with rail)		21 months
Jump in place		24 months
Pedal tricycle		30 months
Walk down stairs, alternating feet		3 years

the same age. This approach avoids an unconnected series of statements about individual milestones. An allowance can be made for the range of normal at the end of the assessment, and at the same time other factors (such as prematurity) can be conveniently adjusted for as well.

Example: A 12-month-old is seen for well child care. By history he pulls up to stand (9 months) and cruises around furniture (10 months). His mother demonstrates that he will walk fairly well when she holds both hands, but when she lets one go, he loses his balance and falls over (Table 6-3). This is a child with a gross motor age of 10 months and a chronologic age of 12 months. This clearly identifies him as behaving, from a motor standpoint, like an average 10-month-old, 2 months behind the average. Is this something to be concerned about, or is he "within normal limits"? (Mother may already be concerned, especially if her neighbor's baby is already walking!) To decide, one must proceed to calculate a motor quotient (MQ):

$$MQ = \frac{\text{motor age}}{\text{chronologic age}} \times 100$$

In the example, the MQ would be 10/12, or roughly 83. The motor age and the motor quotient are both good descriptions of the child and have more meaning than trying to plot the individual milestones and decide whether each falls into the range of normal or not. What, then, is the "range of normal" for a developmental quotient? The lower limit is 70, and this will be addressed in more detail in the following sections. The upper limit is not of particular value to the parent or pediatrician unless one has an interest in identifying above-average individuals. Whether athletically or intellectually gifted children can be identified early by this method is thought provoking but speculative at present.

The child's mental age can be derived in a similar fashion using language and problem-solving milestones to provide the mental age. A developmental quotient for intelligence (consider it an estimated IQ) can then be calculated.

A. Assessment of Motor Development

1. Purpose: The purpose of this procedure is to determine whether the child's level of motor function is appropriate for his age.

2. Selection of Patients:

a. Indications: This procedure should be performed during well child screening and in response to specific concerns such as poor sitting, delayed walking, handedness before 18 months of age, etc.

b. Contraindications and Precautions: There are no contraindications except possible unreliability when the patient is acutely ill, acutely hungry, or already upset for some reason.

3. Equipment and Supplies (See Appendix for equipment and supplies manufacturers and suppliers. Appendix is keyed to italicized words in the equipment and supplies lists):

    · Reflex *hammer*

    · One-inch *cube* (or some other item the patient can grasp)

4. Description of Procedure:

Making a sound statement about a child's motor competence is always easier than trying to do the same for cognitive competence. This is due mostly to the fact that physicians are more comfortable with motor milestones and motor portions of the neurologic examination than they are with the assessment of intelligence. Parents also tend to focus on motor development in infancy and are much less aware of cognitive milestones. Hence, an accurate history of the child's motor milestones is usually easy to obtain, and it is ordinarily just as easy to observe the child's motor skills in the examining room. Motor milestones, arrived at by a combination of historic information and examination, should be separated into gross motor and fine motor abilities (Tables 6-3 and 6-4). Although it is recognized that there are slight differences in the attainment of motor milestones between sexes and among races, for the purpose of screening this is inconsequential.[3]

In addition to milestones, the motor part of the neurologic examination (the evaluation of muscle tone, muscle strength, deep tendon reflexes, and coordination of movement) is an essential component of the motor screen. The neurologic examination is rather difficult in the first 2 years of life because one usually is dealing with an uncooperative subject. The elicitation of reflexes (one is often swinging at a moving target) and the distinction between tone and strength are challenging and can be time consuming. In this age group, especially in the patients between 6 and 18 months of age, milestones alone can easily and precisely identify the delayed infant. After 2 to 3 years of age, the neurologic examination becomes easier and more meaningful as the patient becomes more cooperative. The third aspect of motor assessment, the elicitation of primitive reflexes and postural reactions, has its greatest value in young infants. Because these reflexes and reactions undergo dramatic changes in the first 6 months of life, they are highly useful in the very early recognition of significant motor impairment. However, they are for the most part beyond the scope of screening. Two excellent references are listed in the bibliography for those who are interested in further pursuit of this topic.[4,5]

5. Interpretation: Interpretation is based on a simple calculation of the motor quotient (MQ) (as previously defined) from the child's motor age and chronologic age. Any quotient above 80 is clearly within normal limits and anything below 70 should be considered abnormal until proven otherwise. One can add to this quantitative expression the qualitative impression of the neurologic examination and any other important clinical features. Those children who have MQs in the suspicious range, which lies between 70 and 80, do well as a rule. Although they may be somewhat clumsy in later childhood, they do not warrant a motor diagnosis. Very occasionally, a child with mild but classic cerebral palsy will have normal motor milestones. This situation only occurs in mild spastic diplegia or mild spastic hemiplegia, and the neurologic findings are always unequivocal, thus allowing for the diagnosis despite the fact that the child is compensating well enough to achieve normal milestones.

A great value in specifying a separate developmental age and developmental quotient for motor and intellectual areas at each clinic visit is the possibility of recognizing early a child whose rate of progress is slowing. This can occur with

Table 6-4. Fine Motor Development

Retain ring (rattle)	1 month
Hands unfisted	3 months
Reach	3–4 months
Hands to midline	3–4 months
Transfer	5 months
Take 1-inch cube	5–6 months
Take pellet (crude grasp)	6–7 months
Immature pincer	7–8 months
Mature pincer	10 months
Release	12 months

any chronic illness, and it may be an important factor in raising one's level of concern about other symptoms. Poor growth, especially poor weight gain, odd behavioral changes, etc., combined with a deceleration in developmental progress, may help alert the physician to early failure to thrive or to some serious and hidden family stress. In the rare situation of a child with a degenerative neurologic or muscle disease, the sequence of events is initially a slowing in the rate of developmental progress, then a plateau where the child is making no gain over time, and finally a period of developmental regression. Although these diseases are rare, the value of making a diagnosis early is considerable. The outcome for the involved child may not be altered much, but genetic counseling done sooner rather than later can avoid the added tragedy of a second involved child.

B. Assessment of Intellectual Development

A concise definition of intelligence is difficult because intelligence is represented by so many things, but it is probably best thought of in terms of an individual's ability to reason, to comprehend, to learn, to use judgment. In children, it relates to *potential* for acquiring and using adult-style comprehension, reasoning, and judgment. Early language development is the single best indicator of ultimate intellectual potential.[6] Problem-solving skills are second best.

Assessment of language development

1. Purpose: The purpose of this procedure is to determine if the child's language development is appropriate for his age.

2. Selection of Patients:

a. Indications: The procedure should be performed during well child screening and in response to specific concerns such as delayed speech, hearing loss, etc.

b. Contraindications and Precautions: There are no contraindications, even if the child is uncooperative, as a good language history provides a reliable mechanism for assessment.

3. Equipment and Supplies:
   · Bell, baby rattle
   · Picture book for infants (from any children's bookstore)
   · The Peabody Picture Vocabulary Test (PPVT) is a test of single-word comprehension routinely employed by speech pathologists, and a few pediatricians are familiar with its use. It requires a bit more time to complete and is only scorable down to 18 months of age, but it provides an excellent measure of receptive language capability in toddlers and preschoolers. For practitioners who like it, the PPVT represents a sophisticated addition to the simple equipment above.

4. Description of Procedures:

Language items refer to what the child says (expressive language) and what the child hears and understands (receptive language). Infants and some young children are generally not inclined to talk during clinic visits, so obtaining a meaningful history is critical to pinpointing language milestones. The specific meaning of each milestone is not intuitively obvious either to physicians or to parents, so it is essential that the physician clearly understand the milestones and be able to explain (or, even better, imitate) the items for the parent. Table 6-5 and Figure 6-1 represent combined expressive and receptive milestones (the CLAMS), and Table 6-6 provides a concise description of each milestone and how best to obtain it by history.[7,8] Table 6-7 is an abbreviated list of items collected from a number of sources indicating specific language milestones after 2 years of age. With repetition, it does not take long to get these items clear in one's mind. Keeping a table handy for quick reference eliminates the need to try memorizing each milestone. For example, "cooing" is a distinct noise ("ooh" or "aah") that babies begin to make at about 2 months of age and is different from "babbling," referring to repetitive consonant sounds ("ba-ba," "ga-ga," etc.). The easiest lead-in to expressive language assessment for the child under 24 months of age is simply to ask "Does he talk to you?" If so, "What does he say?" At that point, if mother or father need a little prompting, then all you have to do is speak the baby's language: "Does he say mostly soft sounds like ooh-ooh, aah-aah, or is he saying ba-ba, da-da, ga-ga, and things like that?" Often you may get an intermediate response: "Well, he says ah-good sometimes." This is, of course, not really an expression of the concept "good" but rather a transition between cooing and babbling—"ag-goo" (which occurs at 4 months). Once the child starts saying real words, vocabulary increases at an exponential rate and becomes almost impossible to keep track of after about 18 months of age. Thus, language comprehension items become easier to use and therefore are emphasized in Table 6-7. After 5 years of age, abilities become so complex that it is easier

Table 6-5. Clinical Linguistic and Auditory Milestones (CLAMS)

Milestone	Months
Alerting	1 week
Social Smile	1½
Cooing	2
Orient to voice	4
Orient to bell (I)	5
"Ah-goo"	5
Razzing	5
Laugh	4–5
Babbling	6–7
Orient to bell (II)	7
Gestures	9–10
"Mama/dada" (inappropriately)	8
Orient to bell (III)	9–10
"Dada/mama" (appropriately)	10
One word	11
One-step command (with gesture)	12
Two words	12
Three words	14
One-step command (without gesture)	15
Four–six words	15
Immature jargoning	15
One body part	15
Seven–twenty words	17
Mature jargoning	18
Five body parts	18
Two-word combinations (N + N)	21
Fifty words	24
Two-word sentences (S + P)	24
Pronouns (inappropriate)	24
Pronouns (appropriate)	30

Capute AJ, Shapiro BK, Palmer FB. Marking the milestones of language development. Contemp Pediatr 1987; 4:24–41; Capute AJ, Accardo PJ. Linguistic and auditory milestones during the first two years of life. Clin Pediatr 1978; 17:847–53. Adapted with permission.

(and probably more reliable) to use school performance as a screening indicator of verbal development.

5. Interpretation: After pinpointing as best as possible a single age or narrow age range for language development, interpretation is best done in combination with problem-solving milestones (next section). A separate feature to keep in mind is the important distinction between speech and language. Speech refers to the vocal production of language. A child may have perfectly normal abstract language capability (im-

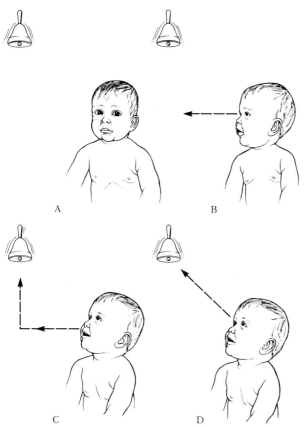

Figure 6-1.
Orienting to sound of bell. In the first stage (5 months), when a bell is rung at one side of the infant's head (**A**), the infant turns horizontally to the correct side (**B**). In the second stage (7 months), when a bell is rung at one side of the head (**A**), the infant localizes the sound by a compound visual maneuver consisting of a horizontal followed by a vertical component (**C**). In the third stage (9½ months), when a bell is rung to one side of the head (**A**), the infant localizes the sound by a single visual movement (**D**). (Reprinted with permission from Capute and Accardo)

plying normal cognitive function), but for one reason or another is unable to talk clearly. Receptive language ability, which is usually easier to ascertain than expressive in most children, especially younger ones, is the best reflection of language competence in the child who can not or will not speak. Hence, in sorting out the differential diagnosis of the child with delayed or absent speech, pinpointing receptive langauge is one critical piece of information. Another very useful assessment in this regard is a simple statement of the child's general intelligibility; that is, what the examiner, as a stranger, can understand of what the child says. Family members, especially the mother, can always understand more than a stranger. Intelligibility can be expressed by estimating the percentage of what you can understand. Speech intelligibility should be at least 65% for 2-year-olds, about 85% for 3-year-olds, and about 95% for 5-year-olds. Anything less than this suggests an articulation disorder and most of the time warrants referral to a qualified speech pathologist.

The pre-linguistic and linguistic milestones discussed herein can be thought of as the foundation of verbal intelligence. Beyond about 3 years of age, formal psychological testing describes individuals quantitatively in terms of an overall intelligence quotient (IQ). This IQ is a composite of two major elements—the verbal IQ (VIQ) and the performance IQ (PIQ). VIQ is the direct extension of infant language milestones, and PIQ is similarly the logical extension of problem-solving abilities. Hence, it should come as no surprise that in early childhood language and problem-solving milestones are the best predictors of adult intellectual potential.

Assessment of problem-solving abilities

1. Purpose: The purpose of this procedure is to determine if the child's nonverbal cognitive abilities are appropriate for his age.

2. Selection of Patients:

a. Indications: The procedure should be performed during well child screening and in response to specific concerns such as speech delay, poor vision, fine-motor clumsiness, etc.

b. Contraindications and Precautions: There are no contraindications except possible unreliability when the patient is acutely ill, acutely hungry, or already upset for some reason. The child with known visual impairment or motor disability will be at a disadvantage performing these tasks.

3. Equipment and Supplies (See Appendix for equipment and supplies manufacturers and suppliers. Appendix is keyed to italicized words in the equipment and supplies lists):

A complete kit that would be used for a thorough developmental assessment is hardly necessary for the screening situation. The items most useful for screening are those that also are most generally available:

- Tin *cup*
- Six 1-inch *cubes* (even better, 10)
- Crayon (pencil for patients over 5 years of age)
- Paper

4. Description of Procedure:

Problem-solving items are referrred to by many names—adaptive (Gesell), fine motor/adaptive (DDST), visual-motor, perceptual-motor, etc. They are sometimes misnamed "fine motor skills." Fine motor should refer purely to manipulative ability with the extremities. Fine motor competence is a component of problem-solving ability, but is only one of three essential components, vision and general intellect being the other two. These three functions must be working well and in concert for the child to accomplish a problem-solving task.

Table 6-6. Sequential Milestone Items

Alerting response to sound. Although many newborns overtly respond to sound, others will respond only with a change in heart rate, respiratory rate, or rate of sucking. By 1 month of age, all babies should produce a visible alerting response.

Social smile. The social smile is a maturational phenomenon that appears at 6 weeks of age. The true social smile is a response that can readily be elicited by the parent or examiner and needs to be distinguished from earlier spontaneous "smiles" in response to feeding, flatus, elimination, or other endogenous stimuli.

Cooing. Cooing is defined as long pure vowel sounds ("ooh," "aah") with variations other than those observed in crying or yawning. It needs to be distinguished from the earlier use of short vowels ("ah," "eh," "uh"), sighs, grunts, and throaty noises. It is best characterized as being somewhat musical or playfully repetitive. When attempting to elicit information on the early stages of infant vocalization, the pediatrician should always ask the parent to imitate the baby's actual sound productions. This reduces misunderstanding and sensitizes the parent to more careful observations of the succeeding stages.

Orienting to voice. In this response, the infant should turn immediately to the side of the room from which the mother is speaking. The infant who does not consistently look first to the correct side is evaluated as not orienting to voice. If this is not demonstrable during the examination, the parent's report should be carefully evaluated.

Orienting to bell. A bell is rung, at a distance between 1 and 2 feet at one side of the infant's head, and his ability to turn horizontally to the source of the sound is observed. Repeat trials should randomly vary from one side to the other, so that the examiner can be certain that the response is not due to chance alone. Care should be taken that the infant does not receive any visual cues! This is best done by the examiner facing the baby who is lying supine with his head in the midline and the examiner's hands symmetrically placed on each side of the head (Figure 6-1).

Ah-goo. This is looked on as a specific vocalization and has been described as appearing at about age 20 weeks; it seems to mark the transition between cooing and early babbling.

Razzing. The child is able to place his tongue between his lips and produce a "raspberry" (bubbles and spray are optional).

Babbling. Mature babbling involves the playful repetition of consonant sounds (syllables including short vowels, e.g., "bada," "gaga," etc.). The child's repertoire should consist of at least 2–4 different consonants able to be repeated in a string. In a severely hearing-impaired child, the production of spontaneous vocalizations usually progresses normally up to the stage of babbling, then advances no further, and in several months falls off.

Gesture. The child either spontaneously (to verbal cues) or imitatively (to motor cues) engages in meaningful gestures such as waving bye-bye, playing pat-a-cake, etc.

"Dada/Mama" inappropriately. Babies begin to vocalize "words" like "dada" fortuitously. Lack of comprehension is demonstrated by the indiscriminate application of "dada" to persons of either sex as well as to inanimate objects or in a vacuum. This usage marks the most mature end of the babbling spectrum.

"Dada/Mama" appropriately. At about 10 months of age, the infant begins to use "dada" and "mama" appropriately. His power of discrimination at this age is only slightly impaired by the presence of multiple caretakers (e.g., "mama" may be applied to both mother and grandmother and babysitter).

One-word vocabulary. When estimating a young child's spontaneous expressive vocabulary, two rules need to be followed throughout: 1) "Dada," "Mama," and the names and nicknames of family members and pets do not count as words; 2) until the child's vocabulary exceeds two dozen words, the parents should be requested to list all the words that the child actually uses. Such an enumeration not infrequently reveals the first estimation of vocabulary size to be too large or too small.

One must always be careful to assess the qualitative sequence of language development and not just several age-appropriate milestones. Not uncommonly, retarded children begin to say single words at about 12 months of age and then, after infrequent usage, discontinue speech. When their earlier pattern of language development is examined, it will be found deviant—certain milestones skipped, first word other than "Dada" or "Mama," etc.

One-step command (with gesture). By history, the child is able to correspond appropriately to simple commands such as "Give me ____," "Bring me ____"; these will need to be accompanied by a gesture for them to be understood. ("No" may be considered a simple command if it is obeyed even when spoken in a normal tone of voice.)

One-step command (without gesture). The child follows simple one-step commands such as "Give me ____," or "Bring me ____" without an accompanying gesture.

Immature jargoning. Jargoning is vocalization with the rhythm and patterns of conversational speech except that the "words" that are run together are unintelligible; the child appears to be trying to speak a sentence using gibberish or some foreign language. Immature jargon does not include any true words.

Mature jargoning. Mature jargoning presents the same vocalization patterns as immature jargoning, except that several intelligible words are mixed in the child's otherwise unintelligible patois.

One body part. When one compares the normative data from different psychometric tests, there appear to be differences between the ability to identify the same body part on the subject, the examiner, a doll, or a picture. Attempts should be made to try to corroborate parental report of body part identification by use of such testing variations.

(continued on next page)

Table 6-6. Sequential Milestone Items *(Continued)*

Two-word combinations (noun + noun). Two-word combinations rarely begin before the child's vocabulary reaches 20 words. When a parent claims two-word combinations with a total of less than 20 words, the child's entire vocabulary should be listed. The words in two-word combinations (frequently both are nouns) must refer to separate concepts; thus, combinations such as "bye-bye" and "all gone" are taken as single words.

The child who has at least a 50-word vocabulary is starting to put two words together. If the parent describes the child's dictionary as much greater than 50 words, with no two-word combinations, the child's vocabulary should be specifically enumerated.

Two-word sentences (subject + predicate). At about 2 years of age, the child's two-word utterances begin to take on the grammatic structure of telegraphic sentences with a subject and a verb (e.g., "daddy go," "me like"). Again, with a 2-year-old child, the parent should be requested to list all the child's two-word combinations.

Pronouns (I, me, you; inappropriately). The child is beginning to use three pronouns (I, me, you), but not necessarily with grammatic correctness.

Caute AJ, Accardo PJ. Linguistic and auditory milestones during the first two years of life. Clin Pediatr 1978; 17:847–53. Adapted with permission.

The child who fails a given problem-solving item may do so because of fine motor impairment (such as with cerebral palsy), because of a visual impairment (perhaps he has cataracts), or because he is not intellectually up to age level for the developmental task (mental retardation, learning disability). The terms visual-motor and perceptual-motor are used interchangeably, especially in reference to older children. These problem-solving items tested in infants are simpler versions of later perceptual-motor test items found on formal intelligence tests that yield the performance IQ.

Problem-solving tasks are defined as situations in which the child must solve a simple problem. An object is placed in the child's environment, and one observes what he does with it. Typical behaviors in response to these items correlate with specific developmental ages. For example, using a 1-inch cube as a stimulus, an average 3-month-old will watch it, will follow it when you move it around, and will often get very animated with this activity; but he will not reach for it. At 4 months of age, he will reach in a very ineffective manner and will not attain the cube unless you actually place it in his hand. By 6 months of age, he will reach in a nicely directed fashion toward the cube and grasp it with great consistency. If you offer him a second cube, however, he will either ignore it or attend to it briefly without reaching. If he accidentally drops the first cube, he will then take the second and interact with that one but will ignore the first. By 7 to 8 months of age, he will reach for and grasp the one and then consistently reach for and grasp the second, maintaining interest in and grasp of both cubes. Each baby is solving the problem of what to do with a cube placed in his environment (Table 6-8 and Figure 6-2). The test items become increasingly com-

Table 6-7. Language Milestones After 24 Months

Milestone	Years
Pronouns (I, you, me: inappropriate)	2
Pronouns (appropriate)	2½
Boy/girl recognition	2½–3
250+ word vocabulary	3
3+ word sentences	3
Plurals	3
Understands 3 prepositional commands	3½
Tells stories with complete syntax	4
Recognizes 4 colors	4
Differentiates bigger/smaller	4
Understands number concepts	5

Table 6-8. Problem-Solving Milestones: One-Inch Blocks

Behavior	Age (mos)
Regards	3
Attains	6
Approaches second	6–7
Takes second	7–8
Attempts third	10
Releases one in cup	12
Takes third	14
Builds tower (two)	15
Releases nine in cup	15
Builds tower (three to four)	18
Builds train	30
Builds tower (ten)	36
Builds bridge	36
Builds gate	48
Builds steps	60

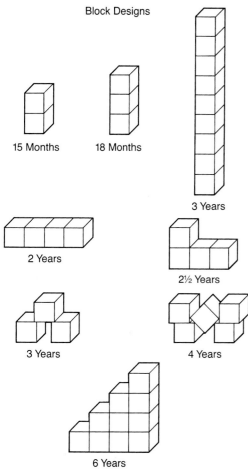

Block Designs

15 Months

18 Months

3 Years

2 Years

2½ Years

3 Years

4 Years

6 Years

Figure 6-2.
Age norms for block figure imitation. Add ½ year to the age levels for the train, bridge, and gate figures when copied (child shown finished figure) rather than imitated (child shown construction of figure). The steps are only presented for copying. (Adapted with permission from Capute and Accardo)

Gesell Figures

15 Months	Imitates scribble.
18 Months	Scribbles spontaneously.
2 Years	Imitates vertical line within 30 degrees.
2½ Years	Perseverative circle

3 Years

3½ Years

4 Years

5 Years

6 Years

6 Years

7 Years

8 Years

9 Years

12 Years

Figure 6-3.
Gesell figures.

plex as the infant gets older—introducing a cup at 11 or 12 months of age, crayon and paper at 14 or 15 months of age, and others (See Table of Developmental Milestones in the Appendix to this chapter).

The Table of Developmental Milestones provides a comprehensive table of all the problem-solving and perceptual motor items from birth to 13 years of age. The block designs are done by demonstration. The examiner constructs one design, for example, the bridge, and the child with a separate set of cubes is directed to make one "just like mine." For the pencil and paper tasks (Figure 6-3) the child is given a piece of paper with the figure already on it and is directed to copy

it: "Draw me a circle" or "Draw me one just like that," etc. It is wise to provide some positive encouragement whether he gets it correct or not: "That's good, now do a better one. . . make it just like mine." The intent is to get the child to demonstrate the best that he can do.

A variety of pencil and paper tests are available to the pediatrician to use in the screening situation. It is important to keep in mind that these are all variations on the same theme of visual-motor copying tasks. The Bender-Gestalt figures, the Goodenough Draw-A-Person, the Rey-Osterrieth complex figure, and the Gesell figures are all good examples. The Gesell figures are the quickest for the child to do and are the easiest for the examiner to score; hence, they have the most applicability to screening. Because they are so simple, the Gesell figures may be less discriminating than the other more complex drawings. A number of pediatricians are familiar with the Draw-A-Person and enjoy using it with their pediatric patients. It provides good information and certainly can be used instead of or in addition to the Gesell figures.

5. Interpretation: This section provides direction for the interpretation of intellectual development, which, as stated before, includes both language and problem-solving abilities.

The next step is to do the arithmetic to arrive at an estimation of the child's relative intellectual competence. Using the tables provided, one should be able to arrive at a fairly narrow age range for the child's language and problem-solving abilities. Usually these ages will be very close. If they are widely separated, this may be indicative of problems in one sphere (e.g., hearing or language comprehension) or the other (for example, vision or perception) that would require further evaluation. The estimated mental age is compared with the chronologic age, yielding a ratio that then is multiplied by 100. Hence:

$$\text{DQ (or estimated IQ)} = \frac{\text{developmental age}}{\text{chronologic age}} \times 100$$

By convention, 85 and above can be passed as normal. Below 70 is significantly low and warrants further investigation. Between 70 and 85 represents a suspicious or uncertain range, and may warrant no special investigation or may warrant immediate referral for further evaluation, depending on the circumstance. Some children truly do fall in a borderline category. It is up to the practitioner to balance his clinical judgment with the parents' comfort or discomfort in determining what to do. In one situation, the best plan might be to reevaluate things in a few months. In another, the only acceptable alternative might be referral for a more thorough evaluation by a subspecialist. Sometimes uncertainties can be cleared up by a quick telephone consultation.

Example: A 12-month-old comes to your office for well child care. By history she says three words: "ma-ma," "da-da," and "up." She will follow a simple command such as "give it to me" or "come here" most of the time. She readily recognizes the word "no" (but probably does not always stop what she is doing). She feeds herself with a spoon (it is messy but mother tolerates it), but she is a little too clumsy to manage her cup alone (See psychosocial milestones, Table 6-9). Stranger anxiety is readily apparent. She has just begun walking independently in the last week, and she can pick up a raisin with two fingers without difficulty.

The child is functioning at a 12-month level of ability in terms of language, gross motor, and psychosocial mile-

Table 6-9. Psychosocial and Self-care Milestones

Approximate Age	Milestones
6–8 mos	Person permanence; stranger anxiety/separation anxiety
8–10 mos	Object permanence
12 mos	Solitary play, helps with dressing
12–15 mos	Spoon feeding, cup drinking
2 years	Parallel play Attempts to wash self in tub or shower
2½ years	Adequate attempt to wash hands Partially dries hands
2½–3 years	Toilet trained day and night
3–4 years	Dries hands (without reminder) Group play
4–4½ years	Brushes teeth Washes and dries face
6–7 years	Combs and brushes hair adequately Blows and cleans nose independently
7–8 years	Bathes independently Keeps nails clean Team play

stones. The developmental screen is complete at this point without the examiner having touched the child, at least providing you trust the mother's history. It would be fun to go ahead and offer her a couple of blocks to see if she will bang them together in imitation and then see if she will place them into a cup. She may even comply with a request to "give it (a block) to me" if you have established a little rapport with her. She will probably stand up and walk a few steps if she is not too anxious about the setting. Of course, if she has had her belly poked and her ears checked already, you probably will get only refusals.

Example: A 4-year-old boy who is healthy and has been developing normally is brought in for a routine checkup. He is talkative and strikes you as rather active. Mother is thinking about starting him in kindergarten in the Fall, although he will be a bit on the young side. On testing he draws a poor-quality circle, despite several attempts, and barely copies a cross. His square is unacceptable. Only with urging can he build the block bridge, and the gate is too much for him. All language and motor skills are age-appropriate.

This boy may be mildly hyperactive, but definitely has some problem-solving (visual-motor) delays and would not likely do well in kindergarten. Further evaluation or perhaps a preschool program would be a wiser course to follow. The physician also needs to review the child's vision screening and eye examination, and perhaps refer to an ophthalmologist if there are any suspicious findings.

These principles of assessment of intellectual development apply to all age groups. The principles are most easily applied to the youngest children, namely infants and preschoolers. In thinking about the measurement of intelligence over the span of childhood, it is worth reflecting on the relative balance of language and problem-solving milestones at different times in a child's life. During the first 2 years, prelinguistic and early language milestones are very important but more often than not are impossible to obtain by direct observation because of the younger child's reluctance to talk and the fact that infants tend to vocalize intermittently and only when they are in a mood to do so. The good news is that these milestones are easy to obtain by history, provided the physician knows what to ask (See Table 6-6). In contrast, problem-solving skills generally are easy to examine at any age. They provide a wonderful opportunity to establish rapport with the infant and young child, because the tasks involve simple "toys." During the preschool years (2–5 years of age), language and problem-solving items are well balanced and relatively easy to obtain in the examining room, providing no invasive events have preceded the developmental screening effort. Once children are ready for school, language becomes increasingly complex and more difficult to screen accurately. Hence, one tends to rely on problem-solving (now referred to as perceptual-motor) items more and more as children get older. One also has the advantage of a school history for clues regarding academic strengths and weaknesses. With adolescents, the issues move beyond language skills into how the child makes use of his or her innate judgment and reasoning abilities. Likewise, perceptual-motor skill evolves into artistic capability, vocational interests, and so forth. In other words, psychosocial development achieves relatively greater significance in older children and adolescents.

One issue that physicians for children often find vexing is the school referral for an "LD (learning disability) physical." In this situation, a child has either failed a grade in school, done poorly in some specific area of academic performance, or failed some sort of screening evaluation. Fortunately, the child has been referred back to the physician for further consideration. As the patient has *already failed* some form of screening, the pediatrician may become uncertain of his role. Further "screening" is inappropriate. What is most needed is to review the child's general medical history and the family and social situation and to perform a good physical and neurologic examination. Thorough intellectual evaluations (educational academic testing, psychological/psychometric testing, etc.) are most likely indicated, and the physician should assert himself or herself as an advocate for the patient by becoming involved in the referral process for this testing. The physician also should request summary reports to assist in their review and analysis, especially if a major alteration in academic placement is to be considered.

C. Assessment of Psychosocial Development
1. Purpose: The purpose of this procedure is to determine whether the child's personal interactions and activities of daily living are appropriate for his age.
2. Selection of Patients:
a. Indications: The procedure should be performed during well child screening and in response to specific concerns about a child's behavior and affect.
b. Contraindications and Precautions: None. Observation of the child's behavioral interactions is meaningful if viewed in concert with the history.
3. Equipment and Supplies: None
4. Description of Procedure:

Psychosocial, sometimes called affective, developmental milestones, fall into two somewhat distinct categories of function: 1) the activities of daily living (ADL), which refer to dressing, bathing, and other self-care skills; and 2) interpersonal communication and interaction. In the office setting, ADL skills are observed to a limited degree, especially in infants and younger children, but a good history should be easy to obtain (Table 6-9). Physician, parent, sibling, and peer interactions and communication style can be observed to some extent in the office and also should be sought by history.

Assessments of temperament and other formal behavioral questionnaires are time consuming and highly subjective. As with other developmental screening questionnaires, they are mainly useful for initiating conversation on a topic. Nothing supplants the value of a long-standing, open, and positive relationship between doctor and patient. As the pediatric patient grows older, this rapport sets the tone for probing questions about behavior, love, sex, drugs, aspirations, and so forth. Good open-ended questions, proffered in a relaxed and confidential atmosphere, can best tap into behavioral and psychosocial adjustment issues. This is important to do but is difficult to formalize, and one needs to be committed to following up on positive responses. In the absence of an established or a trusting relationship, questions should still be asked, but the responses may be considerably less candid. At least one open-ended question ought to be asked and, if necessary, pursued at each clinic visit as part of the general developmental screening examination. This could simply be a question about behavior, an introduction to the concept of temperament, something fairly specific about sleep or getting along with siblings, a question about peer groups or smoking, and so forth (Table 6-10).[9] The main point about psychosocial screening is for the physician to develop his own inquisitive style and achieve a good level of comfort with that.[10]
5. Interpretation: Social milestones are in general the weakest in terms of providing information about innate intelli-

Table 6-10. Examples of Open-ended Questions

Parents

Is he a happy baby?

How would you describe his personality?
    Is he happy . . . fussy . . . irritable?

How does he get along with his brothers or sisters?

Does he have playmates?
    How do they get along?

How is he doing in school?
    Does he pay attention . . . work well?

Is he usually pretty safe?

Do you have any concerns about schoolwork
    (drugs, self-esteem . . .)?

Adolescents

Do you get along well with your parents . . . teachers?

What do you and your friends do for fun?

Do you have close friends?
    A best friend?

Do you smoke?

Do you ever drink alcohol? What do you know about other drugs
    like marijuana, cocaine?

Have you had some type of sex education course in school?
    Have you talked about sex (drugs) with your friends? . . . with
    your parents?

gence. ADL milestones have a very strong environmental component. For example, eating with a spoon depends to a large extent on when the spoon is introduced and how much mess caretakers are willing to tolerate. If they are intolerant, spoon-feeding will be delayed. Conversely, many social items can be taught to young children purely by rote and may not represent a good estimate of the child's true cognitive competence. They may, however, offer some insights into the quality of parent–child interactions and the child's behavioral style.

Pursuit of behavioral concerns is straightforward, which is not to say easy. Interpretation is not so much an issue as is where one can find advice for problems. This will vary greatly among individual practitioners and will depend on the availability of local resources such as mental health clinics, school counselors, young peoples clubs, etc., and more distant referral networks. Written resources can be especially helpful for the more standard behavioral issues with younger children (sleep, behavior management, and the like).[11]

Conclusions

For physicians, the "curbside consult" is a most important and valuable tool. Despite (or perhaps because of) its informality, it may be one of the most efficient things we do. Every practitioner should have well-identified resources in various subspecialties, including developmental and behavioral pediatrics, with whom he can communicate in such a fashion. Every consultant should be available for and receptive to just such interactions. It is especially valuable in situations where the urgency or even the need for referral (a time-consuming, expensive, often anxiety-provoking process) is not clear.

Developmental disabilities, regardless of when they are identified, are lifelong. In most circumstances, early identification should lead to early intervention, resulting in some improvemnt in functional outcome for the patient. It is hard to deny the benefits of early identification and intervention in terms of lessening frustration with and improving psychological adjustment to a disability. This holds true for patients and their parents and may extend to other family members as well. Furthermore, before completing high school, the child with a disability may go through four, five, or more school placements, each with a different principal and guidance counselor; his teachers may change annually; and he will experience any number of different professionals such as occupational therapists, speech therapists, special educators, etc. over the years. The pediatrician stands out as the only professional both able and available to provide the necessary continuity of care and advice that the family will most certainly need. The value of a consistent, reliable, knowledgeable advocate for the family should not be underestimated. Every transition will be a crisis point. It is important that physicians for children be willing to take on this responsibility and acquire the basic developmental assessment skills to provide the needed support.

References

1. Gesell A, Amatruda C. Developmental Diagnosis. New York: Paul Hoeber, 1941.
2. Knoblock H, Stevens F, Malone AE. Manual of Developmental Diagnosis. Hagerstown: Harper and Row, 1980.
3. Capute AJ, Shapiro BK, Palmer FB, et al. Normal gross motor development: The influences of race, sex, and socioeconomic status. Dev Med Child Neurol 1985; 27:635–43.
4. Capute AJ: Identifying cerebral palsy in infancy through study of primitive reflex profiles. Pediatr Ann 1979; 8:589–95.
5. Capute AJ, Accardo PJ, Vining EPG, et al. Primitive Reflex Profile. Baltimore: University Park Press, 1978.
6. Capute AJ, Palmer FB, Shapiro BK, et al. Clinical linguistic and auditory milestone scale: Prediction of cognition in infancy. Dev Med Child Neurol 1986; 28:762–71.
7. Capute AJ, Shapiro BK, Palmer FB. Marking the milestones of language development. Contemp Pediatr 1987; 4:24–41.
8. Capute AJ, Accardo PJ. Linguistic and auditory milestones during the first two years of life. Clin Pediatr 1978; 17:847–53.
9. Guidelines for Health Supervision, manual published by the American Academy of Pediatrics, PO Box 927, Elk Grove Village, IL 60007.
10. Goldenring JM, Cohen E. Getting into adolescent heads. Contemp Pediatr 1988; 5:75–90.
11. Schmitt BD. Your Child's Health: A Pediatric Guide for Parents. New York: Bantam Books, 1987.

Appendix

Table of Developmental Milestones

Age (mos)	Gross Motor	Fine Motor	Problem Solving	Language
0			Visual fixation Auditory alerting	Social smile (2–6 weeks)
1	Prone—lifts chin up		Follows face	
2	Prone—lifts chest up		Red ring, tracks horizontally/vertically	Coos
3	Prone—props on elbows	Unfisted >50%	Visual threat, tracks circularly	
4	Prone—extends elbows Rolls: prone to supine	Removes rattle from chest Hands move to midline	Reaches/bats objects, increased activity	Orients to voice Laughs out loud "Ag-goo"
5	Rolls: supine-prone Anterior protection Parachute Sits—propped	Transfers Ulnar rake Unfisted 100%	Grasps 1 block	Razz Orient I (See Table 6.5)
6	Attains 4-point stance	Radial rake	Mirror—smiles at and touches	Babbles
7	Sits—unsupported Belly crawls Lateral protection		Attains 2 blocks Pegboard, takes 2 out	Orient II (See Table 6.5) Echolalia (7–30 months)
8	Creeps (all fours) Comes to sit Pulls to stand	Attains pellet	Inspects bell Person permanence/ separation anxiety (6–10 months) Pulls string to get ring	"Dada" (inappropriate) "Mama" (inappropriate) Non-reduplicative babble Imitates
9	Cruises	Immature pincer (scissors grasp) Finger feeds	Rings bell Combines blocks Bangs spoon	Gesture games
10	Walks—two-handed support	Mature pincer	Combines cup/block Object permanence (searches)	"Mama" (appropriate) "Dada" (appropriate) Recognizes name
11	Walks—one-handed support		Uncovers toy	Orient III (See Table 6.5) First word
12	Walks independently Posterior protection (12– 18 mos)	Releases into cup	Cooperates with dressing	Command with gesture
13			Glass frustration: solves	Immature jargon, 2–3- word vocabulary

(continued on next page)

Table of Developmental Milestones *(Continued)*

Age (mos)	Gross Motor	Fine Motor	Problem Solving	Language
14	Stands without pulling up	Solitary play	Pill-in-the-bottle-test, finger bottle—imitates solution Pegboard, one in/out Blocks, attain third Marks with crayon Tower, 2	Command without gesture
15	Climbs on furniture Creeps up steps	Spoon feeding Cup drinking	Blocks, 10 in cup Imitates scribble	4–6 words One body part
16	Runs		Pill-in-the-bottle—solves spontaneously Round pegboard, finishes (urged) Formboard circle ●△□	
18	Stoops and recovers Stairs, walks up hand-held		Round pegboard, finishes (spontaneously) Spontaneous scribble	10–25 words Mature jargon Three body parts
20	Kicks ball		Finishes square pegboard Formboard square ○△■	Six body parts
22	Stairs, walks down, hand-held Throws overhand		Tower, 6 Horizontal train Completes formboard	Picture identification—2 Two-word phrase (noun + noun) 50+ words
24		Parallel play		Two-word phrase (noun + verb)
27			After demonstration /	Picture identification—6 Repeats 2 digits
30	Walks up stairs with rail alternating feet Jumps in place	Strings large beads Folds paper Washes hands	Perseverative circle Tower, 10 Formboard, reversed ●▲■ Train with stack	"I" Concept of "just one" End of echolalia
36	Walks up stairs, without rail, alternating feet Heel walks Toe walks Pedals tricycle	Independent eating Cuts with scissors Strings small beads	Draws ○ Builds bridge	Age Boy/girl First and last name Uses plurals correctly Three-word sentences What sleep in? write with? hear with?

Table of Developmental Milestones *(Continued)*

Age (yr)	Gross Motor	Social-Adaptive	Visual Motor	Language
3.5		Buttons Group play	Draws + (cross)	Bigger/smaller Longer/shorter Repeats 3 digits Prepositions, 3
4	Walks down stairs, alternating feet Hops on 1 foot, 5–8 times Skips (4.5 years)	Washes face and hands Zippers Uses straw	Draws □ (square) Gate	Colors, 4 Counts by rote Number concepts to 2
5	Balances on 1 foot (>10 sec) Finger-to-nose test, arm free	Spreads with knife Uses bathroom alone	Draws △ (triangle)	Different Number concepts to 3+ Heavier/lighter Birthday, month, day Repeats 4 digits Day/night (5.5 years) Identifies coins (5.5 years)
6	Tandem walks	Ties shoes Combs hair Cuts with knife	Draws ⊠ (crossed rectangle) Staircase (from memory)	Left vs. right, self (5–7 years) Days of week Seasons of year Telephone number Number concepts to 10 Simple addition
7	Rides bicycle	Bathes alone	Draws ◇ (diamond) House (from memory)	Tells time, hour and half-hour Digits: 5 forward, 3 reversed
8	Reverse tandem walks	Team play	Draws + (plus/cross)	Birth year Cross-midline command Tells time, 5 minutes Left vs. right, examiner (7–9 years) Simple multiplication (8–9 years) Months of year
9			Draws (cylinder)	Simple division Digits: 4 reversed
10				Digits: 6 forward
12			Draws (cube)	
13			Draws (3-D geometric figure)	

This table has been adapted from many sources, the most notable including Gesell A, Amatruda C. Developmental Diagnosis. New York: Paul Hoeber, 1941; Knoblock H, Stevens F, Malone AE. Manual of Development Diagnosis. Hagerstown: Harper and Row, 1980; Capute AJ, Shapiro BK, Palmer FB, et al. Normal gross motor development: The influences of race, sex, and socioeconomic status. Dev Med Child Neurol 1985; 27:635–43; Capute AJ, Shapiro BK, Palmer FB. Marking the milestones of language development. Contemp Pediatr 1987; 4:24–41; Capute AJ, Accardo PJ. Linguistic and auditory milestones during the first two years of life. Clin Pediatr 1978; 17:847–53; Thorndike RL, Hagen EP, Sattlen JM. Stanford-Binet Intelligence Scale, 4th ed. Chicago: The Riverside Publishing Company, 1986; Wechsler D. Wechsler Preschool and Primary Scale of Intelligence. New York: The Psychological Corp, 1967.

Chapter 7

Pediatric Skin Procedures

Gregory F. Hayden

Kenneth E. Greer

I. Diagnostic Procedures

A. Wood's Lamp Examination

1. Purpose: The purpose of this procedure is to provide additional clinical evidence about the presence or absence of certain skin conditions.

2. Selection of Patients:

a. Indications: Wood's lamp examination is indicated for patients who might have one of the medical conditions noted in Table 7-1.

b. Contraindications and Precautions: None

3. Equipment and Supplies (See Appendix for equipment and supplies manufacturers and suppliers. Appendix is keyed to italicized words in the equipment and supplies lists):

A Wood's *lamp* (Figure 7-1) emits a filtered band of long-wavelength ultraviolet light that under normal circumstances is transmitted into the dermis and absorbed by melanin. In the conditions noted in Table 7-1, Wood's lamp examination demonstrates an abnormal color or highlights the differentiation of two adjacent colors.

4. Description of Procedure:

· Turn the lamp on for a minute or 2 before use to insure optimum ultraviolet light output.

· Before turning out the room light, briefly demonstrate the procedure to the child and parent to put them at ease. Reassure them that the ultraviolet light is not harmful to the skin or eyes.

· Hold the lamp 4 to 5 inches from the area to be examined and observe for color change and fluorescence.

5. Side Effects and Complications: None

6. Interpretation: See Table 7-1. Common sources of confusion with pathologic conditions include lint, scales, dandruff, serum exudate, ointments containing petrolatum, and fluorescent ingredients in cosmetics. Wood's lamp examination

Table 7-1. Characteristics of Skin Conditions Identified by Wood's Lamp Examination

Skin Condition	Color	Comments
Tinea capitis	Blue-green	1. Only ectothrix infections, e.g., those due to *Microsporum* spp., fluoresce. 2. The hairs fluoresce rather than the skin; fluorescent hairs can be preferentially selected for KOH examination or fungal culture. 3. Success of treatment can be confirmed by nonfluorescence of hair that regrows.
Tinea versicolor	Golden yellow	1. Fluorescence is not consistent but may be helpful in determining the extent of the disease.
Erythrasma	Coral red	1. Fluorescence may be absent if the affected area has been washed recently.
Pseudomonas aeruginosa infection	Yellow- to blue-green	
Nonpigmented skin	Bluish-white	1. Useful in detecting ash-leaf lesions in children with tuberous sclerosis.
Pediculosis capitis	Greyish	1. Nits glow.
Porphyria cutanea tarda	Pink-orange	1. Urinary fluorescence.
Tetracycline	Yellow	1. Nails and areas of active inflammation (e.g., acne papules) can fluoresce.

is not helpful for the diagnosis of tinea corporis, which does not fluoresce.

B. Scabies Retrieval

1. Purpose: Laboratory confirmation of the clinical diagnosis of scabies is desirable for clinical and epidemiologic reasons in persons of all ages. Confirmation is especially desirable in infants and young children so as not to expose them unnecessarily to therapy with potential side effects.

2. Selection of Patients:

a. Indications: The diagnosis of scabies should be considered in any child with pruritic, excoriated papules, vesicopustules, burrows, or eczematous dermatitis. The typical distribution of lesions in an older child may include interdigital webs, wrists, arms, axillae, belt line, areolae, genitalia, and buttocks. In infants, the trunk, extremities, head, neck, palms, and soles also may be involved. The presence of similar pruritic lesions in a family member heightens the clinical suspicion of scabies.

b. Contraindications and Precautions: None

3. Equipment and Supplies (See Appendix for equipment and supplies manufacturers and suppliers. Appendix is keyed to italicized words in the equipment and supplies lists):

- Ink (optional)
- Fluorescein *strips* (Figure 7-2)
- Wood's *lamp* (See Figure 7-1, left) (optional)
- Mineral or immersion *oil* or potassium hydroxide *solution* (10%) (KOH)
- No. 15 scalpel *blade* (Figure 7-2)
- Clean glass microscope *slide* and *coverslip*
- Microscope

4. Description of Procedure:

- The selection of the site for scraping is crucial. In general, the mites prefer acral areas with a thin stratum corneum, so examine very carefully the patient's hands, wrists, and elbows for suitable lesions. Select several lesions for scraping to maximize the chance of success.
- An undamaged burrow with a tiny black or white speck (the female mite) at one end is ideal. If a small amount of ink is spread over a suspicious area, it will flow into a burrow and outline it nicely after the surface ink is washed off with water (Figure 7-3). Alternatively, a dilute solution of fluorescein, made by dipping a fluorescein ophthalmic strip into a few milliliters of water, can be applied and then washed off in similar fashion, followed by Wood's lamp examination (See Wood's

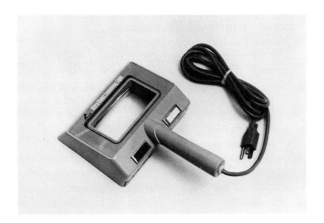

Figure 7-1.
Wood's lamp examination. Equipment and supplies: Wood's lamp.

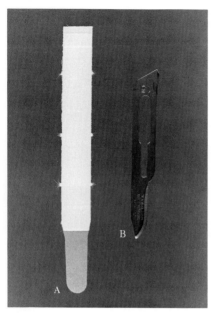

Figure 7-2.
Scabies retrieval. Equipment and supplies: **A,** Fluorescein strips; **B,** No. 15 scalpel blade.

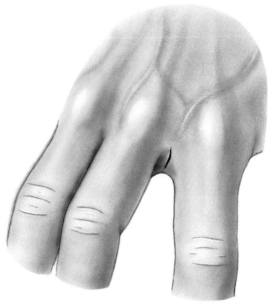

Figure 7-3.
Scabies retrieval. Mite burrow (highlighted with ink).

Lamp Examination, page 58) to highlight fluorescence within the burrow.

· If an undisturbed burrow is not found, select an early papule or vesicle that has not been excoriated.

· Apply a drop or two of mineral or immersion oil over the lesion(s) to be scraped. Some clinicians prefer KOH as an alternative.

· Scrape the lesion gently with a sterile no. 15 scalpel blade (Figure 7-4). A burrow should be repeatedly scraped along its longitudinal axis, with the goal of dislodging the mite at the end of the burrow. A papule or vesicle should be scraped so as to remove the top. When scraping a burrow, papule, or vesicle, stop at the first site of blood, as the mites are located superficially in the epidermis.

· Transfer the scraped material and oil to the glass slide.

· After scraping several lesions in like fashion, cover with a coverslip and examine microscopically under low power.

5. Side Effects and Complications: Local discomfort is usually minimal. Mild bleeding, easily controlled by local pressure, occasionally occurs.

6. Interpretation: Examine the glass slide microscopically for mites, transparent oval eggs, and irregularly shaped clumps of yellowish-brown fecal pellets. An air bubble in the oil may sometimes resemble an egg, but will change shape when

gentle pressure is applied to the coverslip. Dispose of the slide carefully because survival of mites in mineral oil for up to 1 week has been reported.

If the scraping is positive, the diagnosis of scabies is established. A negative scraping does not rule out scabies. Multiple scrapings are sometimes required, so consider repeated scrapings of the child's lesions or of any close contacts with suspicious lesions.

C. Fungal Culture and Potassium Hydroxide (KOH) Preparation

1. Purpose: Because fungal skin infections may closely resemble a number of different cutaneous disorders, the possibility of misdiagnosis of yeast or dermatophyte infection is substantial. The purpose of this procedure is to provide laboratory evidence to confirm or reject a clinical impression of superficial fungal infection.

2. Selection of Patients:

a. Indications: The procedure is particularly useful in situations in which the clinical diagnosis is uncertain at the outset or is being questioned because the response to treatment has been unsatisfactory. Correct diagnosis is essential for tinea capitis, as the usual course of oral therapy is prolonged, expensive, and potentially toxic.

b. Contraindications and Precautions: None

3. Equipment and Supplies (See Appendix for equipment

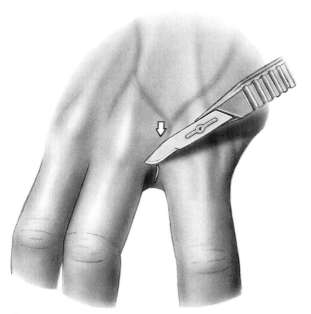

Figure 7-4.
Scabies retrieval. Technique.

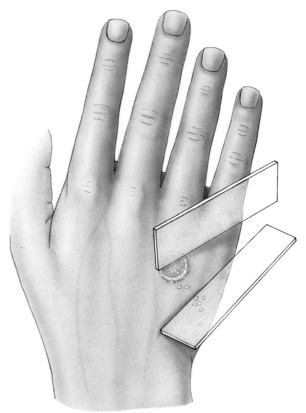

Figure 7-5.
Fungal culture and potassium hydroxide preparation.
Technique.

and supplies manufacturers and suppliers. Appendix is keyed to italicized words in the equipment and supplies lists):

- Clean glass microscope *slides* and *coverslip*
- No. 15 scalpel *blade* (See Figure 7-2, page 60)
- Dermatophyte test *medium*
- Potassium hydroxide *solution* (KOH)
- Alcohol *lamp* for heating (optional)
- Microscope

4. Description of Procedure:
- Use the edge of a glass slide (or a sterile, no. 15 scalpel blade) held parallel to the skin surface to scrape the outer active edge of the lesion adjacent to normal-appearing skin (Figure 7-5). Wetting the scraping edge or the lesion lightly with water may help to prevent the scales from becoming airborne.
- Place another glass slide under the lesion to catch the falling scales.
- The collected scales can be divided into two groups.
- Transfer one group of scales into a jar containing dermatophyte test medium (DTM).
- With a coverslip, push the remaining group of scales toward the center of the slide. Add one to two drops of potassium hydroxide (KOH) (10–20% solution) and cover with the coverslip. Warming the slide (without boiling) will accelerate the activity of KOH in dissolving keratin from the epithelial cells. The slide is warmed for 10 to 15 seconds by gently passing the underside back and forth through the flame of an alcohol lamp. Let the

slide cool for a few minutes, then press the coverslip gently to push out air bubbles. Examine under the microscope using low-power magnification and low illumination.

5. Side Effects and Complications: None
6. Interpretation: DTM is a fungal culture medium that contains a color indicator that changes from yellow to red over 3 to 14 days in the presence of a dermatophyte. Candida colonies appear in 3 to 4 days as cream-colored, puttylike colonies with no associated color change of the underlying medium. Dropping a steel blade onto DTM may cause a false-positive result with red color change of the medium. If more definite identification of a fungus is desired, other media such as Sabouraud's or Mycosel can be used. A wet mount preparation with KOH provides a more rapid answer. Under microscopic examination using a low ($10\times$)-power lens, the hyphae of dermatophytes have a dull green color, are thicker than epithelial cell walls, and have a characteristic branching

pattern. Lesions of candidiasis will yield budding yeasts with or without pseudohyphae, which often closely resemble the hyphae of dermatophytes. Differentiation between candidiasis and a dermatophyte infection solely on the basis of a KOH preparation may be impossible. Lesions of tinea versicolor will reveal short and long hyphae with clusters of spores ("spaghetti and meatballs"). Frequent sources of confusion include: pieces of lint, which are characterized by their variable size and irregular diameter; pieces of fiberglass, which are rigidly straight, have a uniform diameter, extend across cell walls, and do not branch; salt crystals, which often are seen if the specimen is dried or overheated; and overlapping epithelial cell walls. A positive test establishes the diagnosis of a fungal infection, but gives no reliable information concerning the specific organism causing the process. Clinical features may be more helpful in suggesting a specific organism, especially for candida and tinea versicolor. A single negative test does not exclude the diagnosis, but repeated negative scrapings provide some presumptive reassurance that the process is not fungal in origin. A negative fungal culture helps to reinforce the reliability of a negative KOH preparation.

D. Vesicopustule Evaluation

1. Purpose: The purpose of this procedure is to help establish a laboratory diagnosis for patients with vesicopustules of uncertain origin.

2. Selection of Patients:

a. Indications: This test is especially applicable for the rapid diagnosis of herpetic infections, superficial blistering fungal infections, and, in the neonate, erythema toxicum neonatorum.

b. Contraindications and Precautions: None

3. Equipment and Supplies (See Appendix for equipment and supplies manufacturers and suppliers. Appendix is keyed to italicized words in the equipment and supplies lists):

- Isopropyl alcohol *pad*
- No. 15 scalpel *blade* (See Figure 7-2, page 60) or iris *scissors* (See Figure 18-2, page 220)
- Clean glass microscope *slide*
- Microscope
- Potassium hydroxide *solution* (10–20%) (KOH)
- Dermatophyte test *medium* (ACU-DTM)
- Gram staining materials
- Wright's or Giemsa stain
- Bacterial culture media
- Viral culture media
- *Methanol* (95%)
- Immersion *oil*

4. Description of Procedure:

- Depending on the clinical setting, careful attention

should be paid to one or more components of the vesicopustule: the roof, the fluid contained within, and the base.

- Select an intact vesicopustule and begin by cleansing the overlying skin and the surrounding area with isopropyl alcohol.
- Gently remove the roof of the lesion with a no. 15 scalpel blade or, if the lesion is sufficiently large, with a pair of small scissors.
- Place the roof of the lesion upside down on a clean glass slide. Under high-power magnification, microscopically examine the underside of the roof of the lesion for fungal elements. Perform a KOH preparation and a fungal culture as outlined in this chapter (See pages 60 to 62).
- Obtain swabs of the liquid contents for microscopic analysis, including Gram stain, Wright's stain, and scabies preparation, and appropriate bacterial and viral cultures.
- The base of the lesion then may be scraped with a no. 15 scalpel blade. Scrape firmly enough to obtain tissue but avoid bleeding.
- Transfer the scrapings to another slide for microscopic analysis (Tzanck's test). To prepare a Tzanck's smear, make a thin smear of the scrapings on the glass microscope slide. After air drying, fix the slide with methanol (95%) for 1 minute and then stain with Wright's or Giemsa stain. Examine under high-power magnification with a microscope. Occasionally, examination under oil immersion is useful.

5. Side Effects and Complications: Local discomfort is the only complication.

6. Interpretation: The roof of the lesion can be evaluated microscopically under high-power magnification, especially for fungal elements. The fluid contents can be analyzed in several fashions. Gram stain and bacterial cultures will evaluate the possibility of bacterial disease such as bullous impetigo, especially due to *Staphylococcus aureus*. Wright's stain will evaluate the presence of polymorphonuclear leukocytes as encountered, for example, with bacterial impetigo, infantile acropustulosis, or transient neonatal pustular melanosis. Wright's stain also may show eosinophils, as may be seen in lesions of a newborn infant with erythema toxicum neonatorum. A scabies preparation with oil will help evaluate the possibility of scabies (See Scabies Retrieval, page 59). A KOH preparation may show spores and pseudohyphae, as seen with candidiasis. Viral cultures may disclose evidence of herpes virus. On the Tzanck's preparation, lesions of herpes simplex (including Kaposi's varicelliform eruption), herpes zoster, and varicella contain multinucleated giant cells that, on rare occasions, contain intranuclear inclusions. Balloon degeneration of epidermal cells also may be seen. Lesions of pemphigus will show numerous rounded, detached, acantholytic epidermal cells with large nuclei and peripheral, condensed cytoplasm.

E. Cellulitis Culture

1. Purpose: The purpose of this procedure is to obtain fluid that may establish a precise microbiologic diagnosis so that antimicrobial therapy may be as specific as possible.

2. Selection of Patients:

a. Indications: Lesions in most anatomic sites may be cultured, although the yield of positive cultures from this procedure is low (10–20%).

b. Contraindications and Precautions: Do not aspirate lesions involving the eyelids or immediately surrounding the orbit because of the possibility of spread of infection to the orbit (orbital cellulitis) through penetration of the protective membranes located in each eyelid. Direct injury to the globe by the needle can occur in this same setting.

3. Equipment and Supplies (See Appendix for equipment and supplies manufacturers and suppliers. Appendix is keyed to italicized words in the equipment and supplies lists):

- 18-, 20-, or 22-gauge *needle* (See Figure 20-7, page 262)
- 3-mL *syringe* (See Figure 20-7, page 262)
- Povidone–iodine *solution*
- Isopropyl alcohol *pads*
- Sterile *non*bacteriostatic saline *solution*
- Gram staining materials
- Bacterial culture media
- Microscope

4. Description of Procedure:

- Attach an 18- or 20-gauge needle to a 3-mL syringe (A smaller needle, e.g., 22-gauge, may be used for a facial lesion).
- Sterilize the overlying skin with povidone–iodine followed by alcohol.
- Advance the needle into the active inflamed area of the lesion and attempt to aspirate. To prevent the sampling needle from becoming occluded by a skin plug, some authorities recommend puncturing the skin first with a separate needle before inserting the sampling needle. If the advancing margin of the lesion is sharp and inflamed, as in erysipelas, aspirate this leading edge. In most instances, the advancing margin is indistinct and probably represents edema extending from the central area of more active infection. In this case, aspirate the inflamed central portion of the lesion (Figure 7-6).
- If no material can be aspirated, warn the patient about additional local discomfort, inject 0.1 to 0.3 mL of sterile *non*bacteriostatic saline solution, and then aspirate the saline immediately back into the syringe.
- Take the aspirated material to the medical laboratory for Gram stain and bacterial culture. If fluid was aspi-

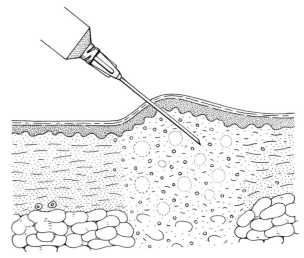

Figure 7-6.
Cellulitis culture. Technique.

rated, rinse the needle and syringe with culture medium and perform the appropriate microscopic analysis and culture.

5. Side Effects and Complications: Local discomfort is the only significant complication.

6. Interpretation: A positive test helps to establish the cause of the cellulitis; but because of the difficulties inherent in the procedure, expect a success rate of only 10% to 20%. If a microbiologic diagnosis is crucial, consider skin biopsy with culture.

F. Abscess Aspiration

1. Purpose: The purpose of this procedure is to obtain material that may allow for a precise microbiologic diagnosis so as to guide the selection of appropriate antimicrobial therapy.

2. Selection of Patients:

a. Indications: In clinical settings that are not urgent, initial therapy often can be selected empirically to treat the pathogens commonly isolated from similar lesions. If the abscess fails to respond to this treatment, however, aspiration may be helpful in directing a change in antimicrobial coverage. Aspiration also will have therapeutic value in some instances, but incision and drainage may be necessary for larger lesions (See Minor Pediatric Surgical Procedures, Incision and Drainage, page 227). Lesions suitable for aspiration will be fluctuant to the touch. Ultrasound examination of a hard lesion may be useful to show an area of central fluctuance, which then can be aspirated.

b. Contraindications and Precautions: Remember that most abscesses that occur after an intramuscular vaccination are sterile and do not require aspiration or antimicrobial treatment. Do not aspirate a cervical abscess when it may be due to atypical mycobacteria, because of the tendency for such lesions to form draining sinus tracts. Obtain a negative tuberculin skin test before aspiration in such instances.

3. Equipment and Supplies (See Appendix for equipment and supplies manufacturers and suppliers. Appendix is keyed to italicized words in the equipment and supplies lists):

- 18- or 20-gauge *needle* (See Figure 20-7, page 262)
- 5-mL *syringe* (See Figure 20-7, page 262)
- Povidone–iodine *solution*
- Isopropyl alcohol *pads*
- Can of ethyl chloride *spray* (optional)
- Gram-staining materials
- Bacterial culture media
- Microscope

4. Description of Procedure:

- Attach an 18- or 20-gauge needle to a 5-mL syringe.
- Prepare the overlying skin with iodine followed by isopropyl alcohol.
- The area may be sprayed with ethyl chloride to provide light local anesthesia.
- At an approximately 45° angle to the skin, advance the needle into the fluctuant portion of the abscess and withdraw the purulent material (Figure 7-7).
- Transport this material to the clinical laboratory for appropriate examination, usually to include Gram stain and bacterial culture.

5. Side Effects and Complications: Local discomfort, which varies considerably, is the only significant complication.

II. Therapeutic Procedures

A. Tick Removal

1. Purpose: The purpose of the procedure is to remove the tick as soon as it is discovered so as to reduce the chance of the child's developing a tick-borne illness.

2. Selection of Patients:

a. Indications: The procedure is indicated for patients with ticks that are attached (i.e., embedded head parts).

b. Contraindications and Precautions: There are no contraindications. Attempts to get a tick to release its hold by subjecting it to a heat source (match head or cigarette) usually meet with failure and may lead to a thermal burn on the patient. Covering the tick with occlusive material (petroleum jelly, cold cream, etc.) is not effective in promoting the tick's release, as the tick has a very slow respiratory rate.

3. Equipment and Supplies (See Appendix for equipment and supplies manufacturers and suppliers. Appendix is keyed to italicized words in the equipment and supplies lists):

- Isopropyl alcohol *pads*
- *Forceps*

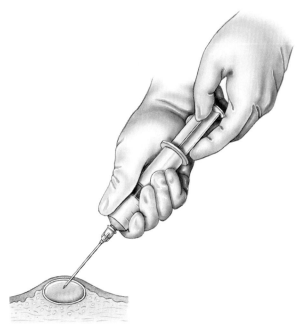

Figure 7-7.
Abscess aspiration. Technique.

- Sterile *gloves* or tissue paper
- *Lidocaine* (1%)

4. Description of Procedure:

- Disinfect the bite site with an isopropyl alcohol swab.
- Grasp the tick as close to the skin surface as possible, using blunt curved forceps or tweezers.
- If no instruments are available and fingers must be used, protect them with gloves, a paper towel, or a tissue. Do not handle the tick with your bare hands.
- Pull upward on the tick with firm, steady pressure, taking special care not to twist, jerk, squeeze, crush, or puncture the tick. Rupture of an engorged tick can lead to inoculation of infectious material.
- Try not to leave any mouthparts in place; if this does occur, any remaining parts can be removed using local anesthesia with lidocaine solution and light currettage. (See Expressing the Core of Molluscum Contagiosum, page 65).
- Conclude by disinfecting the bite site with alcohol.
- Dispose of the tick by placing it in a container of alcohol or flushing it down a toilet.

5. Side Effects and Complications: Tick bite granulomas can develop if embedded parts remain in the skin.

B. Comedone Removal

1. Purpose: The purpose of this procedure is to provide temporary cosmetic benefit by extruding the central keratin plug from comedonal lesions of acne. For closed comedones ("whiteheads"), the procedure may theoretically prevent the eventual formation of inflammatory lesions.

2. Selection of Patients:

a. Indications: This practice is not as common as it once was because of the availability and effectiveness of topical isotretinoin; but the procedure can be useful for patients with multiple comedones.

b. Contraindications and Precautions: The procedure should be used with caution, as careless or overly vigorous attempts at comedone extraction may result in rupture of the pilosebaceous duct, which can lead to an iatrogenic inflammatory papule with cosmetic deterioration rather than benefit. This procedure should be used only as part of a comprehensive plan for acne therapy, as without additional treatment, pilosebaceous plugging will recur.

3. Equipment and Supplies (See Appendix for equipment and supplies manufacturers and suppliers. Appendix is keyed to italicized words in the equipment and supplies lists):
- Comedone extractor (Figure 7-8)
- No. 11 scalpel *blade* (Figure 7-8)

4. Description of Procedure:
- Begin by asking the patient to wash his or her face with soap and water.
- Explain the procedure, demonstrate the instrument to be used, and warn that the procedure may be moderately uncomfortable.
- Apply the loop end of the comedone extractor over an open comedone ("blackhead") and press down gently until the central plug extrudes from the lesion (Figure 7-9).
- For closed comedones ("whiteheads"), gently nick the follicular opening carefully with a no. 11 scalpel blade, then proceed as for open comedones.
- Have the patient wash his or her face with soap and water after the extractions.

5. Side Effects and Complications: Local discomfort is common, and pressing down on skin lesions over orthodontic braces can be particularly painful and may cause oral bleeding. In treating lesions near the eye, the extractor may slip over the orbital rim and injure the eyelid or globe.

C. Expressing the Core of Molluscum Contagiosum

1. Purpose: This procedure can be therapeutic and also can provide laboratory confirmation when a clinical diagnosis of molluscum contagiosum is uncertain.

2. Selection of Patients:

a. Indications: Modes of therapy may include: cryotherapy with liquid nitrogen; curettage with a small sharp curette after light local anesthesia; and destruction by topical application of an agent such as podophyllin. As most lesions of molluscum

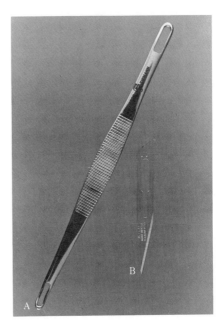

Figure 7-8.
Comedone removal. Equipment and supplies: **A,** Comedone extractor; **B,** No. 11 scalpel blade.

contagiosum regress spontaneously within 6 to 12 months, no treatment is required in many instances. Multiple lesions may develop, however, because of autoinoculation of the virus.

b. Contraindications and Precautions: None

3. Equipment and Supplies (See Appendix for equipment and supplies manufacturers and suppliers. Appendix is keyed to italicized words in the equipment and supplies lists):
- Isopropyl alcohol *pads*
- 20-gauge *needle* (See Figure 20-7, page 262) or no. 11 scalpel *blade* (See Figure 7-8, above)
- Comedone *extractor* (See Figure 7-8, above) or a small skin *curette* (Figure 7-10)

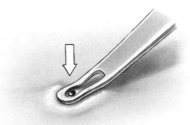

Figure 7-9.
Comedone removal. Technique.

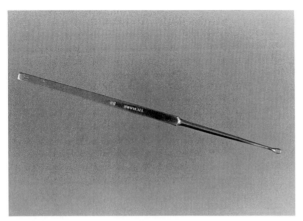

Figure 7-10.
Expressing the core of molluscum contagiosum. Equipment and supplies: small skin curette.

- Clean glass microscope *slides*
- Wright's stain
- Microscope

4. Description of Procedure:
- Select a typical dome-shaped, pearly papule with a small central umbilication and clean the surface with alcohol.
- Puncture the surface with a sterile 20-gauge needle or the tip of a no. 11 surgical blade.
- Express the contents of the lesion with the needle or with the help of a comedone extractor (See Comedone Removal, page 64). The core of a molluscum contagiosum is a cheesy, whitish plug.
- As an option, the papule may be removed with a small curette.
- Press the expressed material between two microscope slides, stain with Wright's stain, and examine under a microscope with low power.

5. Side Effects and Complications: Complications include mild discomfort and minimal bleeding (if the curette is used).
6. Interpretation: The presence of large intracytoplasmic viral inclusion bodies within a lobulated, adhesive mass of epidermal cells confirms the diagnosis of molluscum contagiosum.

D. Cryotherapy of Verruca Vulgaris with Liquid Nitrogen

1. Purpose: The purpose of this procedure is to remove a common wart.
2. Selection of Patients:
a. Indications: Several alternative therapies are available, including the use of such topical agents as salicylic acid, cantharidin, and podophyllin, as well as electrodessication, cur-

ettage, and watchful waiting. Choice of therapy depends on many factors including: the number, size, and location of lesions to be treated; the age and level of cooperation of the patient; cost; the amount of pain and disability produced by the wart; and the availability of liquid nitrogen to the clinician. Cryotherapy with liquid nitrogen is particularly well suited for the treatment of a limited number of smaller warts in an older cooperative child who can tolerate some degree of discomfort.

b. Contraindications and Precautions: The freezing of periungual warts is very painful and largely unsuccessful. Large warts greater than 1 cm in diameter are also poorly suited to freezing in their entirety because of pain and the potential for developing a large hemorrhagic blister. Use cryotherapy only with great caution in darkly pigmented individuals, especially on the face, because of the potential for pigmentary changes.
3. Equipment and Supplies (See Appendix for equipment and supplies manufacturers and suppliers. Appendix is keyed to italicized words in the equipment and supplies lists):
- No. 15 scalpel *blade* (See Figure 7-2, page 60)
- Cotton-tipped *applicator* (See Figure 18-17, page 231)
- Liquid *nitrogen* tank
- Polystyrene foam (Styrofoam®) cup

4. Description of Procedure:
- Before freezing, gently pare down a thick wart with a sterile no. 15 scalpel blade; stop when superficial bleeding occurs or this procedure becomes painful.
- Shape the tip of a cotton-tipped applicator stick into a point smaller than the wart to be frozen. A standard, prepackaged cotton-tipped applicator swab can be used, but persons who perform this procedure often usually prefer to make their own applicators by wrapping a cotton ball loosely around a wooden stick.
- Liquid nitrogen may be transferred from a storage tank to a polystyrene foam cup for use at the exam table, or the applicator can be dipped directly into the storage tank.
- Warn the patient that the freezing will be uncomfortable.
- Dip the applicator in the liquid nitrogen, then apply directly to the wart with minimal pressure (Figure 7-11). The necessary time of freezing averages about 30 seconds, but will vary from 2 to 10 seconds for very superficial lesions up to 30 to 40 seconds for deeper lesions.
- Look for the white freezing front to cover the wart and then to extend 1 to 3 mm onto the margin of adjacent normal skin.
- No dressing is required when completed.
- Warn the patient that the lesion will hurt again over the next few minutes as it thaws. Tell the patient that a blister will likely form within a few hours at the site of the freezing, and that the blister may be large, hemor-

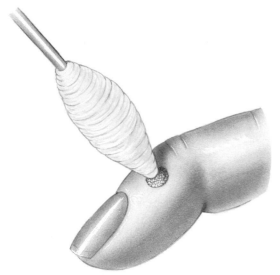

Figure 7-11.
Cryotherapy of verruca vulgaris with liquid nitrogen.
Technique.

rhagic, and somewhat painful. To prevent undue extension of the blister, it is sometimes helpful for the child or parent to puncture, but not unroof, the blister with a sterile needle or blade. Explain that it is hoped the blister will "lift off" the wart.

· A follow-up appointment for possible retreatment may be scheduled in 10 to 14 days.

5. Side Effects and Complications: Complications of the procedure are unusual, but may include scarring and superinfection. Special attention should be given to warts over bony prominences to avoid overfreezing and resulting necrosis of the skin, superficial nerves, and bone.

E. Podophyllin Application for Condylomata Acuminata

1. Purpose: The purpose of this procedure is to treat condylomata acuminata occurring in moist areas in children. The possibility of sexual abuse should be considered in every young child with this condition.

2. Selection of Patients: Other modalities sometimes used include electrocoagulation, liquid nitrogen, surgical excision, and in rare instances, laser therapy.

a. Indications: This procedure is a reasonable choice for treating the patient with condylomata acuminata.

b. Contraindications and Precautions: The procedure should be performed only by a physician, and he or she should exercise extreme caution in handling this caustic chemical. Because of the pain associated with the application of podo-

phyllin, the procedure can be challenging in young children. The only absolute contraindication is pregnancy.

3. Equipment and Supplies (See Appendix for equipment and supplies manufacturers and suppliers. Appendix is keyed to italicized words in the equipment and supplies lists):

· *Petrolatum* or zinc oxide *ointment* (optional)
· Cotton-tipped *applicator* (See Figure 18-17, page 231)
· *Podophyllin* (10–20%) in tincture of benzoin
· Talc

4. Description of Procedure:

· Apply a thick layer of petrolatum or zinc oxide over the normal uninvolved skin surrounding the condylomata (optional).

· Carefully apply a 10% to 20% solution of podophyllum resin in benzoin to the lesions, using a cotton-tipped applicator. Take great care not to spill the solution on normal skin because of a severe irritant effect.

· After the solution dries, powder the area with talc so as to prevent unintended spread of the podophyllin to adjacent normal skin.

· For younger children, instruct the parent to wash off the area thoroughly by local cleansing or by immersing in a bathtub 30 to 60 minutes after the first application. For older children and young adults, a longer first application of up to 2 to 3 hours is usually well tolerated.

· Additional treatments may be needed at weekly intervals; the duration of application for subsequent treatments may be lengthened up to 4 to 6 hours as tolerated.

· Lesions that surround the anus completely should not be treated at the same visit; resulting inflammation, if marked, may lead to significant pain when defecating. Treat lesions on one side at the first visit and on the other side the following week.

· Do not treat extensive areas because of potential toxicity of drug absorption.

· The presence of perianal lesions suggests the possibility of rectal lesions, which can be diagnosed and treated via proctoscopy.

5. Side Effects and Complications: Local discomfort can occur and may be severe if inflammation is marked. Systemic toxicity with renal involvement has been reported rarely after excessive application.

F. Ear Lobe Piercing

1. Purpose: The purpose of this procedure is to perform this minor cosmetic surgery in the safest possible manner.

2. Selection of Patients:

a. Indications: We prefer to treat only children beyond the age of reason who themselves wish to have their ears pierced.

b. Contraindications and Precautions: The procedure can be performed on young infants, but ingestion and aspiration of

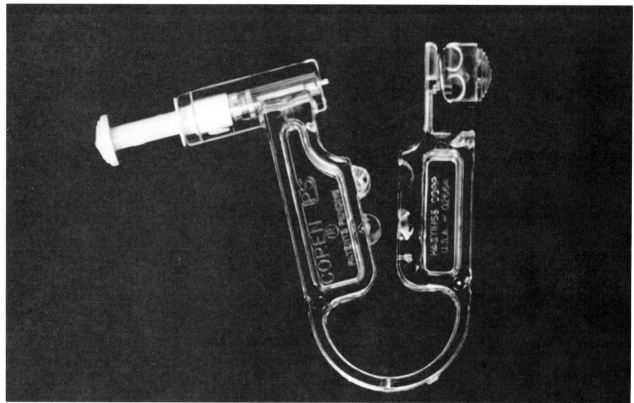

Figure 7-12.
Ear lobe piercing. Equipment and supplies: Spring-loaded ear-piercing gun.

earrings have been reported in this very young age group. The procedure should be avoided in keloid formers and in patients with recurrent cysts of the earlobes.

3. Equipment and Supplies (See Appendix for equipment and supplies manufacturers and suppliers. Appendix is keyed to italicized words in the equipment and supplies lists):

· Isopropyl alcohol *pads*
· Can of ethyl chloride *spray* or an ice cube (optional)
· Spring-loaded ear-piercing *gun* (Figure 7-12)
· Earring with gold or stainless steel post

4. Description of Procedure:

· Clean the ear lobe with isopropyl alcohol.
· No anesthesia is required for this relatively painless procedure. If the patient is nevertheless anxious about the prospect of pain, light anesthesia with ethyl chloride or a cloth-covered ice cube is optional.
· Have the patient indicate the desired site of puncture.
· We use a spring-loaded ear-piercing gun, but alternative instruments and techniques are available.
· After the wound has been created, use an earring with a gold or surgical stainless steel post (to reduce the

likelihood of contact dermatitis). Leave it in place for 10 to 14 days to allow healing and preservation of the created canal.

· During this time, have the patient put a drop or two of isopropyl alcohol on the end of the post twice daily and then rotate the post gently to keep the track open.

5. Side Effects and Complications: Ingestion and aspiration of earrings can occur in young infants as noted above. Local infection, superficial cervical lymphadenopathy, pseudocyst formation, and keloid development are other possible complications.

References

1. Arndt KA. Manual of dermatologic therapeutics. 3rd ed. Boston: Little, Brown and Company, 1983.
2. McBurney EI. Diagnostic dermatologic methods. Pediatr Clin North Am 1983; 30:419–34.
3. Pariser DM, Caserio RJ, Eaglstein WH. Techniques for diagnosing skin and hair disease. 2nd ed. New York: Thieme, 1986.
4. Todd JK. Office laboratory diagnosis of skin and soft tissue infections. Pediatr Infect Dis 1985; 4:84–7.

Chapter 8

Eye Procedures

Bruce T. Carter

I. Screening Procedures

A. Vision Testing

1. Purpose: The purpose of visual testing is to assess the monocular visual status of a child of any age.

2. Selection of Patients:

a. Indications: Visual acuity testing can be a part of any well child examination. Further, it should be performed any time a patient presents with an ocular injury or symptoms referable to the visual system.

b. Contraindications and Precautions: None

3. Equipment and Supplies (See Appendix for equipment and supplies manufacturers and suppliers. Appendix is keyed to italicized words in the equipment and supplies lists):

There are numerous devices available for visual acuity testing. None is superior. A projected chart, self-illuminated chart, or hanging wall chart are all quite adequate.

- Visual acuity *charts* (Figure 8-1)
  - Letters
  - Picture optotypes
- Occluder or adhesive patch (Figure 8-2)

4. Description of Procedure:

- Place the occluder before one eye. Be certain that the eye is completely covered so that the child can not peek around the occluder (Figure 8-3) (Also see Figure 8-12, page 77).
- Ask the patient to read each horizontal line on the visual acuity chart down to the smallest line completely visible to him. From this result, record the acuity.
- Repeat the procedure for the fellow eye.
- Because children generally have excellent accomodative reserves, you need not routinely check near acuity unless there is a specific complaint of difficulty with near vision.

5. Side Effects and Complications: None

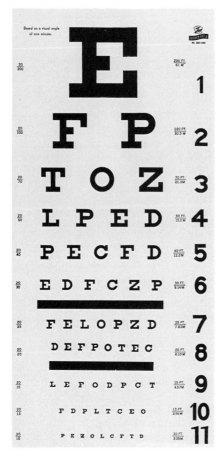
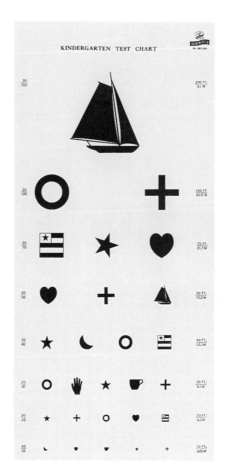

Figure 8-1.
Vision testing. Equipment and supplies: Snellen charts.

6. Interpretation: The preverbal child's vision is judged by his fixation preference (use of a preferred eye) and his objection to or reaction to monocular occlusion. For example, the infant with strabismus whose fixation alternates from one eye to the other will have equal vision and will be free of amblyopia (decreased vision without a detectable organic lesion of the eye). Conversely, if the child with strabismus consistently fixates with one eye and will not fixate with the other eye, the examiner can assume poor visual acuity in the nonfixing eye.

The verbal child begins to participate actively in vision testing at the age of 2 to 2½ years. The examiner shows the patient the eye chart and records the acuity as that which corresponds to the smallest full line of horizontal figures or letters the child is able to identify or read completely. It is important for accuracy that the child read horizontally grouped optotypes (letters or symbols on an eye chart) rather than vertically oriented or single optotypes; the amblyopic eye is able to identify or read isolated or vertically oriented optotypes more readily than horizontally oriented optotypes of the same size. Often a child with amblyopia will read the first and last letters of a horizontal line but miss the center letters. This observation is known as the "crowding phenomenon." Any child in the amblyopia-susceptible age group (birth to 9 years) should be checked more for equality of vision than for an absolute level of acuity. A visual acuity of 20/40 in each eye is far more acceptable than an acuity of 20/30 in one eye and 20/50 in the fellow eye. Usually, bilaterally reduced acuity in the preschool-aged child is a function of immaturity and will result in subsequent normal acuity. Conversely unequal acuity (two lines or more difference between eyes) is highly suggestive of amblyopia and warrants referral.

II. Diagnostic Procedures

A. Strabismus Testing
1. Purpose: The purpose of strabismus testing is to assess ocular alignment.

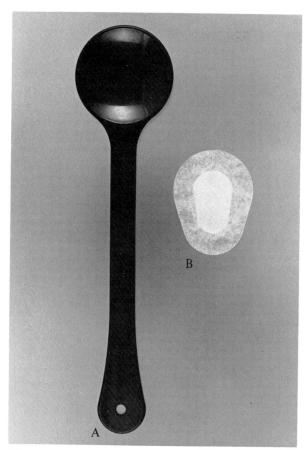

Figure 8-2.
Vision testing. Equipment and supplies: **A,** Occluder; **B,**
Adhesive patch.

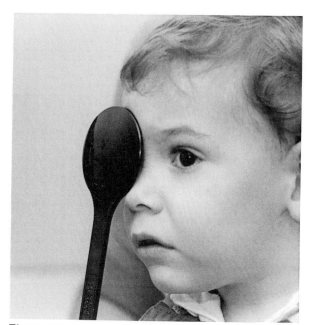

Figure 8-3.
Vision testing. Technique.

2. Selection of Patients:
a. Indications: The procedure should be a part of any well
baby or well child examination. In addition, it should be
performed any time the patient complains of diplopia or the
parent or examiner suspects an ocular deviation.
b. Contraindications and Precautions: None
3. Equipment and Supplies (See Appendix for equipment
and supplies manufacturers and suppliers. Appendix is keyed
to italicized words in the equipment and supplies lists):
  · *Occluder*
  · Fixation targets
    — Near: small finger puppets (Figure 8-4A) or small
    figures pasted on a tongue blade (Figure 8-4B)
    — Far: stuffed animals that make sounds
4. Description of Procedure:
  · Perform the cover test at both 13 inches (0.33 m) (near
  fixation testing) and 20 feet (6 m) (distant fixation testing).

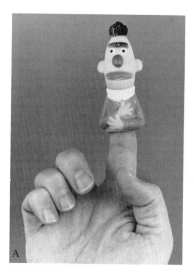

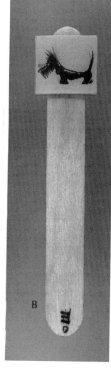

Figure 8-4.
Strabismus testing. Equipment and supplies: **A,** Finger puppet;
B, Small figure pasted on a tongue blade.

· It is essential for you to have the patient fixing on the target; therefore, present to the patient a fixation target of some interest or amusement. Small finger puppets or small figures pasted on a tongue blade serve well as near fixation targets. Larger toys or stuffed animals that make sounds serve as good distant fixation targets.

· While the patient is fixing on the distant fixation target (Figure 8-5A), place the occluder in front of one eye (Figure 8-5B). Direct your attention to the uncovered eye and note movement or the lack thereof.

· Then place the occluder in front of the other eye (Figure 8-5C). Observe the newly uncovered eye for movement or the lack thereof.

· Present a toy or some other accomodative target for near fixation and repeat the cover test at 13 inches (0.33 m).

· Remember that a light source is an unacceptable fixation target. Because it does not stimulate accommodation, it will not precipitate any abnormal deviation.

5. Side Effects and Complications: None

6. Interpretation: If during cover testing, the uncovered eye does not move, the examiner concludes that 1) the fovea (area of clearest vision) of the eye was directed at this object

of regard, and 2) the eyes are normally aligned for that test distance. If, however, as the occluder is placed in front of one eye, the uncovered eye moves out (abducts) to pick up fixation, then it must have been turned in or esotropic (Figure 8-6A). Similarly, if the uncovered eye moves in (adducts) to pick up fixation, then it must have been turned out or exotropic (Figure 8-6B). Generally, esotropias are greater at near fixation and may be present only at near. Frequently, they are only observed during accommodation (the act of focusing the lens). Exotropias, however, are more often greater at distant fixation, and therefore observed when the cover test is done during distant fixation. If an exotropia is suspected, a small examining room is insufficient for this test and one must have the child observe a target at the end of a long hallway or even outside through a clean window. One will occasionally see an intermittent exotropia at near associated with a remote near point of convergence (10 cm or more). This would suggest a convergence insufficiency, which is one of the most common ophthalmic causes of headache in the school-age child. Referral is indicated for orthoptic therapy.

B. Fluorescein Staining

1. Purpose: The purpose of fluorescein staining is to assess corneal epithelial integrity.

2. Selection of Patients:

a. Indications: This procedure should be performed on any

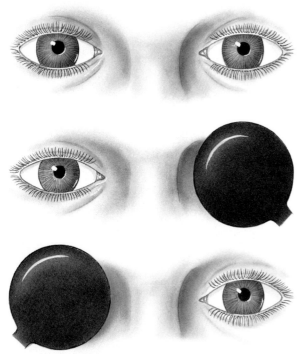

Figure 8-5.
Strabismus testing—Normal cover test. Technique.

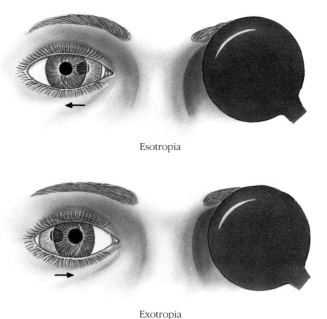

Esotropia

Exotropia

Figure 8-6.
Strabismus testing—Abnormal cover tests. Technique.

patient complaining of foreign body sensation, any patient with an inflamed or injected conjunctiva, and any patient with a corneal opacity.

b. Contraindications and Precautions: An open globe is a contraindication for performing the procedure.

3. Equipment and Supplies (See Appendix for equipment and supplies manufacturers and suppliers. Appendix is keyed to italicized words in the equipment and supplies lists):

· Fluorescein *strips* (Figure 8-7)

· Light source (pen light or transilluminator) (Figure 8-8)

· Cobalt *filter* (Figure 8-8)

· Ophthalmic irrigating *solution* or sterile saline *solution*

· Magnification (hand-held *magnifier*) (optional) (Figure 8-7)

4. Description of Procedure:

· Perform fluorescein staining after the visual acuity has been measured and the globe inspected for intactness.

· Moisten the fluorescein strip with ophthalmic irrigating solution or *sterile* normal saline. Alternatively, moisten the strip with the patient's own tears by momentarily holding the strip in the inferior cul-de-sac (the fold formed by the junction of the bulbar conjunctiva and palpebral conjunctiva of the lower eyelid).

· Touch the moistened fluorescein strip to the conjunc-

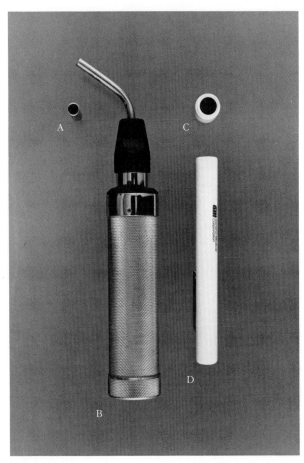

Figure 8-8.
Fluorescein staining. Equipment and supplies: **A,** Cobalt filter; **B,** Otoscope/ ophthalmoscope with transilluminator; **C,** Cobalt filter; **D,** Pen light.

tiva of the lower eyelid of the eye being inspected. This is not painful for the chid and normally does not require restraint.

· Ask the patient to blink his eye.

· Illuminate the eye with the cobalt blue light and inspect for patterns of fluorescence.

5. Side Effects and Complications: A corneal abrasion could potentially occur if the edge of the strip touched the cornea.

6. Interpretation: On illuminating the cornea with the cobalt blue light, the epithelial defect will be obvious as a fluorescent yellow-green area whose size and pattern depend on the nature and extent of the injury. One characteristic pattern is that of faint vertically oriented striae that suggest the presence of a foreign body trapped on the conjunctival surface of the upper lid (Figure 8-9).

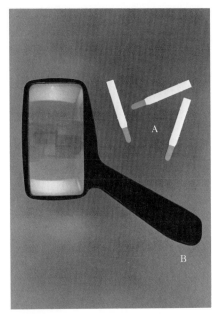

Figure 8-7.
Fluorescein staining. Equipment and supplies: **A,** Fluorescein strips; **B,** Hand-held magnifier.

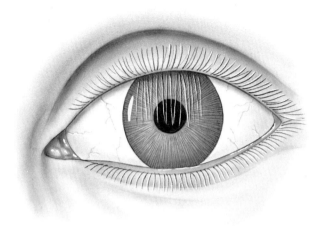

Figure 8-9.
Fluorescein staining. Vertical striae characteristic of retained foreign body under upper lid.

C. Upper Eyelid Eversion

1. Purpose: The purpose of eyelid eversion is to inspect the conjunctival surface of the upper lid and superior cul-de-sac.
2. Selection of Patients:
a. Indications: The procedure should be performed on anyone complaining of foreign body sensation.
b. Contraindications and Precautions: None
3. Equipment and Supplies (See Appendix for equipment and supplies manufacturers and suppliers. Appendix is keyed to italicized words in the equipment and supplies lists):
   · Cotton-tipped *applicator* (See Figure 14-5, page 167)
   · Hand-held *magnifier* (See Figure 8-7, page 73)
   · *Sterile* saline *solution* or ophthalmic irrigating solution
4. Description of Procedure:
   · Instruct the patient to look down.
   · Grasp the eyelashes of the upper lid between the thumb and index finger.
   · Pull the lid out and down (Figure 8-10).
   · Place the tip of a cotton-tipped applicator in the middle of the lid at the lid crease, and depress the applicator (Figure 8-10). The superior tarsal plate (the firm network of connective tissue that gives shape to the upper eyelid) will then evert, exposing the conjunctival surface.
   · Inspect the conjunctiva for the presence of a foreign body (Figure 8-10). Without magnification, identification and localization of a foreign body may be difficult.
   · If a suspected foreign body is not found, moisten a cotton-tipped applicator with *sterile* saline or ophthalmic irrigating solution and gently swab across the surface to remove any unnoticed foreign body (Figure 8-10).

D. Specimen Collection—Lid Margin and Conjunctival Culture Technique

1. Purpose: The purpose of specimen collection is to obtain material for bacterial, viral, chlamydial, and cytologic studies.
2. Selection of Patients:
a. Indications: Any case of neonatal conjunctivitis, hyperacute (grossly purulent) conjunctivitis at any age, membranous conjunctivitis, or chronic conjunctivitis should have conjunctival cultures. Opinions vary regarding the need for culturing the conjunctivae of patients with acute uncomplicated conjunctivitis.
b. Contraindications and Precautions: The conjunctival bacterial cultures should be performed without prior topical anesthesia because of the possible bacteriostatic effects of the preservatives in the anesthetic solutions.
3. Equipment and Supplies (See Appendix for equipment and supplies manufacturers and suppliers. Appendix is keyed to italicized words in the equipment and supplies lists):
   · Sterile *applicators* (dacron-tipped or calcium alginate-tipped) (See Figures 14-5 and 13-12, pages 167 and 153).
   · *Sterile* saline *solution*
   · Platinum *spatula* (Figure 8-11)
   · Clean glass microscope *slides*
   · Bacterial culture media (blood agar, chocolate agar, and Thayer-Martin media)
   · Stains (Giemsa, Gram, Hansel)
   · Topical anesthetic (e.g., *proparacaine HCl* [0.5%] Ophthetic)
4. Description of Procedure:
   · Premoisten a dacron-tipped or calcium alginate-tipped swab with *sterile* saline before use.
   · Evert the unanesthetized lower lid (See Upper Eyelid Eversion, this page).
   · Wipe the moistened swab along the conjunctival surface of the lower lid, avoiding large aggregates of pus and mucus. Take care to avoid contamination from the skin of the lower lid.
   · Plate the specimen onto a blood or chocolate agar plate and onto Thayer-Martin media if gonococcal conjunctivitis is a consideration.
   · Wipe the lid margin with an applicator and streak it on the same plates.
   · If a chlamydial fluorescent antibody test is desired, obtain a second specimen with a dacron-tipped or calcium alginate-tipped swab and transport it to the laboratory.
   · Sterilize the platinum spatula by holding it in a flame until it glows red and then allow it to cool to room temperature. The cooling process usually takes 15 to 20 seconds.
   · Instill a drop of topical anesthetic in the cul-de-sac.
   · Pull the lower eyelid downward with the index finger

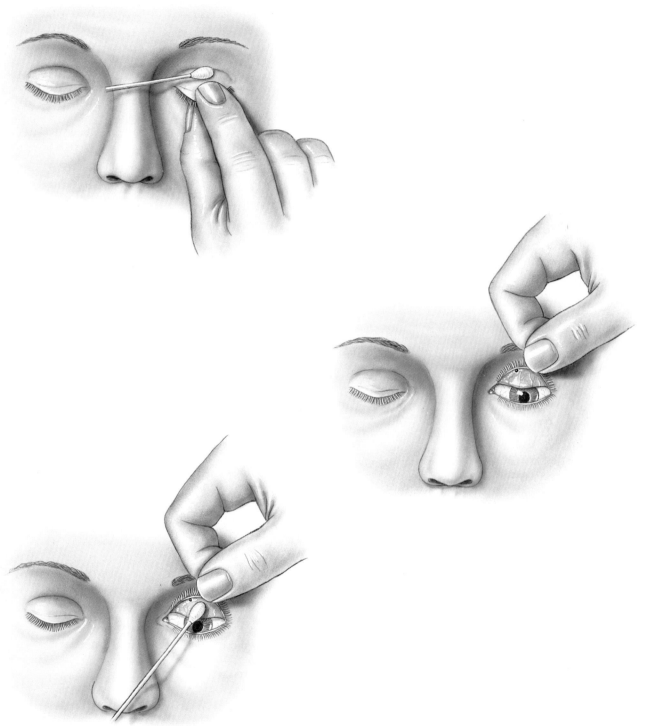

Figure 8-10.
Upper eyelid eversion. Technique.

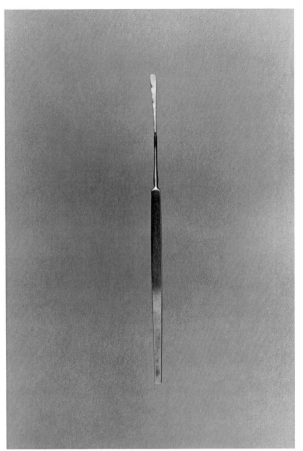

Figure 8-11.
Specimen collection—Lid margin and conjunctival culture.
Equipment and supplies: Platinum spatula.

or a cotton-tipped applicator, everting the lower eyelid.
• Gently scrape the conjunctival surface. Care should be taken to avoid conjunctival bleeding.
• Spread the specimen on a precleaned glass slide and stain it appropriately.
5. Side Effects and Complications: If care is not taken to allow the platinum spatula to cool before use, a conjunctival burn could occur. A conjunctival or corneal abrasion may rarely occur if a swab is carelessly or too forcefully used.
6. Interpretation: The Giemsa stain is used to provide information concerning the inflammatory cell type, the condition of epithelial cells, and the presence or absence of cytoplasmic inclusion bodies. As a general rule, the Giemsa stain provides more useful information regarding the cause (viral, bacterial, or allergic) of the conjunctivitis. The Gram stain gives information regarding bacterial origin and also may give information about fungal elements on the slide. The Hansel stain

is a simple and quick stain. Its major usefulness is in ocular cytology for identification of an eosinophilic response. This stain is not recommended, however, for the identification of cytoplasmic granules.

III. Therapeutic Procedures

A. Patching for Amblyopia
1. Purpose: The purpose of this procedure is to restore normal visual acuity to an amblyopic eye by occlusion of the uninvolved eye.
2. Selection of Patients:
a. Indications: Amblyopia can be detected either through a child's fixation preference (See Vision Testing, page 69) or through conventional visual acuity measurement. The fixation preference, as previously mentioned, represents simply which eye the child prefers to use. The child with amblyopia will not choose to use the worse eye. When the better eye is covered, the amblyopic child will usually resist, cry, attempt to pull the patch off, or push the examiner's hand away.
Three basic types of amblyopia exist:
(1) Anisometropic—This type results from a significant difference in the refractive state of the two eyes (e.g., one eye is severely myopic and the other eye is hyperopic or one eye is hyperopic and the other eye is astigmatic).
(2) Strabismic—This type results from malalignment of the eyes. When strabismus is present, the eyes may alternate fixation such that amblyopia does not develop. However, if a child prefers one eye, the fellow eye may lack sufficient visual stimulation and develop amblyopia.
(3) Form deprivation—The severest form, this amblyopia results from such significant unilateral visual deprivation that either no vision is allowed (e.g., complete ptosis from an upper lid hemangioma) or minimal vision is allowed (e.g., a unilateral congenital cataract).
b. Contraindications and Precautions: The use of a black tie-on patch is less effective than the method described below because the patch does not fit flush to the skin, allowing the child to peep out through the side. For the same reason, patching, painting, or frosting of spectacle lenses are less than optimal means of amblyopia therapy.
3. Equipment and Supplies (See Appendix for equipment and supplies manufacturers and suppliers. Appendix is keyed to italicized words in the equipment and supplies lists):
• Flesh-colored, adhesive-backed *patches* are available commercially in two sizes (adult and junior). Generally, the junior size is adequate for children of all ages (See Figure 8-2, page 71).
• Tincture of *benzoin*
4. Description of Procedure:
• Ask the patient to close the eye to be patched.

· Apply tincture of benzoin to the area of skin to which the patch will be attached. This process will aid in securing the patch after its application.

· Apply the patch so that the eye is totally occluded (Figure 8-12).

· Generally, the eye is patched during waking hours 1 week for every year of age and then is seen in follow-up. Subsequent patching instructions may vary according to the patient's initial response.

5. Side Effects and Complications: Minor skin breakdown and excoriation are frequently seen. In these cases, the application of a moisturizing lotion at night followed by slight decentration of the patch the following morning will allow uninterrupted patch therapy as well as resolution of the skin breakdown.

For the child with dense amblyopia, patching of the normal seeing eye may meet with strong objection and behavioral problems. The child may withdraw, cry, and tax the parents patience in any number of ways. The most frequent problem is the constant removal of the patch by the child. To maintain the patch in place, cut the fingernails, use tincture of benzoin, and splint the elbows to prevent bending of the arms (Figure 8-13).

Occlusion amblyopia may result from excessive or unmonitored patch therapy in the eye with previously normal vision. This form of amblyopia usually is easily reversed.

B. Patching for Corneal Abrasion

1. Purpose: The purpose of this procedure is to immobilize the upper eyelid to reduce the discomfort associated with the constant movement of the upper lid over the epithelial defect and at the same time to aid in the closure of the epithelial defect.

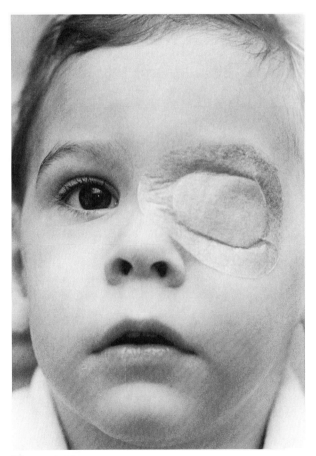

Figure 8-12.
Patching for amblyopia. Technique.

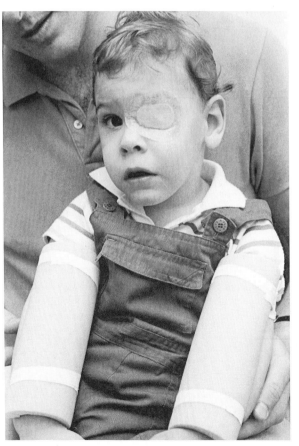

Figure 8-13.
Patching for amblyopia—Splinting of elbows. Technique.

2. Selection of Patients:

a. Indications: The presence of an epithelial defect is an indication for an eye patch, with few exceptions. However, not all patients will tolerate an eye patch. Children under 3 years of age often will remove the patch at their first opportunity; therefore, instilling antibiotic solution or ointment is usually all that can be accomplished and is sufficient in this age group.

b. Contraindications and Precautions: Epithelial disruptions from a caustic agent and corneal ulcers are best left unpatched and should be managed by an ophthalmologist on an emergency basis.

3. Equipment and Supplies (See Appendix for equipment and supplies manufacturers and suppliers. Appendix is keyed to italicized words in the equipment and supplies lists):

- Topical antibiotic solution or ointment (e.g., *Polymyxin B-bacitracin*)
- Sterile oval eye *pads* (Figure 8-14)
- One-half-inch or one inch paper *tape*

4. Description of Procedure:

- Instill an antibiotic solution or ointment (See Instillation of Ointments and Solutions, page 81).
- Ask the patient to close his eyes. Then place an oval eye pad over the injured eye (Figure 8-14).
- Place a strip of tape from the glabella across the patch to the zygoma while the skin over the zygoma is pulled nasally (Figure 8-14). Further secure the patch with additional strips as illustrated.

    As the tape adheres to the skin and the skin relaxes, the patch tightens and holds the eyelids firmly closed. In the case of a deep orbit, a second oval eye pad may be necessary to give adequate pressure.

5. Side Effects and Complications: It is important that the patch be firm and tight such that the eye can not be opened beneath it; otherwise, the patient may find the patch quite uncomfortable with an immobilized upper lid and a partially opened eye beneath.

If a topical anesthetic is used to relieve blepharospasm at the time of the examination, it is important to warn the patient that the anesthetic will wear off in 15 to 20 minutes and there may be some return of discomfort. This anticipatory guidance will prevent an unnecessary return visit to the office or the emergency room as the discomfort returns. Mild analgesics with codeine are usually prescribed for the discomfort.

The patient is followed every 24 hours until the corneal epithelial defect has healed. Time to healing depends on the size of the abrasion, but generally occurs within 24 to 72 hours.

C. Corneal/Conjunctival Foreign Body Removal

1. Purpose: The purpose of this procedure is to remove a foreign body from the cornea or conjunctiva.

2. Selection of Patients:

a. Indications: Any patient with a foreign body resting on the surface of the cornea or conjunctiva may benefit.

b. Contraindications and Precautions: Any foreign body appearing to penetrate the globe or associated with hemorrhage should be examined and removed under magnification by an ophthalmologist.

3. Equipment and Supplies (See Appendix for equipment and supplies manufacturers and suppliers. Appendix is keyed to italicized words in the equipment and supplies lists):

- Topical anesthesia [e.g., *proparacaine HCl* (0.5%) Ophthetic]
- Sterile cotton-tipped *applicators* (See Figure 14-5, page 167)
- Ophthalmic irrigating *solution*
- 25-gauge *needle* (See Figure 20-7, page 262)
- *Spud* (blunt-tipped instrument) (Figure 8-15)
- Sterile oval eye *pad* (See Figure 8-14, page 79)
- ½ or 1-inch paper *tape*
- Antibiotic solution or ointment (e.g., *polymyxin B-bacitracin*)

4. Description of Procedure:

a. *Foreign body:*

- Instill a topical anesthetic solution.
- Once the eye is anesthetized, gently swab the area of the foreign body with a moistened cotton-tipped applicator in an attempt to dislodge it (Figure 8-16).
- If the foreign body will not move from the cornea or conjunctiva, use the spud or needle to dislodge and remove the foreign body (Figure 8-17).

b. *Dislocated contact lenses:*

- In the case of a dislocated or decentered contact lens, initially inspect the globe in primary or straight-ahead position.
- If the lens is resting on the nasal or temporal conjunctiva, simply place the tip of the index finger on the lens and slide the lens back on the cornea. This process may be slightly uncomfortable and may need to be done after the instillation of a topical anesthetic.
- If the lens is not in view, instruct the patient to look up and down while the inferior and superior cul-de-sacs are inspected. Many contact lens wearers who initially do not understand orbital anatomy fear the loss of the contact lens behind the eye. Reassure them by explaining that the contact is limited to the front of the eye by the conjunctival reflection on itself (cul-de-sac). Extreme up or down gaze will demonstrate the lost lens, at which time the lens may be teased into position with a clean finger.

c. *Adherent contact lenses:*

- Occasionally, you will encounter a hard contact lens that has been pressed against the conjunctiva and is tightly adherent to the conjunctiva by suction. Using

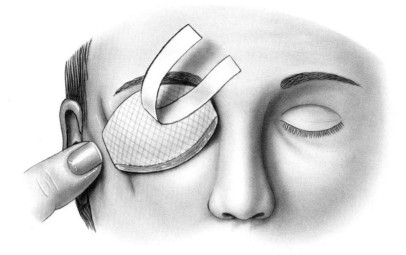

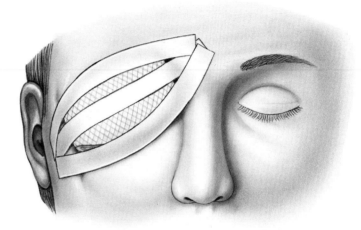

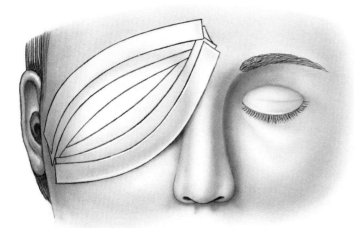

Figure 8-14.
Patching for corneal abrasion. Technique.

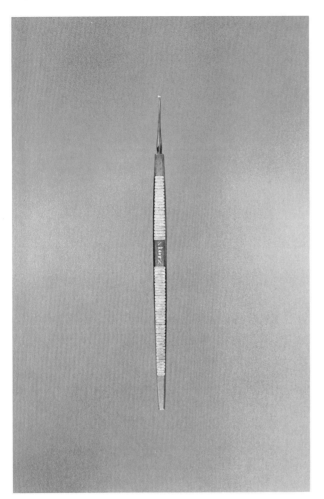

Figure 8-15.
Corneal foreign body removal. Equipment and supplies: spud.

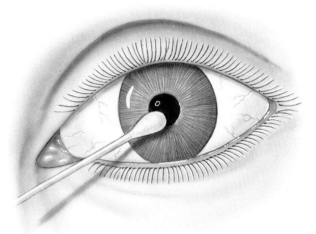

Figure 8-16.
Corneal/conjunctival foreign body removal. Technique using cotton-tipped applicator.

dure, and if the foreign body appears embedded, the use of a spud rather than a needle is advisable.

If you obtain the history of the patient striking metal against metal (e.g., hammering a nail) at the time of injury, remove any obvious foreign body and proceed with orbital

topical anesthesia (See Instillation of Ointments and Solutions, page 81) and a clean hand, break the suction by placing a fingernail (or a blunt-tipped instrument) beneath the edge of the lens. The lens can then be removed and cleaned. Should a lens be fractured, you must carefully inspect the globe under magnification for fragments. At no time should a chipped or damaged lens be worn.

5. Side Effects and Complications: The presence of a residual rust ring after the removal of a metallic foreign body necessitates referral of the patient to an ophthalmologist for removal of the stained tissue (Figure 8-18).

The young child is often less cooperative for this proce-

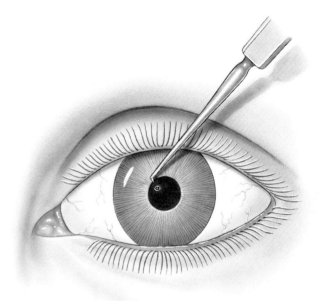

Figure 8-17.
Corneal foreign body removal. Technique using spud.

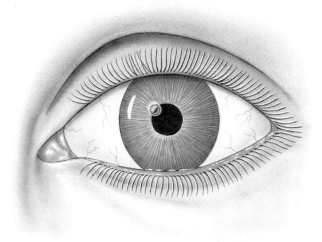

Figure 8-18.
Corneal/conjunctival foreign body removal. Residual rust ring following metallic foreign body removal.

radiographs to rule out the presence of an intraorbital or intraocular metallic foreign body.

On completion of the evaluation of the patient and removal of the foreign body, treat the patient for the corneal epithelial defect in the conventional manner (See Patching for Corneal Abrasion, page 77).

D. Flushing for Chemical Irritants

1. Purpose: The purpose of this procedure is to provide immediate and copious irrigation of the cul-de-sacs, bulbar conjunctiva, and cornea to reduce or eliminate damage from noxious chemicals.

2. Selection of Patients:

a. Indications: The procedure is indicated for any patient who has an irritating substance brought into contact with the eyes. The patient should be instructed to irrigate copiously at home or on the job with tap water before being seen in the office or emergency room.

b. Contraindications and Precautions: The use of a neutralizing substance in the case of a chemical injury is contraindicated.

3. Equipment and Supplies (See Appendix for equipment and supplies manufacturers and suppliers. Appendix is keyed to italicized words in the equipment and supplies lists):

· Topical anesthetic (e.g., *proparacaine HCl* [0.5%] Ophthetic)

· Ophthalmic irrigating *solution,* if available, or normal saline or lactated Ringer's *solution*

· *Intravenous* set with tubing

· Cotton-tipped *applicators* (See Figure 14-5, page 167)

4. Description of Procedure:

· Instill a topical anesthetic solution (See Instillation of Ointments and Solutions, page 81).

· Hold the eye open and irrigate the eye and cul-de-sacs with at least 1 liter of solution over 15 to 20 minutes (Figure 8-19).

· Inspect both cul-de-sacs for particulate debris (e.g., lime granules going into solution).

· Evert the upper lid, with attention to the uppermost aspect of the superior cul-de-sac.

· Swab away any debris with a cotton-tipped applicator and continue copious irrigation.

· Once the basic irrigation procedure has been completed, refer the patient to an ophthalmologist for damage assessment and treatment.

E. Instillation of Ointments and Solutions

1. Purpose: The purpose of this procedure is to topically medicate the eye or eyelids.

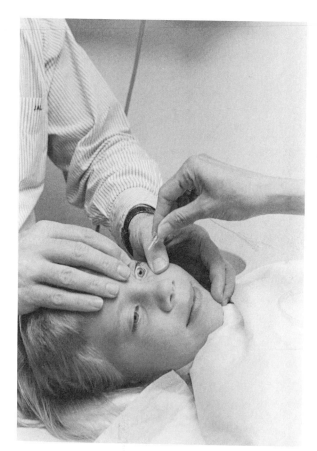

Figure 8-19.
Flushing for chemical irritants. Technique.

2. Selection of Patients:

a. Indications: Any infection or inflammation of the eye or ocular adnexa.

b. Contraindications and Precautions: Topical medication should never be instilled when the possibility of an open globe exists.

3. Equipment and Supplies (See Appendix for equipment and supplies manufacturers and suppliers. Appendix is keyed to italicized words in the equipment and supplies lists):

- The selected solution or ointment

4. Description of Procedure:

- Ask the patient to lie down in a supine position.
- Ask the patient to look up.
- Place gentle but firm traction on the lower lid, thereby pulling it down and out from contact with the globe (Figure 8-20).
- Place the solution or ointment in the inferior cul-de-sac (Figure 8-20). In the case of the instillation of ointment, hold the lid in this position for a matter of seconds until the body temperature melts the ointment. Some topical medications are more uncomfortable than others. By having the patient look up and placing the medication in the inferior cul-de-sac, direct contact with the highly innervated cornea is postponed until the lid is released.
- If you are treating a lid infection, do not place the medication in the cul-de-sac. Instead, brush it on the lid margin with a cotton-tipped applicator laden with the antibiotic ointment.

5. Side Effects and Complications: When a topical anesthetic is used it is important to caution the patient not to rub the eyes. The anesthetic effect lasts approximately 15 to 20 minutes. During that time the child may inadvertently abraid the cornea if he rubs his eyes.

F. Massage of the Lacrimal Sac in the Treatment of Nasolacrimal Duct Obstruction

1. Purpose: The purpose of this procedure is to break the obstruction of the nasolacrimal duct.

2. Selection of Patients:

a. Indications: Any infant with signs of nasolacrimal duct obstruction such as chronic recurrent conjunctivitis since birth or shortly thereafter or chronic mucopurulent discharge. Chronic tearing is highly suggestive of nasolacrimal duct obstruction, but infantile glaucoma needs to be ruled out.

b. Contraindications and Precautions: None

3. Equipment and Supplies: None

4. Description of Procedure:

- Instruct the parent to closely trim the fingernails of

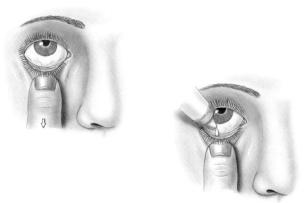

Figure 8-20.
Instillation of ointments and solutions. Technique.

both of his or her index fingers so as not to cut into the skin of the medial canthal region during the massage.

- Have the parent locate his own medial canthal ligament by placing the index finger in the medial canthus and identifying the small "bump" of the medial canthal ligament (Figure 8-21).

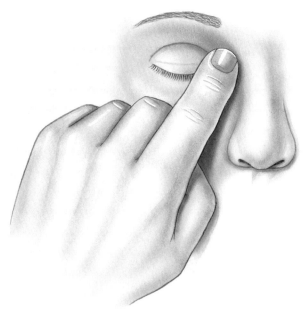

Figure 8-21.
Massage of the lacrimal sac in the treatment of nasolacrimal duct obstruction. Palpation of underlying medial canthal ligament.

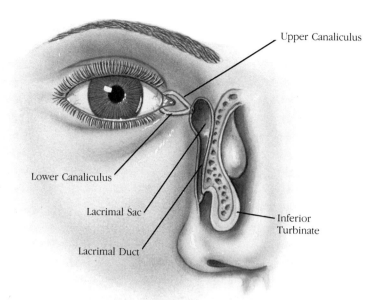

Upper Canaliculus

Lower Canaliculus

Lacrimal Sac

Lacrimal Duct

Inferior Turbinate

Figure 8-22.
Massage of the lacrimal sac in the treatment of nasolacrimal duct obstruction. Anatomy of nasolacrimal system.

· Familarize the parent with the anatomy of the naso-lacrimal system. Parents tend to massage the side of the nose, thinking the duct runs externally rather than its normal interosseous path from just below the medial canthal ligament to beneath the inferior turbinate (Figure 8-22).

· Instruct the parent to place the tip of his or her index finger over the child's medial canthal ligament and with gentle but firm pressure rock the finger pad vertically for 10 to 15 seconds.

· Instruct the parent to repeat this action several times daily at home. During the child's feeding is a convenient time. The pressure over the lacrimal sac serves to express residual stagnant fluid from the sac and presumably allows for a transient increase in the hydrostatic pressure within the nasolacrimal duct, thereby effecting the eventual rupture of the obstructing membrane.

5. Side Effects and Complications: Massage of the lacrimal sac and instillation of topical antibiotics is not always successful in opening the duct. Probing and irrigation of the

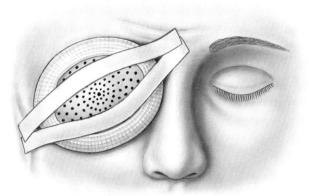

Figure 8-23.
Management of the open globe. Placement and taping of Fox shield.

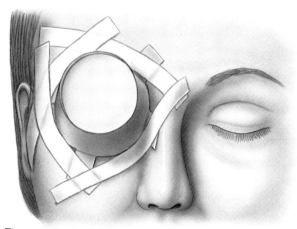

Figure 8-24.
Management of the open globe. Placement and taping of modified paper cup "shield."

nasolacrimal system may be required. The timing of this procedure remains somewhat controversial. However, most ophthalmologists would agree that the duct should be probed by 12 months of age.

G. Management of the Open Globe

1. Purpose: The purpose of this procedure is to protect the open globe and prevent extrusion of intraocular contents.

2. Selection of Patients:

a. Indications: Any patient with an open globe or the possibility of an open globe is a candidate.

b. Contraindications and Precautions: Avoid external pressure to the ruptured globe, because the contents may be extruded under pressure.

3. Equipment and Supplies (See Appendix for equipment and supplies manufacturers and suppliers. Appendix is keyed to italicized words in the equipment and supplies lists):

- Fox *shield* (Figure 8-23)
- Paper or Styrofoam® cup, modified to become a shield (Figure 8-24)
- 1-inch paper *tape*

4. Description of Procedure:

- Place the Fox shield or modified shield fashioned from a cup over the eye, taking care not to exert pressure on the globe.
- Tape the shield or cup into place (Figures 8-23 and 8-24).

5. Side Effects and Complications: Many patients who have sustained severe eye injuries have also suffered head injuries and are in varying states of consciousness. It is important that these patients be protected from additional self-inflicted eye trauma such as that from flailing limbs or other forms of external pressure to the injured eye.

Chapter 9

Ear, Nose, and Throat Procedures

Gregory F. Hayden

Paul R. Lambert

I. Screening Procedures

A. Audiometry

1. Purpose: Audiometry can be used to assess hearing quantitatively and to help define or localize a hearing loss (e.g., middle ear conductive loss, cochlear loss, or retrocochlear loss).

2. Selection of Patients:

a. Indications: Because screening audiometry is a behavioral test requiring the patient's cooperation, it is most accurate for children older than 3 years. Behavioral observation audiometry, visual reinforcement audiometry, and play audiometry can provide information on hearing acuity for younger children, but these tests should be conducted by an audiologist.

b. Contraindications and Precautions: None

3. Equipment and Supplies: Precise audiometric assessment requires a sound isolation room, sophisticated instrumentation, and the expertise of an audiologist. In the office setting, however, screening audiometry to detect the presence or absence of a hearing loss can be performed by non-audiologists using less sophisticated equipment. A number of portable audiometers are commercially available. Theoretically, thresholds for both air and bone conduction can be tested using many of these instruments. The inability to mask bone-conducted tones makes interpretation of these thresholds problematic, so only air conduction measurements are practical for the non-audiologist in the office setting.

4. Description of Procedure:

- Have the child sit comfortably in a chair or on his parent's lap.
- Keep ambient noise to a minimum.
- Present air-conducted tones at 1000, 2000, and 4000 Hz to each ear through the head phone at a 25- to 30-db level. The usual ambient noise in an office precludes

accurate measurement of sensitivity to lower frequencies. Based on the child's response to these three tones, a qualitative assessment of hearing can be made and recorded (Figure 9-1). Attempting to define threshold levels more precisely is inappropriate and unnecessary in the office setting, as this procedure is intended only for screening.

5. Side Effects and Complications: None

6. Interpretation: Cooperative children who fail this screening protocol should have a careful examination of their tympanic membranes. If middle ear effusion is present, testing can usually be repeated after a period of treatment or of watchful waiting. If the effusion persists for more than 2 or 3 months, the child should be referred to an audiologist and otolaryngologist for more complete evaluation.

II. Diagnostic Procedures

A. Pneumatic Otoscopy

1. Purpose: The purpose of this procedure is to improve the accuracy of routine otoscopy in the diagnosis of middle ear disease. Routine otoscopy with careful inspection of the color, luster, and position of the tympanic membrane will often establish a correct otologic diagnosis. Additional assessment of the tympanic membrane to gentle pneumomassage, how-

---

CHILDREN'S MEDICAL CENTER

UNIVERSITY OF VIRGINIA

DEPARTMENT OF PEDIATRICS

Date: _____

Patient Identification

SCREENING AUDIOGRAM

Tone Frequency (in Hertz)	Right Ear		Left Ear	
	Pass	Fail	Pass	Fail
1000	Pass	Fail	Pass	Fail
2000	Pass	Fail	Pass	Fail
4000	Pass	Fail	Pass	Fail

Pass = Responded at screening level of 25 dB hearing level
(American National Standard Institute 1969)

Comments:
Ambient noise:	Low/Normal	Excessive
Child's cooperation:	Good	Poor
Reliability of test:	Good	Poor
Validity of test:	Acceptable	Questionable

Tested by: _____

Audiometer: _____

Figure 9-1.
Audiometry. Screening audiogram record.

ever, can increase the diagnostic accuracy of the routine examination.

2. Selection of Patients:

a. Indications: Pneumatic otoscopy can be employed for all ear examinations in children whether or not ear disease is suggested.

b. Contraindications and Precautions: None

3. Equipment and Supplies (See Appendix for equipment and supplies manufacturers and suppliers. Appendix is keyed to italicized words in the equipment and supplies lists):

- *Otoscope.* Use a 3.5-V halogen-illuminated otoscope and the diagnostic head equipped with a thin rubber tube that can be connected to either a rubber *bulb* or a plastic *mouthpiece* (Figure 9-2). Learn how to replace the light bulb as needed (With frequent daily use, a light bulb will usually last about 2 to 6 months; manufacturers state the light bulb has a 20-hour life span.); keep re-

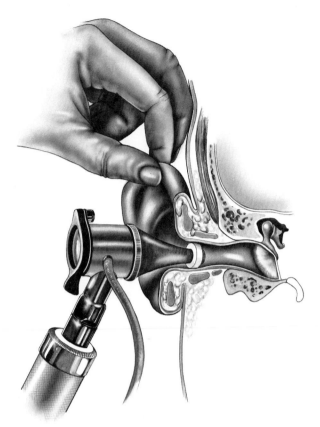

Figure 9-3.
Otoscopy. Technique.

chargeable batteries well charged. Check for an air leak in the system by occluding the tip of the speculum with your finger and then applying positive and negative pressure. A rubber, bulb-type insufflator is suitable for use in older children and provides a reproducible change in air pressure. For the examination of young children, however, most clinicians replace the bulb insufflator with a small plastic mouthpiece to provide a method for better control of the air pressure changes. A normal tympanic membrane will show outward motion with a gentle suck, creating a negative pressure equal to that of a light kiss.

Use the largest speculum that can be inserted into the external auditory meatus, so as to allow the greatest amount of light to pass through and to minimize air leak during the pneumatic examination. Specula with a soft, flexible tip are less painful to use, but because of their relatively large size, are most useful in older children with large canals. Cutting a small (2–3-mm length) piece

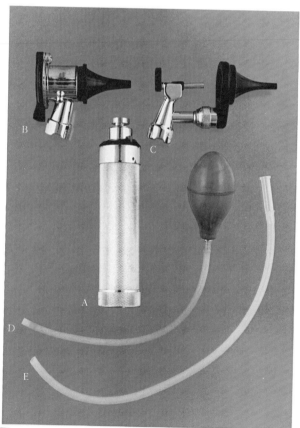

Figure 9-2.
Otoscopy. Equipment and supplies: **A,** Otoscope; **B,** Diagnostic head; **C,** Operating head; **D,** Insufflator bulb and rubber tube; **E,** Mouthpiece and rubber tube.

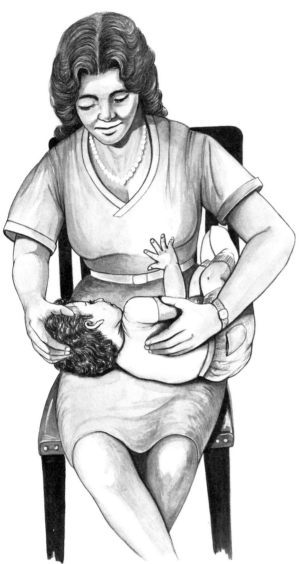

Figure 9-4.
Otoscopy. Restraint of the infant or small child on his mother's lap.

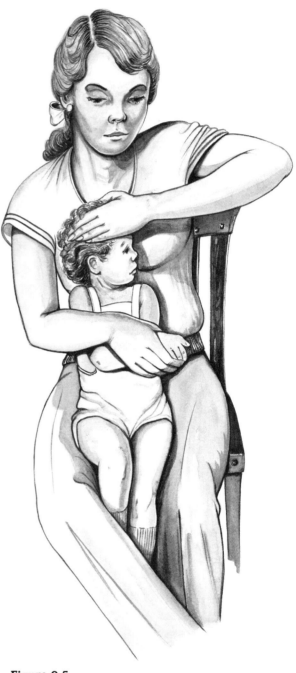

Figure 9-5.
Otoscopy. Restraint of a preschool child on his mother's lap.

of the rubber tubing and placing it about 6 to 8 mm proximal to the tip of the smaller rigid specula makes insertion into the ear less painful and also helps to achieve an airtight seal (Figure 9-3).

4. Description of Procedure:

a. Restraint:

· The infant or small child can be positioned on the parent's lap with the head supported (Figure 9-4). The

patient's body is restrained by the parent's placing one of his or her hands around the child's upper arm, shoulder, and upper back; the parent's forearm lies across the

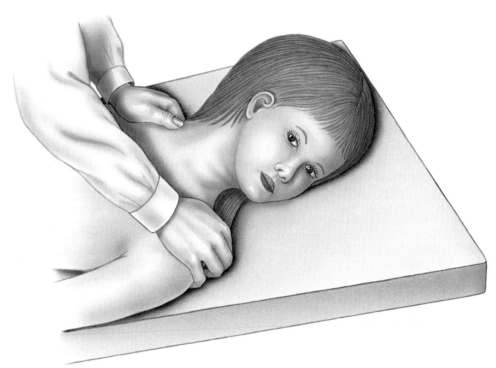

Figure 9-6.
Otoscopy. Restraint of a child on a table.

hip and lower extremities. The parent's other hand is placed around the head to support and restrain it.

· A preschool child may sit in the parent's lap (Figure 9-5). One of the parent's hands is used to hold the child's head against the parent's chest, and the other hand prevents excessive motion of the child's arms and body. The child's legs are placed between those of the parent for further restraint.

· Alternatively, the patient can be placed supine on an examination table and the parent or assistant can provide restraint (Figure 9-6). The shoulders should be held flat against the table to prevent rotation of the trunk. The arms need to be held to prevent the child from reaching up and grabbing the instrument being used by the examiner, who is standing at the end of the examination table. Specially designed restraint boards with Velcro straps to immobilize the arms, body, and legs are occasionally useful for uncooperative younger children.

· The older, cooperative child may sit without restraints on the examination table.

b. Pneumomassage:

· Insert the speculum into the external auditory canal.

· Hold the otoscope more like a pencil than a hammer, and rest the hypothenar aspect of the examining hand

against the child's head (Figure 9-7). In this manner, any unexpected movement of the head will cause a corresponding movement of the otoscope, thus minimizing

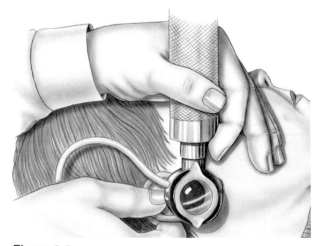

Figure 9-7.
Otoscopy. Technique.

the possibility of trauma to the ear canal. In the illustration, the patient is lying supine on an examination table, and the examiner is standing at the end of the table above the patient's head. If the patient is positioned otherwise (sitting or on the parent's lap), the location of the examiner's hands on the patient's head will need modifying, but the grip on the otoscope should remain the same. Many physicians find it technically easiest to hold the otoscope in the hand opposite to the side of the ear being examined (i.e., holding the otoscope in the right hand while examining the left ear and then switching the otoscope to the left hand to examine the right ear). This method provides the most effective means of restraining the child's head motion by having the heel of the examiner's hand rest directly over the child's cheek.

· Pulling backward and upward on the pinna may help to straighten the natural angle of the canal and allow easier insertion of the speculum.

· Insert the speculum 5 to 10 mm into the canal.

· Identify the bony landmarks of the tympanic membrane, then apply a short suck to the mouthpiece.

· Allow the tympanic membrane to return to its usual position and repeat the sucking.

· Then puff lightly into the mouthpiece.

· Allow the tympanic membrane to return to its usual position and puff again.

5. Side Effects and Complications: Excessive pressure may induce pain.

6. Interpretation: Interpretation of the results depends on the responses of the tympanic membrane to positive and negative pressure. A normal tympanic membrane will move equal distances briskly in response to positive and negative pressure. A tympanic membrane that is retracted because of underaeration of the middle ear space can move outward to negative pressure better than it can move inward to positive pressure. Conversely, a tympanic membrane that is bulging as a result of acute otitis media can move inward slightly with firm positive pressure, but will move outward only very poorly with negative pressure.

Whenever the results of pneumatic otoscopy are uncertain or conflict with other clinical signs and symptoms, tympanometry (See page 92) should be used as a more objective and quantitative means of assessing middle ear pressure and tympanic membrane compliance.

B. Cerumen Removal

1. Purpose: Cerumen removal from the external auditory canal is performed to provide an adequate diagnostic view of the tympanic membrane.

2. Selection of Patients:

a. Indications: The procedure is most often necessary in young children and infants, whose small canals are more easily occluded by cerumen.

b. Contraindications and Precautions: The irrigation procedure is contraindicated if the patient has a tympanostomy tube in place or if a perforated tympanic membrane is suggested clinically because of otorrhea. Some clinicians use a Water-Pik instrument to irrigate cerumen from the external canal, despite concerns that the pressures generated by this instrument can be dangerously high.

Patients with a large amount of cerumen impacted in the canal should be questioned about the use of cotton-tipped swabs (Q-tips). Although such swabs can remove some of the superficial cerumen, they often push cerumen further into the canal. Patients who produce large amounts of cerumen can periodically (once or twice weekly) use cerumen-softening ear drops (such as 3 drops of a homemade solution of 50% hydrogen peroxide and 50% water) to decrease the likelihood of forming an impaction. Several days before an office visit, the same ear drops can be used twice daily to soften any cerumen present and facilitate its removal.

3. Equipment and Supplies (See Appendix for equipment and supplies manufacturers and suppliers. Appendix is keyed to italicized words in the equipment and supplies lists):

· *Otoscope* with either the diagnostic or the operating head (See Figure 9-2, page 87)

· Ear *curette(s)* (Figure 9-8) Plastic *curette(s)* are also available

· 8-oz. cup

· Lukewarm water

· Butterfly *needle* with clear plastic tubing and a connector hub (See Figure 20-7, page 262)

· 10-mL *syringe* (See Figure 20-7, page 262) or dental *syringe* with a curved and tapered end (See Figure 10-2, page 110)

· Small towels

· Kidney-shaped *basin*

4. Description of Procedure: The two techniques used most often are curettage and irrigation.

a. Curettage

· Restrain the child's head carefully (See Figures 9-4, 9-5, and 9-6, pages 88 and 89).

· Warn an older child that the procedure may be uncomfortable and that an "ouch" or a cry is safer and more acceptable than a rapid head jerk.

· Warn the parent of a younger child that removing the cerumen may sometimes provoke a small amount of harmless bleeding from the external canal.

· Ascertain the location of the cerumen in the canal, using your otoscope.

· For cerumen that is very superficial in the canal, the otoscope may not be necessary. Try to reach around the cerumen with a blunt curette under direct vision and tease the cerumen out gently. During the procedure,

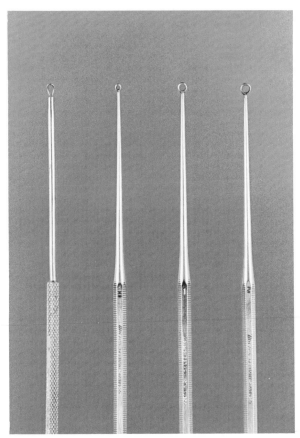

Figure 9-8.
Cerumen removal. Equipment and supplies: Ear curettes.

stabilize the ulnar aspect of your hand on the patient's head so that your hand and the curette will move along with the child's head should the restraint fail.

· Reassess your progress, using the otoscope.

· For cerumen located deeper in the canal, place an operating head on the otoscope and tease the cerumen out under view through the magnifying lens (Figure 9-9). If the diagnostic head is being used, slide the magnifying lens over so that the curette can be introduced beside the magnifying lens and maximum visualization of the cerumen can be maintained.

· Stop the procedure if it is too painful for the child or when your view of the tympanic membrane is adequate for diagnostic purposes.

b. Irrigation

· The older child can usually sit unrestrained on the examination table. The younger child who is uncooperative is placed in a supine position on the examination table and the parent or an assistant provides restraint (See Figure 9-6, page 89).

· Fill an 8-oz. cup with lukewarm (about 36°C) water. Irrigation with cold or hot water may lead to symptoms of dizziness or nausea.

· Cut the needle off the end of a butterfly-type infusion set and attach the hub of the clear plastic tubing to a 10-mL syringe. Alternatively, a plastic dental syringe with a long, gently curved and tapered end can be used.

· Squirt a little water on your wrist to verify that the water temperature is suitable.

· Warn an older child that the procedure may feel "funny" and uncomfortable, but hopefully not painful.

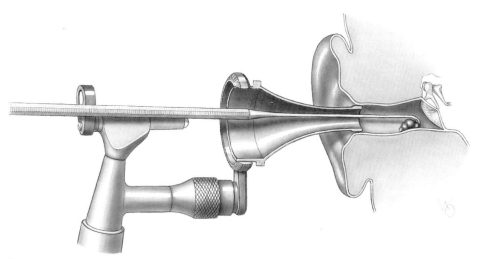

Figure 9-9.
Cerumen removal. Technique.

· Cover the child's shoulders with a towel or gown to keep his clothing dry.

· Place a small kidney-shaped basin under the ear to catch the water and cerumen that will drain out.

· Place the end of the tubing just inside the external auditory meatus and then begin to infuse the water with a moderate, constant force.

· Try to inject some of the water past the plug of cerumen so as to create outward pressure on it.

· Sometimes a large, intact plug of cerumen will flow out into the basin, whereas in other instances the effluent will be tinted yellow but without an obvious plug.

· Reassess the ear examination after infusing several syringes of water. It is often necessary to dry the external canal with an absorbent material, such as gauze, before good visualization can be obtained.

· Stop the procedure if it becomes too uncomfortable for the child or when the view of the tympanic membrane is adequate for diagnosis.

c. Curettage and Irrigation

· Sometimes curettage and irrigation can be used together with a good result.

· Partial cerumen removal with a curette may make subsequent irrigation simpler and more successful.

· Likewise, after irrigation has broken up a plug of cerumen and softened the remaining debris, gentle curettage may be used to complete removal of the cerumen.

5. Side Effects and Complications: An abrasion of the ear canal can result in discomfort or bleeding. Too forceful irrigation can rarely cause a perforation of the tympanic membrane. Irrigation should not be used if a perforation is present or suspected.

C. Tympanometry

1. Purpose: The purpose of tympanometry is to provide objective measurements of the compliance of the tympanic membrane as the air pressure in the external ear canal is altered. Tympanometry is primarily used to confirm middle ear pathology suggested by physical examination, but it has also been used, often together with audiometry, as a screening procedure for hearing loss and middle ear disease.

2. Selection of Patients:

a. Indications: Although tympanometry does not require the same level of cooperation and response as does audiometry, it does require the child to be relatively still and preferably not crying. Therefore, children older than 3 years of age are better candidates for the procedure.

b. Contraindications and Precautions: Tympanometry should not be performed if the patient has had ear surgery in the preceeding 4 to 6 weeks.

3. Equipment and Supplies (See Appendix for equipment and supplies manufacturers and suppliers. Appendix is keyed to italicized words in the equipment and supplies lists):

A number of portable tympanometers are commercially available. In all cases, a probe with three small holes at its tip is inserted into the external meatus (Figure 9-10). A tone (usually 220 Hz) is emitted through one of these holes and the resulting sound pressure in the external canal is conducted through a second hole to a microphone. The third hole is an outlet for an air pressure system that varies the pressure within the external canal slightly above and below atmospheric pressure.

4. Description of Procedure:

· Verify through the otoscope that the external canal is not occluded by cerumen. The presence of some ceru-

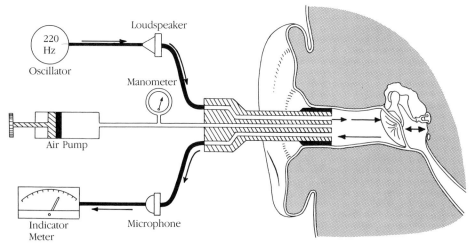

Figure 9-10.
Tympanometry. Variable reflection of probe tone based on compliance.

men will not affect the test, but a large amount should be removed (See Cerumen Removal, page 90).

· Insert the probe tip of the tympanometer and obtain an airtight seal.

· The machine then varies the air pressure within the ear canal from approximately +200 to 300 mm H_2O to −200 to −300 mm H_2O.

· The acoustic energy from the probe tone will either be admitted to the middle ear or reflected back into the external canal, depending on the compliance of the tympanic membrane and middle ear system (Figure 9-11).

· This information is plotted as a tympanogram showing compliance as a function of air pressure (Figure 9-12). Although tympanometry is similar in some respects to pneumatic otoscopy, the amount of air pressure involved is very small compared with that used with the pneumatic otoscope.

5. Side Effects and Complications: None

6. Interpretation: The tympanogram provides information on the pressure in the middle ear, as the compliance will peak when the pressure generated in the external canal equals that in the middle ear (Figure 9-13). The shape of the tympanogram also suggests whether fluid is likely to be present in the middle ear space. For example, a middle ear effusion allows little change in the amount of reflected sound energy as air pressure is varied, resulting in a flat or dome-shaped tympanogram (Figure 9-13). Tympanograms can be broadly classified into three types: Type A shows a peak in the compliance curve near atmospheric pressure and is usually associated

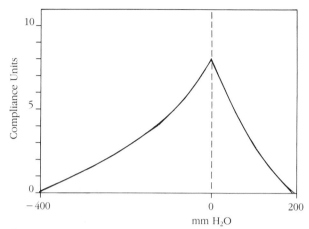

Figure 9-12.
Tympanometry. Normal tympanogram, Type A; abnormal tympanogram, Type B.

with a normal middle ear (Figure 9-13); Type B shows a flat or dome-shaped curve, suggesting a noncompliant middle ear, as found with a middle ear effusion (Figure 9-13); and Type C shows peak compliance in the negative pressure range and most often indicates eustachian tube dysfunction (not shown).

D. Transillumination of the Sinuses

The maxillary sinuses are present at birth and are the most common site of sinusitis in preschool children. The frontal

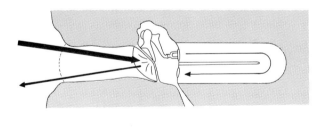

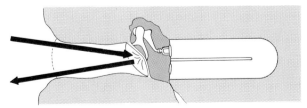

Figure 9-11.
Tympanometry. Equipment and supplies: Schematic of a tympanometer.

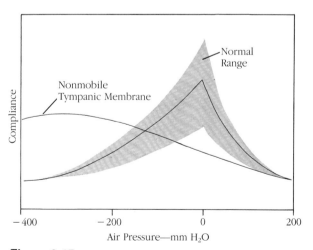

Figure 9-13.
Tympanometry. Tympanogram, showing compliance as a function of air pressure.

sinuses usually appear in the second or third year of life, but remain rudimentary until school age.

1. Purpose: The purpose of this procedure is to assess aeration of the paranasal sinuses.

2. Selection of Patients:

a. Indications: The primary indication for the procedure is the clinical suspicion of maxillary or frontal sinusitis. An adult with sinusitis often presents with fever, headache, and facial pain. Because children with sinusitis often lack these findings, less specific complaints such as chronic purulent rhinorrhea, prolonged daytime cough, headache, swelling of the eyes, and malodorous breath should alert the clinician to the possibility of sinusitis. After sinusitis has been diagnosed, some clinicians also use transillumination to follow the clinical response to antimicrobial therapy.

b. Contraindications and Precautions: None

3. Equipment and Supplies (See Appendix for equipment and supplies manufacturers and suppliers. Appendix is keyed to italicized words in the equipment and supplies lists):

The procedure requires an instrument with a bright light source that emits a narrow beam of light. A special sinus *transilluminator* that attaches to the otoscope power source is a convenient instrument to use (Figure 9-14).

4. Description of Procedure:

· Demonstrate your transilluminator to the child and parent and review briefly with them how you will perform this procedure.

· Turn off all the lights in the examination room and allow your eyes to accommodate to the complete darkness for a few moments.

· To examine the maxillary sinuses, have the child open his mouth and tip his head back slightly. Place the light source over the midpoint of the inferior orbital ridge pointing downward slightly (Figure 9-15). Inspect the amount and symmetry of the blush shining through the hard palate. Try to ignore the light passing through the alveolar ridges. Alternatively, the light source can be

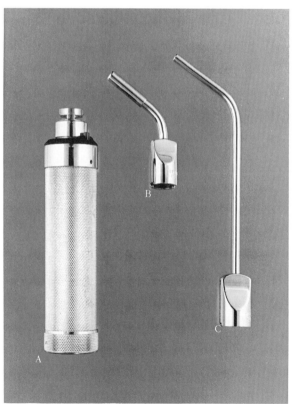

Figure 9-14.
Transillumination of the sinuses. Equipment and supplies: **A,** Otoscope; **B,** Transilluminator; **C,** Transilluminator.

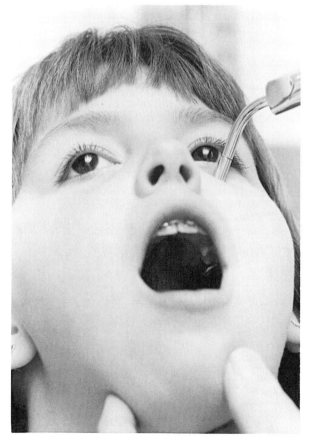

Figure 9-15.
Transillumination of a maxillary sinus. Technique.

placed inside the child's mouth and the child asked to close his mouth and lips around the instrument. The examiner can then assess the amount and symmetry of light passing directly through the maxillary sinuses to the anterior wall of the antrum.

· To visualize the frontal sinuses, place the tip of your instrument just below the medial border of the superior orbital ridge, pointing upward slightly (Figure 9-16). Inspect the amount and symmetry of the blush.

5. Side Effects and Complications: None

6. Interpretations: In general, transillumination is less useful in children than in adults because many of the sinuses are not fully developed and do not transilluminate well. Even among adults, the interpretation of the procedure is subjective, and the predictive value of the test is limited, especially among patients with chronic sinus disease and persistent mucosal abnormalities.

When the procedure shows normal passage of light or completely absent passage of light, the clinical prediction of normality or abnormality, respectively, is moderately accurate. When the light transmission is judged to be only reduced, rather than absent, interpretation is problematic. Important diagnostic or therapeutic decisions should not be made solely on the basis of the results of transillumination.

In many instances, a clinical diagnosis of sinusitis is suggested on the basis of the history and physical examination, irrespective of the results of transillumination, and the child can be begun on oral antibiotic therapy. If necessary, sinus radiography can be obtained to confirm a clinical diagnosis of sinusitis. A single occipitomental (or Waters) view suffices in most instances for the diagnosis of maxillary sinusitis. When a precise microbiologic diagnosis is important to direct the selection of antimicrobial therapy, as in an immunocompromised child, surgical aspiration of the involved sinus is necessary.

E. Specimen Collection—Middle Ear Fluid (Tympanocentesis)

1. Purpose: Tympanocentesis is a needle aspiration of middle ear fluid for diagnostic purposes. This procedure is performed when the diagnosis of acute otitis media is in doubt or when determination of the causative agent is necessary.

2. Selection of Patients:

a. Indications: Specific indications include: 1) otitis media associated with a suppurative complication such as mastoiditis, facial paralysis, or meningitis; 2) otitis media in a newborn or an immunocompromised child in whom an unusual organism such as a gram-negative organism or *Staphylococcus aureus* is suggested; and 3) unsatisfactory response to antimicrobial therapy.

b. Contraindications and Precautions: In most instances, children less than 4 to 6 months of age or any child with a tympanic membrane that is difficult to visualize (e.g., secondary to a narrow external canal) should have the tympanocentesis performed by an otolaryngologist, who will have additional equipment available, such as an otoscopic microscope.

3. Equipment and Supplies (See Appendix for equipment and supplies manufacturers and suppliers. Appendix is keyed to italicized words in the equipment and supplies lists):

· Sterile *swab* with a thin, tightly wrapped fiber tip and a flexible but firm aluminum shaft (calcium alginate swab) (Figure 9-17)
· Isopropyl alcohol (70%)
· Tuberculin *syringe* (Figure 9-17)
· *Otoscope* with an operating head (See Figure 9-2, page 87)
· Eighteen-gauge spinal *needle* attached to a 3-mL *syringe,* a tuberculin *syringe,* or a collection *trap* (Figure 9-17). A 30-degree angle near the midpoint of the spinal needle may improve visualization by helping to remove

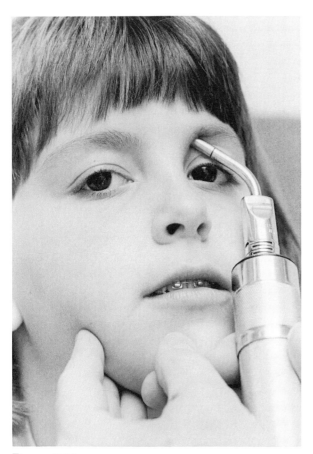

Figure 9-16.
Transillumination of a frontal sinus. Technique.

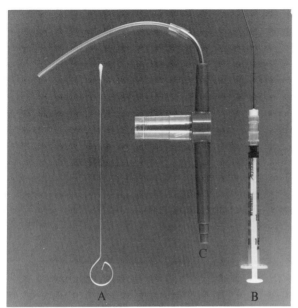

Figure 9-17.
Specimen collection—Middle ear fluid (tympanocentesis).
Equipment and supplies: **A,** Swab with fiber tip and flexible shaft;
B, Tuberculin syringe with attached angled spinal needle; **C,**
Collection trap with attached plastic tubing.

the operator's hand from the visual field at the time of tympanic membrane puncture.
· Sterile *non*-bacteriostatic saline *solution*
· Gram staining materials
· Bacterial and fungal culture media
4. Description of Procedure:
· Begin by insuring proper restraint of the patient (See Figures 9-4, 9-5, and 9-6, pages 88 and 89). In rare cases a sedative, such as chloral hydrate, or even general anesthesia, is required. Local anesthesia of an inflamed tympanic membrane is usually unsuccessful and is not recommended.
· Culture the external ear canal with a single cotton-tipped swab; this will often help in the later intrepretation of the middle ear culture results.
· Instill a solution of isopropyl alcohol (70%) into the canal with a tuberculin syringe. Turn the child's head to allow the alcohol to drain from the canal. Allow the canal to dry for a few minutes.
· Using the largest speculum that will fit the external canal, visualize the tympanic membrane through the operating head of the otoscope (Figure 9-18), and puncture the inferior portion of the tympanic membrane with an 18-gauge needle (Figure 9-19).
· Aspirate any middle ear fluid with either an attached 3-mL or tuberculin syringe or a collection trap.

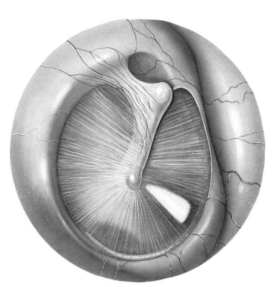

Figure 9-18.
Normal tympanic membrane.

· Withdraw the needle.
· Because the quantity of the aspirated fluid is usually small, it is frequently necessary to draw up a milliliter of sterile, *non*-bacteriostatic saline and flush it through the needle to maximize the sensitivity of the collection.
· The obtained fluid should undergo microscopic anal-

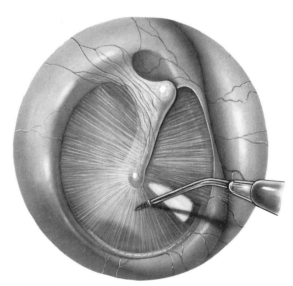

Figure 9-19.
Specimen collection—Middle ear fluid (tympanocentesis).
Technique.

ysis (Gram stain) and bacterial, and occasionally fungal, culture.

· If drainage of the middle ear is also desired, tympano-centesis is followed by myringotomy.

5. Side Effects and Complications: Complications of tympan-ocentesis may include: bleeding, usually minor and transitory; persistent otorrhea, usually resulting from the underlying middle ear disease rather than the procedure itself; damage to the ossicular chain, which can be avoided by making the needle puncture inferiorly; and a persistent perforation of the tympanic membrane or formation of an atrophic scar of the tympanic membrane if the tympanic membrane is torn rather than punctured.

F. Specimen Collection—Throat Swab

1. Purpose: The purpose of this procedure is to provide a specimen for either culture or one of the newer, rapid, non-culture antigen detection tests. In most instances the proce-dure is performed to determine if beta-hemolytic streptococci (BHS) from Lancefield group A are present in the throat of a patient with symptomatic tonsillopharyngitis. Less commonly the throat swab is performed to obtain a specimen for viral culture (e.g., for enterovirus) or for evaluation of less usual bacterial illnesses such as pharyngeal gonorrhea, chlamydia, or diphtheria. This discussion will focus on the usual instance of trying to distinguish streptococcal from viral pharyngitis.

2. Selection of Patients:

a. Indications: The clinical indications for performing a throat culture can vary because the likelihood of obtaining a positive culture is influenced by the patient's age, the month of year, disease patterns in the community, and such clinical variables as fever, cervical lymphadenitis, and tonsillar exudate. For example, because streptococcal pharyngitis is relatively un-usual in children less than 2 years of age, throat cultures are of limited benefit in children this young. The throat swab should be used to confirm clinical judgment rather than to replace it. An accurate diagnosis through clinical judgment and supplementary laboratory studies limits the prescription of antimicrobial therapy to those children who need it. We do not recommend reculturing children completing a course of antimicrobial therapy for culture-proven streptococcal pharyngitis unless they again become symptomatic.

b. Contraindications and Precautions: None

3. Equipment and Supplies (See Appendix for equipment and supplies manufacturers and suppliers. Appendix is keyed to italicized words in the equipment and supplies lists):

· Wooden tongue *blade* (Figure 9-20)
· Fiber-tipped dual swab (Figure 9-20). The choice of fiber (cotton, rayon, etc.) does not influence the culture result, but is important with some of the rapid aggluti-nation methods that prohibit use of cotton fiber.
· Bacterial culture medium

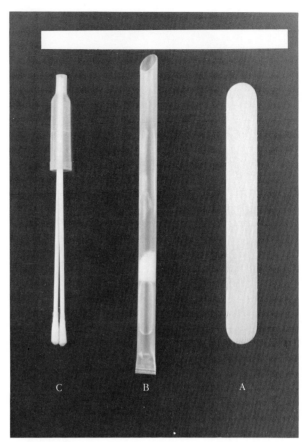

Figure 9-20.
Specimen collection—Throat swab. Equipment and supplies: **A,** Tongue blade; **B,** Swab case; **C,** Fiber-tipped dual swab.

4. Description of Procedure:

· Position the child so that he cannot easily withdraw his head when you obtain the sample. Have a younger child sit in the parent's lap with his chin tilted slightly upward and with his head facing forward and propped against his parent's chest (See Figure 9-5, page 88). An older child can sit on the back of the examination table with his head resting against the wall or can lie down with the back of the head resting on the examination table (See Figure 9-6, page 89). With the child in the latter position, most examiners stand at the head of the examination table and obtain the culture from that po-sition (Figure 9-21). With any of the positions, the child's arms and hands need to be restrained so that he will not reach to cover the mouth or grab the swabs. In the uncooperative child, the torso may also require restraint.

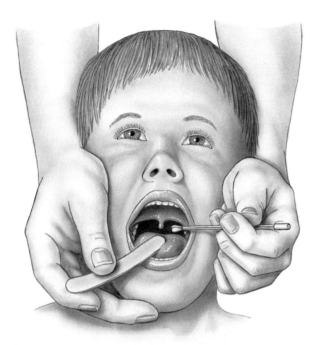

Figure 9-21.
Specimen collection—Throat swab. Technique.

• Use a tongue depressor so as to minimize contamination of the swabs with normal mouth flora.

• Warn the child that the procedure may be somewhat uncomfortable and cause him to gag briefly. With an uncooperative child, a tongue blade may have to be gently inserted between the premolar or molar teeth, then rotated sideways to spread and maintain the upper and lower teeth apart. That tongue blade or a second one can then be advanced toward the back of the tongue to expose the posterior pharyngeal region.

• Proceed to swab the posterior pharynx and tonsillar pillars. Reaching these posterior areas will significantly enhance the detection of streptococci.

• One of the swabs is used for the "quick test." If necessary, the other swab can be inoculated directly onto the culture plate, but a holding medium is often used when a delay of more than 2 hours before plating is anticipated.

5. Side Effects and Complications: None

6. Interpretation: With routine culture, the detection of any colonies of group A BHS in the pharynx of a child with symptomatic pharyngitis is considered a positive test and an indication for antimicrobial treatment. Admittedly, some such patients will not be truly infected but will simply be carriers of these organisms. If carefully obtained and processed, a negative culture for group A BHS is about 90% reliable in excluding this pathogen.

With the newer, rapid agglutination tests to detect group A BHS antigen, a positive test is about 90% to 95% reliable. A patient with a positive rapid test can be treated immediately and a culture need not be processed. A negative rapid test has only 70% to 80% accuracy, however, so it should be confirmed by culture.

G. Specimen Collection—Nasopharyngeal Swab

1. Purpose: The purpose of this procedure is to provide a specimen for culture, rapid antigen testing, or microscopic analysis.

2. Selection of Patients:

a. Indications: Suitable indications include evaluation for the presence of:

(1) Group A beta-hemolytic streptococci in a young child with chronic purulent rhinorrhea ("streptococcosis")

(2) Respiratory syncytial virus via rapid test (such as enzyme-linked immunosorbent assay [ELISA]) in a high-risk (e.g., underlying cardiopulmonary disease) infant with bronchiolitis who is being considered for antiviral therapy with ribavirin

(3) A respiratory virus by culture

(4) Eosinophils in the nasal secretions of a child with possible allergic rhinitis by using Hansel's stain

(5) *Chlamydia trachomatis* in a young infant believed to have chlamydial pneumonia

(6) *Bordetella pertussis* via culture and rapid direct immunofluorescence test in a child with signs or symptoms of whooping cough

The nasopharyngeal culture differs from the anterior nares culture often used to evaluate for colonization with *Staphylococcus aureus* in a patient or hospital employee. For the latter procedure, the specimen is taken from the very anterior part of the nares compared with a much deeper site of swabbing for the nasopharyngeal culture.

b. Contraindications and Precautions: The procedure has sometimes been used to obtain a microbiologic diagnosis in children with otitis media or sinusitis. The rationale in such instances has been that the result of this less invasive alternative to culturing the middle ear or sinus directly will correlate with the organism causing the localized infection in the contiguous middle ear of sinus. Unfortunately, the predictive value of the nasopharyngeal culture is not sufficiently high to be clinically useful in most instances. The clinical correlation is highest when the culture reveals a very heavy growth of a single pathogen.

Detection of an ampicillin-resistant organism in the nasopharynx is also potentially of some clinical value. In most clinical situations, however, the selection of antimicrobial therapy is more appropriately based on the bacteriologic findings in previous large-scale clinical studies than on the results of nasopharyngeal culture in any one particular patient.

3. Equipment and Supplies (See Appendix for equipment and supplies manufacturers and suppliers. Appendix is keyed to italicized words in the equipment and supplies lists):

  • Sterile *swab* with a thin, tightly wrapped fiber tip and a flexible but firm aluminum shaft (See Figure 9-17, page 96)

  • Bacterial culture media, viral culture media, or selected streptococcal, chlamydial, or viral rapid antigen detection test

4. Description of Procedure:

  • Warn the patient about the temporary discomfort of the procedure.

  • Restrain his head so as to prevent withdrawal. Have younger children lie supine on the examining table and restrain their heads, arms, and torso (See Figure 9-6, page 89).

  • Tip the child's head back very slightly.

  • Hold the swab by the wire handle, insert it through the nostril, and pass it along the floor of the nose to the nasopharynx (Figure 9-22). The angle of insertion of the swab will be roughly perpendicular to the examining table for a child who is lying down.

  • Leave the swab in place for a few seconds. The patient will probably cough and possibly gag during this brief period.

  • Gently remove the swab.

  • Inoculate the swab onto appropriate bacterial culture media or use the swab for rapid antigen detection test.

5. Side Effects and Complications: Mucosal abrasions and bleeding may occur, but are self limited.

III. Therapeutic Procedures

A. Nose Bleed Care

1. Purpose: The purpose of this procedure is to stop nose bleeding.

2. Selection of Patients:

a. Indications: Most nose bleeding in children is secondary to an upper respiratory infection or nose picking and originates from the anterior aspect of the nasal septum. When confronted with an otherwise normal child with an acute nose bleed (or when consulted by telephone by an anxious parent caring for such a child), assume that the site of bleeding is from the venous plexus (Kiesselbach's plexus) on the anterior one third of the nasal septum (Figure 9-23).

b. Contraindications and Precautions: None

3. Equipment and Supplies (See Appendix for equipment and supplies manufacturers and suppliers. Appendix is keyed to italicized words in the equipment and supplies lists):

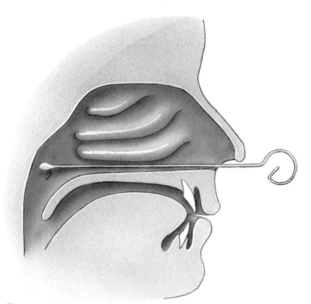

Figure 9-22.
Specimen collection—Nasopharyngeal swab. Technique.

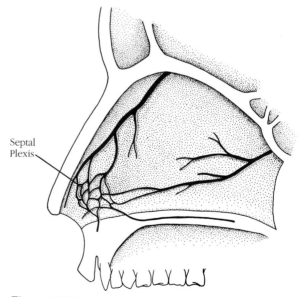

Septal
Plexis

Figure 9-23.
Nose bleed care. Anterior venous plexus.

· *Otoscope* with a nasal *speculum* or bivalved nasal *speculum* (Figure 9-24)

· Vasoconstrictor drops [such as *phenylephrine hydrochloride* (¼%)]

· Topical anesthetic solution or spray (such as *tetracaine* [2%])

· Fiber-tipped *applicators* (Figure 9-25)

· Silver nitrate cautery *sticks* (Figure 9-25)

· Absorbable gelatin *sponge* or oxidized *cellulose* (Figure 9-25)

4. Description of Procedure:

· Tell the child that you are going to press gently on his nose for a few minutes.

· Have him open his mouth and practice a breath or two through the mouth.

· Demonstrate the procedure on yourself briefly, then pinch his nose gently between your thumb and index

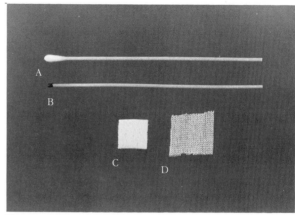

Figure 9-25.
Nose bleed care. Equipment and supplies: **A,** Fiber-tipped applicator swab; **B,** Silver nitrate cautery stick; **C,** Absorbable gelatin sponge; **D,** Oxidized cellulose.

finger so as to put pressure on the anterior aspect of the nasal septum.

· Apply moderately firm pressure for 5 minutes.

· If the bleeding persists, insert the nasal speculum of your otoscope (or a bivalved nasal speculum) into the affected side and try to locate the site of the bleeding.

· If an anterior site is visualized, insert a small cotton pledget moistened with a mild vasoconstrictor (such as phenylephrine hydrochloride [¼%]) and again apply finger pressure to hold the cotton in place for 5 minutes.

· If this is unsuccessful, attempt to cauterize the bleeding site with silver nitrate as follows.

· Restrain an uncooperative, younger child on his back (See Figure 9-6, page 89).

· Place a topical anesthetic solution (such as tetracaine [2%]) on a cotton pledget or fiber-tipped applicator swab and apply to the site for 30 to 60 seconds. Alternatively, spray this medication into the involved nostril.

· Touch the site with a silver nitrate stick for 15 seconds. Repeat the application several times if needed.

· Once the bleeding has been controlled, place a small piece of absorbable gelatin sponge or oxidized cellulose against the site to prevent recurrent bleeding. The cellulose will not require removal, as it typically will fall out or be absorbed.

5. Side Effects and Complications: If the bleeding persists from an anterior site, referral to an otolaryngologist for repeat cauterization or insertion of a nasal pack is advised. If no anterior bleeding site can be visualized, more complicated treatment is required, and again referral to an otolaryngologist is advised. If the bleeding is not stopped easily, consider

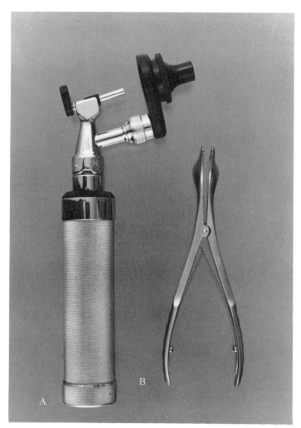

Figure 9-24.
Nose bleed care. Equipment and supplies: **A,** Otoscope with operating head and nasal speculum; **B,** Bivalved speculum.

the possibility that the child may have an underlying bleeding disorder.

B. Myringotomy

1. Purpose: Myringotomy is a procedure in which an incision is made in the tympanic membrane. Its usual purpose is to provide drainage from the middle ear in cases of acute otitis media or to evacuate middle ear fluid in cases of persistent middle ear effusion.

2. Selection of Patients:

a. Indications: Most cases of acute otitis media do not require myringotomy and can be readily treated with medical therapy. Myringotomy is indicated, however, if there is a suppurative complication from the otitis media, such as acute mastoiditis, labyrinthitis, facial paralysis, or meningitis. Myringotomy is also useful to relieve severe otalgia from otitis media. Myringotomy with placement of a ventilation tube is often performed for cases of middle ear effusion persisting longer than 3 months.

b. Contraindications and Precautions: In most instances, children less than 4 to 6 months of age or any child with a tympanic membrane that is difficult to visualize (e.g., secondary to a narrow external canal) should have the procedure performed by an otolaryngologist, who will have additional equipment available such as an otoscopic microscope.

3. Equipment and Supplies (See Appendix for equipment and supplies manufacturers and suppliers. Appendix is keyed to italicized words in the equipment and supplies lists):

· Restraint *board*
· *Otoscope* with an operating head (See Figure 9-2, page 87)
· Myringotomy *knife* (Figure 9-26)
· Suction apparatus (wall suction or portable electric suction machine)
· Flexible plastic suction *catheter* (See Figure 9-28, page 102)

4. Description of Procedure:

· If indicated, diagnostic tympanocentesis should precede myringotomy (See Specimen Collection—Middle Ear Fluid, page 95).
· For the young infant or child with acute otitis media, a restraint board is used; a sedative, such as chloral hydrate, or even general anesthesia may be required for older children. Topical anesthetics applied to an inflamed tympanic membrane are usually inadequate.
· Visualize the tympanic membrane through the otoscope (See Figure 9-18, page 96). Make the incision in the tympanic membrane inferiorly to avoid the malleus and especially the incus and stapes in the posterior superior quadrant (Figure 9-27). The incision should be circumferential, midway between the umbo and the edge of the tympanic membrane, and should extend

approximately one third the length of the tympanic membrane at that level.

· Insert the myringotomy knife just through the tympanic membrane; avoid contact with the underlying bone, to avoid bleeding. Some bleeding from the tympanic membrane, especially one that is inflamed, is to be expected.
· Suction any exudate that extrudes into the external canal, thereby promoting further drainage.
· The myringotomy incision hopefully will remain open for at least several days, during which time antibacterial otic drops are often used.

5. Side Effects and Complications: Complications of myringotomy include: bleeding, usually minor and transitory; persistent otorrhea, usually resulting from the underlying middle ear disease rather than the procedure itself; damage to the ossicular chain, avoided by making the incision inferiorly; and a persistent perforation of the tympanic membrane or

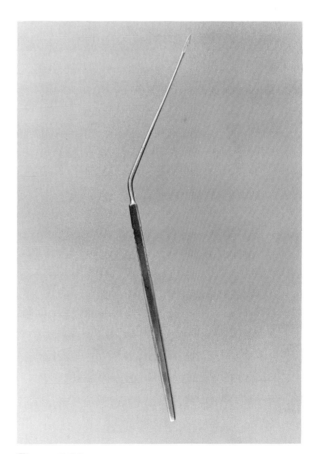

Figure 9-26.
Myringotomy. Equipment and supplies: Myringotomy knife.

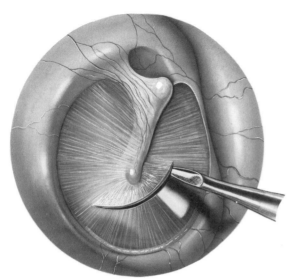

Figure 9-27.
Myringotomy. Technique.

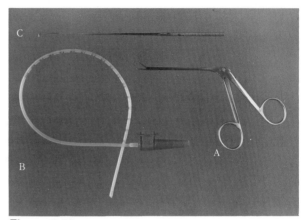

Figure 9-28.
Removal of otic foreign body. Equipment and supplies: **A,** Alligator ear forceps; **B,** Plastic suction catheter; **C,** Right-angled hook.

formation of an atrophic scar on the tympanic membrane if the tympanic membrane is torn rather than sharply incised.

C. Removal of Otic Foreign Body

A large variety of foreign bodies (paper wads, toy parts, earring parts, hair beads, eraser tips, food, insects, and others) can become lodged in the external auditory canal. Occasionally these objects will cause no symptoms and simply be discovered on routine ear examination. More frequently, however, they will be associated with pain and possible infection with otorrhea.

1. Purpose: The purpose of this procedure is to remove a foreign body from the ear canal.

2. Selection of Patients:

a. Indications: Any patient with a foreign body in the ear canal should have it removed.

b. Contraindications and Precautions: None

3. Equipment and Supplies (See Appendix for equipment and supplies manufacturers and suppliers. Appendix is keyed to italicized words in the equipment and supplies lists):

· *Otoscope* with an operating head (See Figure 9-2, page 87)

· Bivalved speculum (See Figure 9-24, page 100)

· Alligator ear *forceps* (Figure 9-28)

· *Suction* apparatus (wall suction or portable electric suction machine)

· Flexible plastic suction *catheters* (Figure 9-28)

· Blunt, right-angled *hook* (Figure 9-28)

· Irrigation equipment as for cerumen removal (See Cerumen Removal, page 90).

· Dropper filled with mineral oil

· Isopropyl alcohol (70%)

4. Description of Procedure:

· The procedure uses techniques similar to those described for cerumen removal.

· Restrain the child as described under pneumatic otoscopy (See Figure 9-6, page 89) or with the use of a restraint board. A general anesthetic may be necessary for children who cannot be calmed or appropriately restrained during foreign body removal.

· Visualize the object through either the operating head of the otoscope or the bivalved speculum.

· Many foreign bodies in the outer one half of the ear canal can simply be grasped with ear forceps and extracted.

· For *round, firm objects* that cannot be grasped easily, touch the tip of a suction catheter to the surface of the object and tease it outward.

· If these methods are unsuccessful, pass a right-angled hook carefully along the canal wall beyond the foreign body, then turn it to engage the backside of the object and gently pull it out.

· Irrigation, as for a cerumen impaction, also can be effective.

· *Insects* should first be immobilized and killed by instilling several drops of mineral oil into the canal. After a few minutes the insect can be flushed out.

· *Organic objects,* such as seeds, that have become swollen by the absorption of water can be dehydrated by the instillation of several drops of alcohol. After several minutes to allow shrinkage, such objects can more easily be removed by forceps or suction.

• For foreign bodies that cannot be removed by these methods or for objects lodged deep within the canal, consult an otolaryngologist.

5. Side Effects and Complications: Fright is a common reaction; discomfort can occur. Significant pain is uncommon. Minor bleeding can occur but is usually self-limited. Damage to the tympanic membrane is rarely a complication.

D. Removal of a Foreign Body from the Nose

1. Purpose: The purpose of this procedure is simply to remove a foreign body from the nasal cavity.

2. Selection of Patients:

a. Indications: Any patient with a foreign body lodged in the nasal cavity should have it removed.

b. Contraindications and Precautions: None

3. Equipment and Supplies (See Appendix for equipment and supplies manufacturers and suppliers. Appendix is keyed to italicized words in the equipment and supplies lists):

• *Phenylephrine* hydrochloride (¼%) or *ephedrine* (2%) solution or spray
• *Tetracaine* (2%) solution or spray
• Fiber-tipped *applicators* (See Figure 9-25, page 100)
• Bivalved nasal *speculum* (See Figure 9-24, page 100)
• Head *mirror* or other strong light source
• Alligator *forceps* (See Figure 9-28, page 103)
• Blunt, right-angled *hook* (See Figure 9-28, page 102)
• A *suction* apparatus (wall suction or portable electric suction machine)
• Flexible plastic suction *catheter* (See Figure 9-28, page 102), usually a no. 8 French with the whistle tip cut off
• Lubricating *jelly*

4. Description of Procedure:

• The ease of the procedure varies tremendously according to many factors, including: the age of the child and the size of his nasal cavity; the size, shape, and consistency of the foreign body (bead, toy part, paper wad, food, and others); the length of time the foreign body has been in the nose and the degree of associated inflammation and swelling; the child's level of cooperation; and the skill and equipment of the operator. General anesthesia may be required for extraction of some nasal foreign bodies, especially from young, uncooperative children and for the removal of objects that have been embedded in the nose for a long time and have a large amount of associated swelling.

• The head should be restrained by having the child rest it against the examination table (supine position) or against the back of a chair or wall (sitting position) (See Specimen Collection—Throat Swab, page 97).

• Either spray or instill a few drops of vasoconstricting agent (such as phenylephrine hydrochloride [¼%] or ephedrine [2%]) into the involved nostril.

• Tetracaine (2%) can be applied for 30 to 60 seconds using a fiber-tipped applicator swab to provide light topical anesthesia. Alternatively, a tetracaine spray can be used.

• Wait about 10 minutes for the maximum decongestant effect of the vasoconstricting agent.

• Ask a cooperative older child to blow his nose in an attempt to dislodge the foreign body without instrumentation. If this fails, or in an uncooperative, younger child, proceed as follows.

• Insert a bivalved nasal speculum into the affected nostril to visualize the object.

• Good illumination is essential and can be obtained from a head mirror or a strong, carefully positioned light source.

• If the object is soft or small enough to be easily grasped, take hold of it with a pair of alligator forceps and gently remove it from the nose.

• If the object is hard, large, and not easily grasped with the forceps, delicately pass a thin probe with a hooked end along the floor of the nose past the object. Rotate the probe so that the hooked end slips behind the object, and then attempt to pull the object out with a constant, gentle force.

• If the end of a probe will not slip past the object, a well-lubricated appropriate size suction catheter can be passed so that the catheter tip makes contact with the object. The suction is then increased so the object is held firmly to the catheter tip. The catheter and object are then removed. This method works best with round objects.

• If these maneuvers fail, consult an otolaryngologist.

5. Side Effects and Complications: Some degree of discomfort ordinarily occurs; significant pain is unusual. Minor bleeding often occurs but is usually self-limited. Damage to the turbinates or the septum is a rare complication.

E. Instillation of Ear Drops

1. Purpose: Ear drops can be used to clean the ear canal or to treat infections in the canal.

2. Selection of Patients:

a. Indications: There are a number of commercially available drops that help dissolve cerumen; some of these are effective within 30 to 60 minutes, while others require 12 to 24 hours. Hydrogen peroxide diluted to 50% strength by water can also be used to help soften and remove a cerumen impaction. Use of hydrogen peroxide on a periodic (several times weekly) basis may help prevent an overaccumulation of cerumen in some patients. Otic drops containing either antibiotics or an acidifying agent are essential for the successful treatment of otitis externa.

b. Contraindications and Precautions: Otic drops for cerumen

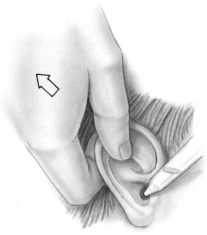

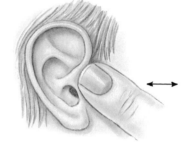

Figure 9-29.
Instillation of ear drops. Technique.

should not be instilled if there is a perforation of the tympanic membrane or if there is pain or drainage from the ear canal. These are not contraindications for the treatment of otitis externa.

3. Equipment and Supplies (See Appendix for equipment and supplies manufacturers and suppliers. Appendix is keyed to italicized words in the equipment and supplies lists):

· Otic drops
· Cotton

4. Description of Procedure:

· Position the patient supine with his head turned so that the involved ear is up. As this procedure is not painful, restraint as for some diagnostic or therapeutic procedures is usually not necessary.
· Pull the pinna posteriorly and superiorly to open the canal fully (Figure 9-29).
· Hold the tip of the dropper at the edge of the external auditory meatus.
· Instill three to five drops and then push the tragus into the canal several times (Figure 9-29). This pumping action forces the medication deeper.
· Place a piece of cotton in the ear canal and keep the child in the same position for several minutes. If further applications will be necessary (e.g., for the treatment of otitis externa), have the parent observe this technique closely so that it can be used at home.

5. Side Effects and Complications: Some otic preparations used for otitis externa can cause a mild stinging sensation, especially if a tympanic membrane perforation is also present.

F. Care of the Infected External Ear Canal

A bacterial or fungal infection within the external ear canal (otitis externa) is a common condition that can be readily

treated in most cases with careful cleaning of the canal, instillation of otic drops, and occasional use of an otic wick. Cleaning the canal increases the effectiveness of otic drops, which can then reach the infected skin more easily.

Cleaning the Ear Canal—Suction Method

1. Purpose: The purpose of this procedure is to remove debris (squamous epithelium, cerumen) and purulent drainage from the ear canal.

2. Selection of Patients:

a. Indications: In very early cases of otitis externa, only erythema and mild swelling of the canal are seen and cleaning is not necessary. Typically, however, purulent drainage and desquamated epithelial debris are present in the canal. Such matter is removed most efficiently by suctioning the ear canal.

b. Contraindications and Precautions: The only contraindication to use of suction is the very uncooperative patient, in whom the possibility of inducing trauma becomes a concern.

3. Equipment and Supplies (See Appendix for equipment and supplies manufacturers and suppliers. Appendix is keyed to italicized words in the equipment and supplies lists):

· *Otoscope* with an operating head (See Figure 9-2, page 87)
· *Suction* apparatus (wall suction or portable electric suction machine)
· Flexible plastic suction *catheter* (See Figure 9-28, page 102)
· Metal suction tips of variable size (e.g., no. 3 and no. 5 French) (Figure 9-30)
· Cup of warm water

4. Description of Procedure:

· Begin by explaining to the patient that he will hear a loud noise, but that the procedure should not be painful

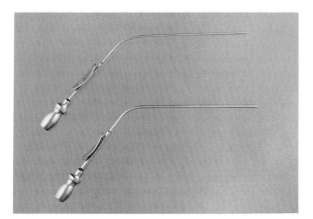

Figure 9-30.
Care of the infected external ear canal. Equipment and supplies: Metal suction tips.

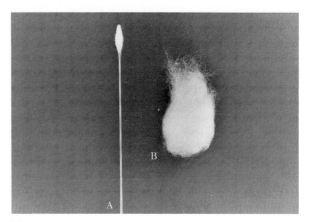

Figure 9-31.
Cleaning of the ear canal—Cotton swab method. Equipment and supplies: **A,** Metal applicator with cotton attached to roughened tip. **B,** Cotton.

if he keeps his head still. Restrain the head of a younger, uncooperative child (See Figure 9-6, page 89).
· Begin suctioning at the canal meatus to let the patient become accustomed to the suction noise.
· Then introduce an appropriate size suction tip into the lateral portion of the canal and aspirate the exudate and debris. Usually a no. 5 suction tip will be appropriate. Occasionally a no. 3 will be necessary for the small child, but its lumen may be easily occluded.
· Intermittently place the suction tip into a cup of warm water to prevent occlusion with the debris.
· Most drainage within the lateral two thirds of the ear can be removed using this method.
· Deeper cleaning within the canal is not advised without the use of an operating microscope.
5. Side Effects and Complications: The only usual complications are discomfort and minor bleeding. Damage to the tympanic membrane is a rare occurrence.

Cleaning the Ear Canal—Cotton Swab Method
1. Purpose: To remove cellular debris or purulent drainage from the ear canal.
2. Selection of Patients:
a. Indications: This method of cleaning the ear canal is appropriate when there is only a small amount of debris or a thin film of purulence within the canal.
b. Contraindications and precautions: In most instances a cotton swab is inadequate to remove a large amount of drainage or debris from the ear canal.
3. Equipment and Supplies (See Appendix for equipment and supplies manufacturers and suppliers. Appendix is keyed to italicized words in the equipment and supplies lists):

· Thin metal *applicator* with a roughened tip (Figure 9-31)
· Piece of cotton (Figure 9-31)
· *Otoscope* with operating head (See Figure 9-2, page 87)
4. Description of Procedure:
· Commercial cotton swabs are too large, so the examiner must prepare his own. A small wisp of the cotton (fingernail size) is twisted around the applicator end, leaving a small tuft at the end, which can be firmed or left loose. A firm tuft is chosen for particulate debris and a loose tuft is selected for fluid contents.
· Insert the swab through the operating head of the otoscope, and gently brush the walls of the ear canal.
· Several pieces of cotton are usually necessary to clean the canal adequately.
5. Side Effects and Complications: Discomfort and minor bleeding are common. Damage to the tympanic membrane is rare.

Use of Otic Drops or Otic Wick
Once the ear canal has been cleaned, otic drops should be instilled. There are a number of commercially available preparations, including some that contain one or more antibiotics with or without hydrocortisone, and others that contain acidifying agents without antibiotics. The acidifying agents are best when there is evidence of a fungal infection (e.g., spores or mycelia within the canal), which occurs in 5% to 10% of cases of otitis externa. The drops are instilled using the method previously described in this chapter (See Instillation of Ear Drops, page 103).

1. Purpose: The purpose of this procedure is to provide effective topical therapy for otitis externa.

2. Selection of Patients:

a. Indications: Occasionally otitis externa will cause significant swelling or even closure of the ear canal. In such instances, instillation of drops is difficult or impossible, and the placement of a commercially available ear wick is necessary. The wick simply serves to stent the canal and act as a vehicle to distribute the drops deeper into the canal.

b. Contraindications and Precautions: There are no contraindications except for an unusual degree of pain on insertion of the wick.

3. Equipment and Supplies (See Appendix for equipment and supplies manufacturers and suppliers. Appendix is keyed to italicized words in the equipment and supplies lists):

· Straight *scissors* (See Figure 18-17, page 231)

· Otic *wick* (Figure 9-32), which consists of a firm but porous material, approximately 2 mm in diameter, which greatly expands when moistened

· An *otoscope* with an operating head (See Figure 9-2, page 87)

· Alligator *forceps* (See Figure 9-28, page 102)

4. Description of Procedure:

· Cut the wick to approximately one half the length of the ear canal (average ear canal length is 25 mm for a person aged 9 years to adult).

· Restrain the child's head (See Figures 9-4, 9-5, and 9-6, pages 88 and 89).

· Using forceps to grasp the wick, insert it such that its distal end is just visible at the meatal opening. This procedure can cause some discomfort, which is usually mild and transient.

· Instillation of otic drops on the visible tip of the wick will spread down the length of the wick and cause the wick to expand. The desired result is application of the otic drops to the inflamed wall of the ear canal.

· As the swelling subsides over several days, the wick usually falls out.

· The wick should be removed in 3 to 4 days if still present; placement of a second wick usually is not required.

5. Side Effects and Complications: When first introduced, the wick can cause transient mild discomfort. If the wick is inserted too deeply, it can impinge on the tympanic membrane and cause more intense and persistent pain. Perforation of the tympanic membrane and damage to the middle ear structures by the wick or the forceps rarely occur.

G. Instillation of Nose Drops

1. Purpose: The purpose of this procedure is to instill drops into a child's nose.

2. Selection of Patients:

a. Indications: Saline drops are often used, especially in infants, just before a rubber nasal aspirator is used to clear excess mucus. In older children, vasoconstrictor drops can be used to shrink the mucous membranes and allow easier flow through the nose. The newer metered nose sprays can deliver a relatively precise volume of medication and may provide a useful alternative to nose drops for some children.

b. Contraindications and Precautions: None

3. Equipment and Supplies (See Appendix for equipment and supplies manufacturers and suppliers. Appendix is keyed to italicized words in the equipment and supplies lists):

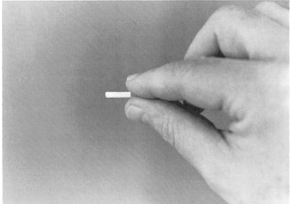

Figure 9-32.
Use of otic drop or otic wick. Equipment and supplies: Otic wick.

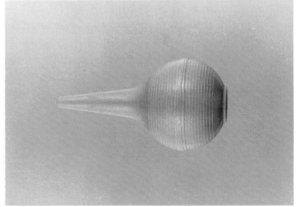

Figure 9-33.
Instillation of nose drops. Equipment and supplies: Rubber bulb aspirator.

- Rubber bulb *aspirator* (Figure 9-33)
- Selected nasal drops

4. Description of Procedure:

- Begin by removing as much nasal mucus as possible. For a young child, apply gentle suction at each nostril with a rubber bulb aspirator; have an older child blow his nose.
- Place a young infant in the supine position either on a parent's lap or on the examination table (See Figures 9-4, 9-5, and 9-6, pages 88 and 89).
- Tip the head back slightly and restrain the head to prevent undue motion. Restraint of the hands may also be necessary.
- Place the dropper tip just inside the nostril and expel the desired number of nose drops or volume of solution.
- Keep the child's head horizontal for a few minutes to prevent the drops from flowing out of the nose too rapidly.
- Repeat gentle suction at each nostril with a rubber bulb aspirator.
- For older children, either of two specialized methods (Proetz or Parkinson) of drop instillation is sometimes used in an attempt to decongest specific sinus openings:

(1) To use the Proetz method, place the child supine on a bed or examining table and gently let his head drop backwards over the edge of the surface with his chin pointed toward the ceiling. Rotate his head to the right, instill the nose drops into the right nostril, and have him keep his head in this position for a few minutes. Then repeat the procedure for the left side. This method is intended to be especially useful in opening the passages to the ethmoid and sphenoid sinuses.

(2) To use the Parkinson method, have the child lie on his side with his shoulder slightly elevated, such as by propping with a folded sheet. Have him tilt his head down laterally and rest it on his arm. Instill the nose drops into both nares and have the child remain in this position for a few minutes. Have him turn over to his other side and repeat the procedure. This method is intended to be particularly useful in opening the passages to the frontal and maxillary sinuses.

Chapter 10

Dental Procedures

Andrew B. Martof

I. Therapeutic Procedures

Even without the armamentarium of the standard dental office, a number of dental procedures can and should be accomplished to treat acute dental injury in children before referral to a dentist. The procedures require only the equipment found in most medical offices where children are treated. These procedures include the reimplantation or reduction of avulsed teeth, the incision and drainage of an acute dental abscess, and the reduction of a dislocated temporomandibular joint.

A. Replacement or Reduction of a Displaced Tooth

When teeth are injured traumatically, they may either be fractured or avulsed. There are four basic types of fractures of teeth (Class I–III fractures and root fractures) (Figure 10-1). Class I–III fractures refer only to coronal injuries. Class I injury involves chipping or fracturing of the enamel only and does not expose any dentin to the oral cavity. This type of fracture requires no care acutely. Class II fractures occur through the crown of the tooth, fracturing the enamel and exposing the dentin of the tooth to the oral cavity. Exposure of the free nerve endings located in the dentin may produce pain, requiring referral to a dentist. Class III fractures occur through the crown of the tooth, directly exposing the dental pulp to the oral cavity. Root fractures also expose the dental pulp. Class III fractures and root fractures will require root canal therapy or extraction and should be referred to a dentist immediately if pain is intense and unrelenting. If pain is not prominent, referral should be made as soon as it is feasible. Nondisplaced root fractures are difficult to diagnose clinically, but in the absence of mobility of the crown probably do not require acute care and should be seen the following day for radiographic diagnosis.

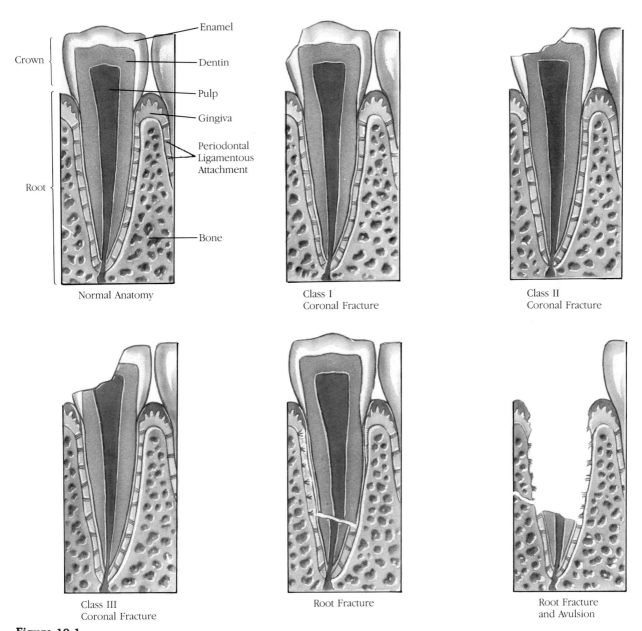

Figure 10-1.
Replacement or reduction of a displaced tooth. Basic types of fractures of teeth.

Teeth may be partially or totally avulsed. Partially avulsed tooth injuries include intruded, extruded, or tipped teeth. Intruded teeth are depressed into the jaw from a force along the long axis of the tooth. Extruded teeth appear as though the tooth has erupted further than normal. Tipping injuries include those that displace the crown of the tooth toward the tongue or palate (the usual case) or toward the lips. Tipping injuries and extrusion injuries usually occur together. An entire tooth or any portion of the tooth can be avulsed, leaving a fractured segment within the alveolar bone. To determine complete avulsion and to rule out fractured segments remaining in the alveolar bone, every effort should be made to locate all pieces of the avulsed tooth. Primary and secondary teeth are treated quite differently. The age of the patient and the appearance of the tooth are helpful in determining the primary or secondary nature of the tooth. Any primary tooth that has been avulsed from the alveolus should not be replaced. Any permanent tooth that has been avulsed should be found and replaced as quickly as possible.

1. Purpose: The purpose of the procedure is to return the displaced tooth to a position as close as possible to its original alignment and to stabilize it in that position. This is a dental emergency: the sooner that the tooth can be replaced, the better the prognosis. Teeth that have been reimplanted within the first 15 to 30 minutes have an 80% survival at 8 to 10 years. Teeth left out of the mouth for over 2 hours have only a 20% chance for 8- to 10-year survival.

2. Selection of Patients:

a. Indications: The patients selected for this procedure should have partially or totally avulsed tooth injuries of the permanent or adult teeth.

b. Contraindications and Precautions: Patients with injuries that include intruded teeth, primary teeth, or any tooth that is severely fractured and displaced should be referred to a specialist. Multiple adjacent loose teeth are difficult to reduce and realign without immediate splinting; therefore, the patient should be referred immediately.

3. Equipment and Supplies (See Appendix for equipment and supplies manufacturers and suppliers. Appendix is keyed to italicized words in the equipment and supplies lists):

- Saline irrigating *solution*
- 10- to 20-mL *syringe* with an appropriate blunt tip (Figure 10-2)
- Suction apparatus (wall-mounted suctioning or portable *suction* machine) or a 10- to 20-mL *syringe* attached to a suction *catheter* (Figure 10-2)
- *Lidocaine* (1%) with or without epinephrine (1:100,000)
- 3- to 5-mL *syringe* (See Figure 20-7, page 262) with a 25-gauge 1-inch *needle* (See Figure 20-7, page 262)
- Nonresorbable *suture* material (Figure 10-3)
- Needle *holder* (Figure 10-3)
- Suture *scissors* (Figure 10-3)
- 2 × 2-inch gauze *pads* or 4 × 4-inch gauze *pads*
- Sterile *gloves*

4. Description of Procedure:

- When a parent calls your office seeking advice concerning an avulsed tooth, tell them to find all of the tooth and place the tooth in the socket. Instruct the parent to properly align the tooth relative to the adjacent teeth. Advise the parent to take care not to scrub, abrade, or further injure the tooth with any cleansing processes other than rinsing the tooth.
- If the parent is unable to replace the tooth quickly,

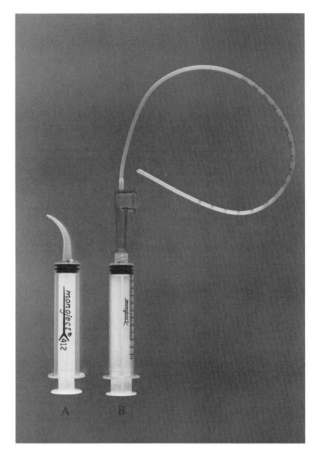

Figure 10-2.
Replacement or reduction of a displaced tooth. Equipment: **A,** Syringe with a blunt tip; **B,** Syringe attached to a suction catheter.

tell the parent to transport the tooth in the mouth of the child (between the buccal mucosa and the lower gum) if the child is of an age when swallowing or aspirating the tooth is not a risk. As an alternative, tell the parent to transport the tooth in saline or even milk.
- On presentation in your office, verify and correct tooth position and alignment.
- Thorough examination of an injured mouth can only be accomplished after wound irrigation with saline and debridement of injured tissues of the lips, teeth, and oral cavity.
- Use suction to remove clots and debris from around the teeth.
- After the wounds have been thoroughly cleaned, inspect the mouth for foreign bodies, exposure of alveolar bone, and fractured or chipped tooth segments.

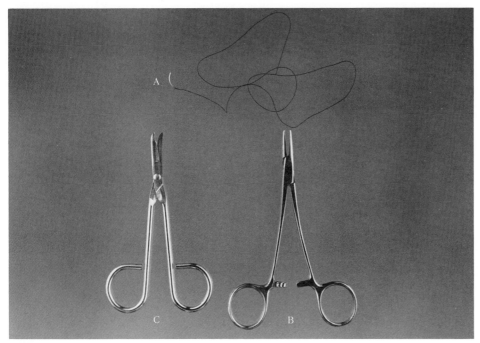

Figure 10-3.
Replacement or reduction of a displaced tooth. Equipment: **A,** Suture material and
needle; **B,** Needle holder; **C,** Suture scissors.

· Palpate each tooth (with a single finger for smaller teeth and between two fingers for larger teeth) and assess for crepitus and mobility (Figure 10-4).

· If a tooth has been totally avulsed, rinse it thoroughly in saline, not tap water, taking care not to scrub and abrade the root surface of the tooth.

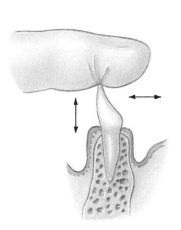

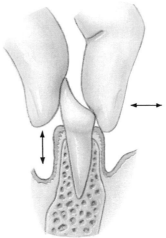

Figure 10-4.
Replacement or reduction of a displaced tooth. Technique for assessment of tooth
mobility.

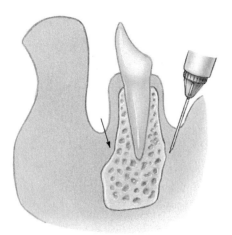

Figure 10-5.
Replacement or reduction of a displaced tooth. Technique for local infiltration of anesthetic into the labial and lingual surfaces of the gingiva.

• Remove any clot from the alveolar space before the tooth is inserted.
• Replace the tooth into the alveolar space. Extreme force is not necessary or beneficial, as it will usually only cause complications.
• If the tooth does not go fully into place because of physical limitation or discomfort, anesthetize the patient locally by infiltration of lidocaine into the labial and palatal or labial and lingual surfaces of the gingiva (Figure 10-5).
• After reimplantation, stabilize the tooth. Accomplish this by either wiring the tooth to the adjacent teeth or by placing a nonresorbable suture through the gum and over the top of the tooth (Figure 10-6). If stabilization is not possible in your office, replace the avulsed tooth and refer the patient for specialized dental care.
• Reduce teeth that have been displaced by using the finger and thumb of a gloved hand to squeeze or press the tooth into alignment.
• After reimplantation or realignment of displaced teeth, firmly squeeze the alveolar process so as to compress any expanded bone.
• Have the patient bite to verify that the alignment of the teeth is appropriate relative to the opposing arch.
• Do not leave a tooth in a position such that it is the only tooth that contacts the opposing dentition. If this occurs, additional realignment is necessary.

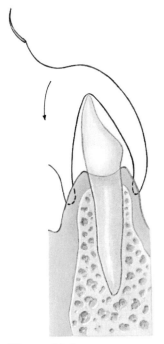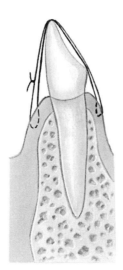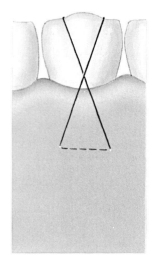

Figure 10-6.
Replacement or reduction of a displaced tooth. Technique for interim stabilization of a displaced tooth using a nonresorbable suture.

· Suture any soft tissue lacerations that expose the alveolar process.

· Apply direct wound pressure to effect hemostasis.

· Prescribe an appropriate analgesic (not aspirin).

· After reimplantation or realignment, refer the patient for definitive dental care as soon as possible. Complete communication with the dentist regarding findings and completed procedures is essential.

5. Side Effects and Complications: Infection is always a concern with any traumatic injury in the oral cavity, and antibiotic therapy for a week postoperatively is recommended. Totally or partially avulsed teeth are likely to have severed the nerve and blood supply at the apical foramen of the tooth, thereby devitalizing the tooth and necessitating root canal therapy.

B. Acute Management of a Dental Abscess

Most patients with acute dental abscesses or pain should be referred to a dentist for dental care. If this is not available for an individual who has a fluctuant swelling adjacent to his or her teeth or jaws, management should include surgical intervention as well as appropriate antibiotic therapy. Surgical management of an acute alveolar or dental abscess involves drainage of pus and removal of pathologic dentition to facilitate wound healing. The removal of the dental pathology may require extraction of the tooth or root canal therapy.

1. Purpose: The purpose of the procedure is to identify the microbial pathogens and expedite resolution of the infection.

2. Selection of Patients:

a. Indications: This procedure is indicated in patients possessing acute dental swelling of a fluctuant nature that is not draining through a spontaneous fistula.

b. Contraindications and Precautions: Contraindications include nonfluctuant cellulitis or any systemic disorder that would complicate a minor surgical procedure.

3. Equipment and Supplies (See Appendix for equipment and supplies manufacturers and suppliers. Appendix is keyed to italicized words in the equipment and supplies lists):

· *Lidocaine* (1%)

· 3- to 5.0-mL *syringe* (See Figure 20-7, page 262) and 25-gauge *needle* (See Figure 20-7, page 262), for administration of local anesthetic

· 5- to 10-mL *syringe* (See Figure 20-7, page 262) with a 1½-inch, 21-gauge *needle* (See Figure 20-7, page 262), for wound aspiration

· Glass microscope *slide*

· Gram stain

· Aerobic and anaerobic bacterial culture media

· A no. 15 scalpel *blade* (Figure 10-7)

· A curved *hemostat* (Figure 10-7)

· Irrigating saline *solution*

· 10- to 20-mL *syringe* (See Figure 20-7, page 262) for irrigation

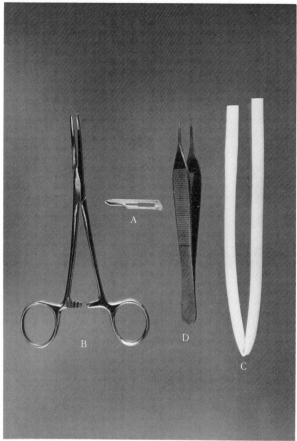

Figure 10-7.
Acute management of a dental abscess. Equipment: **A,** No. 15 scalpel blade; **B,** Curved hemostat; **C,** Latex rubber drain; **D,** Tissue forceps.

· Latex rubber *drain* (Figure 10-7), iodoform *gauze,* or petroleum *gauze*

· 3–0 or 4–0 nonresorbable *suture* material

· Suture *scissors* (See Figure 10-3, page 111)

· Tissue *forceps* (Figure 10-7)

4. Description of Procedure:

· Administer ½ to 1 mL of lidocaine adjacent to the area of fluctuance (See Figure 10-5, page 112)

· Wait a few minutes for the anesthetic to take effect.

· Use the aspirating syringe and needle to explore the swelling for the presence of pus (Figure 10-8). The pus may be in any of the anatomic spaces of the facial region or may be confined to a subperiosteal space adjacent to the infected dentition.

· Gram stain any aspirated purulence and culture the material aerobically and anaerobically for bacteria.

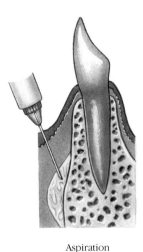
Aspiration

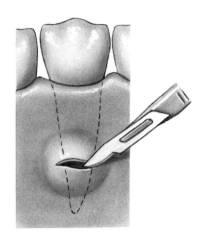
Incision

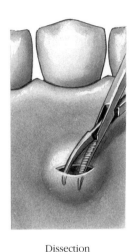
Dissection

Figure 10-8.
Acute management of a dental abscess. Techniques for aspiration, incision, and dissection of a dental abscess.

· After wound aspiration, make an incision through the mucosa adjacent to the fluctuant area (Figure 10-8).

· Once the mucosa has been perforated, perform blunt disection toward the area from which the pus was aspirated (Figure 10-8). This is best accomplished with a curved hemostat. After the hemostat is placed into the incision, spread the beaks. Repeat this action as the hemostat is progressively inserted deeper into the abscess cavity. Explore the wound thoroughly for any multilocular pockets of pus that are present.

· Compress the wound with finger pressure adjacent to the wound to express as much pus as possible.

· Copiously irrigate through the incision with saline solution. Assist adequate drainage of the saline by finger compressions.

· Place a packing or drain to prevent clot formation from sealing the wound orifice. You may use a small piece of rubber latex drain or a gauze packed lightly into the wound to its full depth. You will need to suture the latex rubber drain at the wound–drain interface to prevent the premature removal of the drain. The packed gauze will usually stay by itself and is probably the easier drain to place.

· Leave a drain in place as long as it is productive, but exchange it within 24 to 48 hours to reduce the chances of reinfecting the wound.

· Institute appropriate antibiotic therapy, keeping in mind that most dental alveolar infections are of mixed oral bacterial origin.

5. Side Effects and Complications: Side effects and complications include damage to adjacent anatomic structures, including nerves and blood vessels.

C. Reduction of an Open, Locked Temporomandibular Joint

Individuals who have a locked, open jaw have displaced the head of the condyle anterior to the articular cartilage such that the head of the condyle will no longer return to the glenoid fossa (Figure 10-9). The longer this condition persists, the more likely the pterygoid musculature is to spasm, making subsequent reduction of the dislocation more difficult. When displacement occurs, an individual is usually comfortable in the locked open position, but they may be extremely anxious.

1. Purpose: The purpose of this procedure is to restore function to a dislocated temporomandibular joint.

2. Selection of Patients:

a. Indications: Any patient who has voluntarily opened his mouth or has had his mouth forcefully opened and is unable to close it is a candidate for this procedure.

b. Contraindications and Precautions: Chronic conditions of the temporomandibular joint or muscles of mastication should be referred to appropriate specialists. Other contraindications include jaw fractures, tumors, or infections.

3. Equipment and Supplies (See Appendix for equipment and supplies manufacturers and suppliers. Appendix is keyed to italicized words in the equipment and supplies lists):

· Examining *gloves*
· Numerous tongue *blades*
· Systemic muscle relaxants such as diazapam or benzodiazapam that can be given intravenously or intramuscularly.
· *Lidocaine* (1%)

4. Description of Procedure:

· Have the patient in a sitting, erect position. You stand in front of the patient.

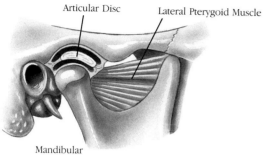

Articular Disc

Lateral Pterygoid Muscle

Mandibular
Condyle

Normal Anatomy,
Mouth Closed

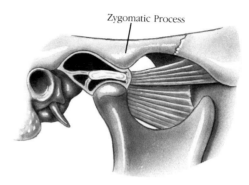

Zygomatic Process

Normal Anatomy,
Mouth Open

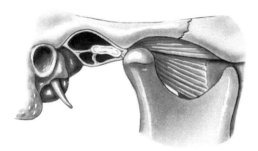

Displaced, Locked
Temporomandibular
Joint, Mouth Open

Figure 10-9.
Reduction of an open, locked temporomandibular joint (TMJ). Anatomy of
normal TMJ and anatomy of displaced TMJ.

· Your elbows should be approximately at the height of the chin of the patient.
· Place the thumbs of each hand on the occlusal surfaces of the lower, posterior teeth while the fingers grasp the inferior border of the mandible (Figure 10-10A).
· Apply downward pressure with the thumbs as the fingers lift upward, thus increasing the joint space in the temporomandibular joint.

· As you apply a slight posterior force, the joints should reduce and close (Figure 10-10C).
· If this maneuver fails to reduce the joint, have the patient open his mouth as far as possible. Insert the tongue blades vertically between the posterior teeth on each side and have the person bite lightly on them (Figure 10-10B). Apply upward force and then backward concurrent force on the anterior portion of the mandi-

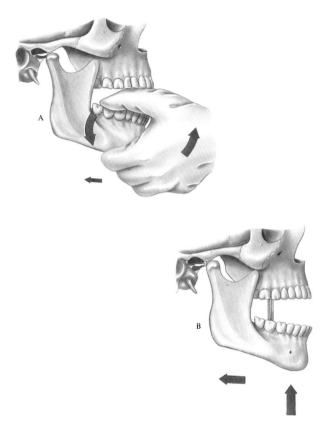

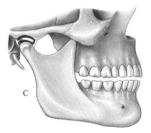

Figure 10-10.
Reduction of an open, locked temporomandibular joint (TMJ). A and **B**, Techniques. **C**, Successfully reduced displacement showing mandibular teeth and mandible in a position posterior to maxillary teeth and maxilla.

ble, allowing reduction to be accomplished (Figure 10-10C).
· If the person is having great difficulty because of

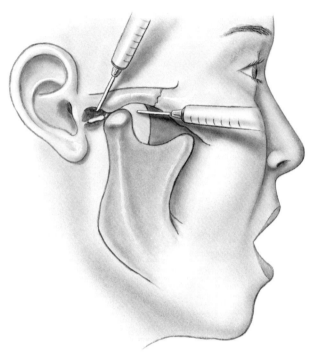

Figure 10-11.
Reduction of an open, locked temporomandibular joint (TMJ). Technique for instillation of anesthetic into several sites adjacent to the TMJ.

preauricular pain, inject a local anesthetic percutaneously in that area (Figure 10-11).
· A third approach is to have another individual stimulate the gag reflex of the patient while you attempt the reduce the jaw joint using one of the described methods.
· After successful reduction by any of the methods, check the occlusion to insure that it is appropriately reduced. In addition, rule out a fracture of the jaw.
· Instruct the patient to limit range of opening, to not yawn, and to consume a soft diet without any excessive or exaggerated chewing motions. An appropriate anti-inflammatory medication (not aspirin) is indicated. Ice applied to the preauricular area on the day of injury is helpful to reduce swelling. To promote healing, heat may be applied beginning 24 hours after the injury.
5. Side Effects and Complications: An inability to reduce the jaw joint necessitates a referral to a specialist.

Chapter 11

Respiratory Tract Procedures

Robert F. Selden, Jr.

I. Diagnostic Procedures

A. Functional Examination of the Respiratory Tract

1. Purpose: Outpatient evaluation of lung function may be used to detect abnormal respiratory function, to monitor the natural course of a known or suspected respiratory problem, or to determine the response to therapy in a patient with a respiratory disorder. In patients who complain of shortness of breath, weakness, or easy fatigability, testing may be of assistance in screening for impairment of lung function or respiratory muscle weakness as part of their evaluation. In the primary care setting, spirometry is the ideal procedure.

Specialized testing through referral to a pulmonary function laboratory can measure various aspects of lung function in terms of volume and rates of air flow. Terminology related to these measures include:

- Total Lung Capacity (TLC) (Figure 11-1): The volume of gas in the lungs after a maximal inspiration.
- Residual Volume (RV) (Figure 11-1): The volume of gas remaining in the lungs after full expiration.
- Functional Residual Capacity (FRC) (Figure 11-1): The volume of gas remaining in the lungs at the end of a normal, resting expiration.
- Inspiratory Capacity (IC) (Figure 11-1): The volume of gas that may be inhaled as one achieves TLC from the end expiratory level (FRC).
- Expiratory Reserve Volume (ERV) (Figure 11-1): The volume of gas exhaled in moving from the end expiratory level (FRC) to RV.
- Vital Capacity (VC) (Figure 11-1): The volume of gas exhaled as one moves from TLC to RV. This may be achieved slowly, Slow Vital Capacity (SVC), or with maximal effort, Forced Vital Capacity (FVC).
- Forced Expiratory Volume in one second (FEV_1) (Fig-

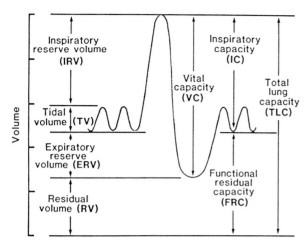

Figure 11-1.
Functional examination of the respiratory tract. Spirogram with divisions of total lung capacity. From Eigen, H. Pulmonary function testing: A practical guide to its use in pediatric practice. Pediatrics in Review 1986; 7:235-45, with permission.

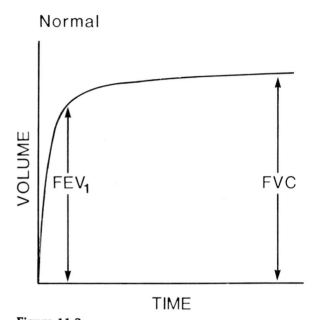

Figure 11-2.
Functional examination of the respiratory tract. Normal forced expiration spirogram. From Eigen, H. Pulmonary function testing: A practical guide to its use in pediatric practice. Pediatrics in Review 1986; 7:235-45, with permission.

ure 11-2): The volume of gas exhaled during the first second while performing an FVC measurement.

· FEV_1/FVC (Figure 11-2): A ratio of two volumes, expressed as a percentage, often used to determine the presence of obstructive lung disease.

· Forced Expiratory Flow between 25% and 75% of FVC ($FEF_{25-75\%}$) (See Figure 11-4, page 120): The volume of gas in liters that would be exhaled in 1 second if done at an average flow rate for the middle 50% of the FVC curve. (Formerly the Maximal Mid-Expiratory Flow Rate, MMEFR).

Spirometry in the office setting is customarily used to obtain the last four determinations (VC, FEV_1, FEV_1/FVC, and $FEF_{25-75\%}$). In young children, cooperative but not yet skilled at spirometry, peak expiratory flow rates (PEFR) may be helpful in assessing the possibility of airway obstruction.

2. Selection of Patients:

a. Indications: The usefulness of pulmonary function measurements obtained by spirometry is directly related to the cooperation of the person tested. The patient should understand what is required and make a maximal effort for the result to be meaningful. Children 6 years of age and older can usually achieve satisfactory results with practice. Acute illness, fatigue, emotional stress, anticipation of an injection, and other factors may alter the patient's desire and ability to perform maximally. These factors must be considered by the clinician requesting the spirometry and assessing the results.

The clinician must use judgment in deciding which patient's evaluation will be aided by testing of pulmonary function. Classic examples would include those patients with re-

active airway disease, cystic fibrosis, and less common disorders such as the immotile cilia syndrome.

b. Contraindications and Precautions: There are few contraindications to spirometry. In the presence of significant respiratory embarrassment, spirometry may be deferred. If chest pain or acute dyspnea is part of the clinical picture, especially in patients with known obstructive airway disease, radiographic studies should be obtained first to rule out a pneumothorax before subjecting the patient to forced inspiratory and expiratory maneuvers that could increase the intrapleural air. Similarly, significant hemoptysis or the suspicion that a foreign body may be present should delay functional studies.

3. Equipment and Supplies (See Appendix for equipment and supplies manufacturers and suppliers. Appendix is keyed to italicized words in the equipment and supplies lists):

A number of *spirometers* are available for use with children. Some are connected to computers that provide prompt results of several measurements. From a practical standpoint, the less expensive volume displacement and bellows types of spirometers are quite suitable for office testing and have the advantage of providing a tracing of the performance that can be studied for flaws in technique and retained in the patient's chart. Even the younger patients can see their record and compare its pattern with an example of optimal performance.

At our institution, two simple spirometers have been used

for routine studies in the outpatient clinics. These are the Breon 2400 and the Vitalograph spirometers. Both of these units allow repetitive tracings on paper graphs, have the convenience of disposable mouthpieces, and are light enough to be moved from a central storage area to the examining room. Models that meet the standards set forth by the American Thoracic Society[1] are available for office use.

It is suggested that clinicians interested in purchasing a spirometer for office use review select literature on spirometry as well as the information provided by the manufacturers of spirometers under consideration. Assuring that supplies and necessary repairs are readily available is important.
  - Mouthpiece (Figure 11-3)
  - Noseclip (Figure 11-3)
4. Description of Procedure:
  - Performance of spirometry requires practice with the technical aspects of the procedure. Patience and an ability to teach are especially valuable traits when dealing with younger children.
  - Perform the testing in a quiet, uncrowded room where the number of people and distractions can be minimized.
  - For the patient who is attempting spirometry for the first time, explain what action is going to be required and how the spirometer will record the results. A demonstration of spirometry either by the tester or by an experienced patient not only may be instructive but may reduce the apprehension that some children have for new experiences at the doctor's office.
  - In the younger patient, it is appropriate to start without any equipment simply by practicing deep breaths in unison with the tester. Repeat the same exercise with the mouthpiece held appropriately between the teeth

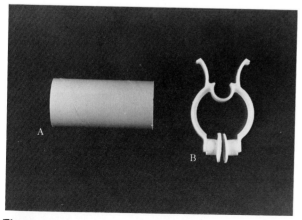

Figure 11-3.
Functional examination of the respiratory tract. Equipment and supplies: **A,** Mouthpiece; **B,** Noseclip.

with the lips tight (preventing air leakage) before the mouthpiece is connected to the spirometer. A useful approach for testing involves placing a cotton ball in the distal end of the mouthpiece and letting the child demonstrate how fast he can expel it and how far he can blow it across a table. This is accomplished with a single deep breath and a forced and prolonged expiration.
  - When practice exercises have been completed, the patient may try spirometry. In childhood it is customary to test the patient in a standing position for maximal volume and with a noseclip blocking nasal airflow. In those over the age of 12 years, there appears to be no significant difference in the vital capacity when performed standing or sitting. When a bellows spirometer is used, have the patient grip the hose attached to the mouthpiece, inhale maximally to achieve TLC, pause briefly while holding this volume in, and after inserting the mouthpiece fully between the lips, exhale forcefully and completely into the spirometer, expelling all air possible until RV is reached. The exhalation phase should last at least 3 seconds. With practice this process becomes a smooth performance. Multiple practice trials may be needed for younger patients who forget their previous training and alternate exhalation and inhalation, causing the spirogram to rise and fall. Words of encouragement assist the performance during both inhalation and exhalation.
  - It is customary to have the patient perform three tracings that are of good technical quality. The best is used for interpretation. Vigorous exhalation may be quite fatiguing, and adequate rest intervals must be allowed, providing an ideal time to discuss the previous tracing and to point out desirable changes.
  - Repeat spirograms altered by coughing. In patients with significant airway disease, coughing may be unavoidable, especially near the end of expiration, and a descriptive summary of the performance should include problems witnessed if that spirogram is retained in the patient's record.
  - When the history or physical examination suggests the diagnosis of reactive airway disease, additional spirometric testing can be helpful. If the patient is symptomatic, spirometry may be performed before and 15 to 20 minutes after an inhaled bronchodilator to detect the presence of reversible airways obstruction. A significant change is considered present when the FEV_1 increases by approximately 10% or the $FEF_{25-75\%}$ by greater than 20%. In the majority of asthmatics who come to the office asymptomatic and have normal pulmonary function tests, bronchoconstriction may be induced by exercise. Controversy exists, however, about the advisability and safety of using this challenge in a routine office setting. The customary challenge is to have the patient

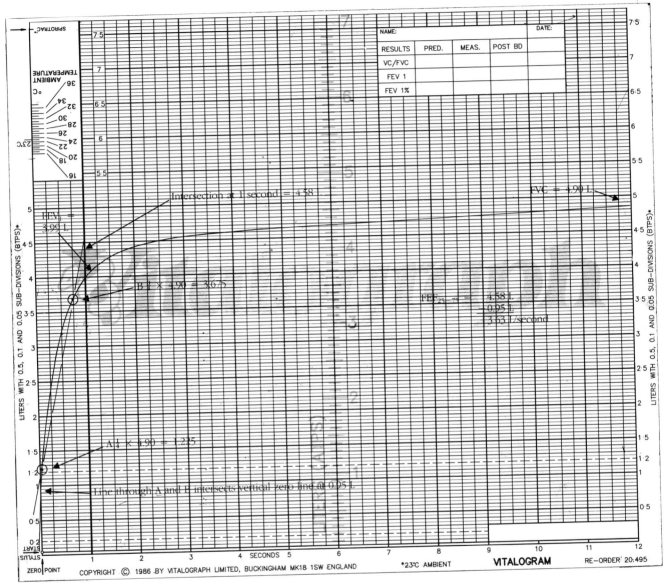

Figure 11-4.
Functional examination of the respiratory tract. Determination of $FEF_{25-75\%}$.

run in a safe area outside of the office for several minutes. The patient then returns to the examining room, where auscultation and spirometry are repeated. This approach is nonstandardized, and the exercising child should be observed by a professional in case severe bronchospasm occurs. A better approach might be to refer the patient to an experienced laboratory where provocation using exercise or an inhaled agent (methacholine or histamine) will document bronchial hyperreactivity safely and accurately. Exercise provocation is

not recommended for the symptomatic patient. A 10% drop in FEV_1 is considered significant evidence of bronchospasm.

5. Side Effects and Complications: There are rarely significant complications from spirometry. Initiation of hemoptysis, facial petechiae, or a pneumothorax have been seen. More commonly, prolonged forced exhalation may cause temporary headache, which may be reduced by avoiding repeat testing if the first tracings appear appropriately performed.

If exercise provocation is performed in an office setting

and the patient possibly has reactive airway disease, both inhalable and injectable bronchodilators should be available to reverse significant bronchospasm.

6. Interpretation: Given a properly performed tracing, it is relatively easy to determine the FVC and FEV$_1$ and calculate the FEV$_1$/FVC ratio. Points may then be placed on the curve where one fourth and three fourths of the FVC have been reached (Figure 11-4). A line drawn through these two points is extended until it crosses two vertical chart lines 1 second apart. From these intersections, the difference in volume readings can be calculated to give the FEF$_{25-75\%}$ in liters per second.

Values obtained from spirometry are usually compared with two references. Charts are available that provide the mean and standard deviation values for normal children of the same height, sex, and race. The values also may be compared with those of previous recordings from the same patient. If measurements are less than before, the clinician must decide if the cause is a change in health or in the effort and technique of the patient.

Children in normal health may exceed the published mean values without concern because this is not a sign of pulmonary disease. Achieving less than 80% of the mean for FVC and FEV$_1$ and less than 65% for FEF$_{25-75\%}$ should usually be considered abnormal. The FEV$_1$/FVC ratio is considered abnormal if less than about 75%.

Examples of a restrictive curve and an obstructive curve are shown in Figure 11-5A. Characteristic patterns for obstruction and for restriction are shown in Figure 11-5B.

B. Sweat Test for Cystic Fibrosis

1. Purpose: The collection of sweat and its quantitative analysis for chloride has been used extensively for over 35 years as the diagnostic test for cystic fibrosis. Quantitation of the sweat sodium also may be performed, but this measurement does not have the diagnostic acceptance that a chloride determination has.

2. Selection of Patients:

a. Indications: The manifestations of cystic fibrosis vary greatly from patient to patient. The entire triad of elevated sweat electrolytes, respiratory tract disease, and pancreatic insufficiency leading to malabsorption is often not present when the first symptoms are witnessed. In some patients, malabsorption and consequent growth failure are not observed. The clinician must have a high index of suspicion and request testing before significant health changes have occurred.

Testing should be done when children and young adults demonstrate:

· Salt loss by sweating. This may lead to profound electrolyte depletion and metabolic alkalosis associated with chronic lethargy, anorexia, and failure to thrive in infants, or a more acute depletion (i.e., heat prostration)

in young and older patients under hot environmental temperatures.

· Respiratory tract manifestations such as chronic sinus disease, nasal polyposis, recurrent or chronic bronchitis and pneumonia, atelectasis, or hyperexpansion of lung tissue due to endobronchial disease and bronchiectasis. Clubbing of the fingers or culture of *Pseudomonas aeruginosa* from respiratory tract secretions also should alert one to the possibility of cystic fibrosis.

· Digestive tract manifestations such as those potentially associated with pancreatic insufficiency: Intestinal obstruction in the newborn with or without the classic appearance of meconium ileus, failure to thrive, excessive hunger, abnormal character and frequency of bowel movements, visible steatorrhea, fat-soluble vitamin deficiencies, hypoproteinemia, distal intestinal obstruction syndrome (meconium ileus equivalent), rectal prolapse,

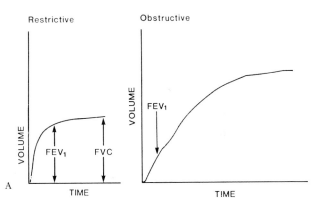

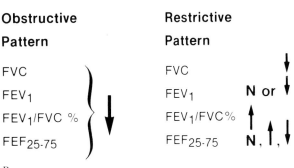

Figure 11-5.
Functional examination of the respiratory tract. A, Restrictive and obstructive spirograms; **B,** Obstructive and restrictive patterns. From Eigen, H. Pulmonary function testing: A practical guide to its use in pediatric practice. Pediatrics in Review 1986; 7:235-45, with permission.

and intussusception. Biliary cirrhosis with splenic enlargement and varices may be a presenting manifestation.

In addition, all siblings of children known to have cystic fibrosis should be sweat tested.

b. Contraindications and Precautions: There are virtually no contraindications to the performance of a sweat test. In the young infant it may be difficult to obtain adequate quantities of sweat for accurate analysis.

Each clinician should ascertain that the sweat test available to his or her practice conforms with the standards outlined below. If only "screening tests," (e.g., those using chloride-specific electrodes, conductivity, or osmolarity analyses) are offered, it would be wise to refer the patient to a medical center where approved methods are used.

3. Equipment and Supplies (See Appendix for equipment and supplies manufacturers and suppliers. Appendix is keyed to italicized words in the equipment and supplies lists):

A sweat test is done in two phases. First, sweat glands are stimulated to produce sweat and the specimen is collected. Second, a quantitative analysis for chloride content is accomplished.

Until recently the only method accepted by the Cystic Fibrosis Foundation as accurate enough for diagnostic use was the *quantitative pilocarpine iontophoresis technique (QPIT)*, described by Gibson and Cooke in 1959. A detailed description of the equipment, technique, and standards necessary was published and remains available from the Foundation.[2] The stimulation and collection process requires:

- A current source to drive the iontophoresis process
- Two *electrodes* with rubber straps
- 2- × 2-inch gauze *pads*
- Pilocarpine *nitrate*
- Sodium *nitrate,* as a second conducting liquid
- Preweighed sealed flasks containing a collection material and protected from surface contamination by a towel cover
- Kelly *clamp* (See Figure 21-7, page 282) or like device for transferring the material in the flask to and from the patient's arm
- 4- × 4-inch gauze *pads*
- Distilled water
- Clean plastic sheeting trimmed in size to cover the collection material while on the patient's arm. Edges must be taped down to avoid evaporation during sweat collection.

In 1986, after comparison with the QPIT, the Cystic Fibrosis Foundation approved the *Macroduct sweat collection system* as equally acceptable. This system is simpler to use and sweat that accumulates in the coiled tubing of the collection device can be seen, thereby identifying the sweat volume as it develops. There is virtually no exposure to air, eliminating concern about evaporation of water content. Explicit instructions are provided to guide the user.

4. Description of Procedure:

- When properly performed, a sweat test should reliably identify the chloride content of the patient's sweat. Every effort should be made to standardize each step of the procedure. It is recommended that a test be the responsibility of one or two experienced technicians who can collect the sweat, analyze it, and record the chloride result and the volume of sweat obtained in proper records. The technician should be able to identify any problem that occurs during collection or analysis.
- Sweat collection is customarily performed on the volar surface of the forearm, on skin that appears normal, without rash or other lesions. The selected site should be far enough away from the elbow to allow freedom of motion without tipping or otherwise disturbing the electrodes or collection device in use.
- First wash the skin to remove surface debris, dry briefly, then place electrodes where iontophoresis is to be performed.
- The detailed instructions regarding the QPIT from the Cystic Fibrosis Foundation or accompanying the Macroduct system from Wescor, Inc., direct the technician through the procedure. After 5 minutes of iontophoresis, cleanse the skin with distilled water, carefully dry it, and begin the collection process.
- The collection time is customarily 30 minutes.
- Once sweat is collected by the QPIT method and the collecting material is sealed in the flask, weigh the flask again on analytical scales in the Chemistry Laboratory to determine the volume of sweat obtained. The analysis process then begins.
- If the Macroduct system is used, carefully remove the collection device from the forearm and transport it to the medical center's laboratory for analysis. We find that the sweat can be collected in field clinic operations, sealed at the entry portal, and transported without fear of evaporation. It has been our policy to collect sweat from both forearms concomitantly and to analyze each specimen at least twice for additional quality control. Our chloride analyzer requires 20 μL of sweat for each analysis, much less than the capacity of the Macroduct collecting tube. Two known chloride standards (10 mEq/L and 100 mEq/L) are routinely analyzed to ascertain technical accuracy.

5. Side Effects and Complications: Even with extreme care some patients may develop small burns beneath an electrode using the QPIT. The Macroduct system of iontophoresis has not been reported to be associated with burns, and children appear to tolerate the period of iontophoresis with less complaint of pain or a burning sensation.

6. Interpretation: In the presence of clinical evidence suggesting the presence of cystic fibrosis or a family history of cystic fibrosis, a sweat chloride value above 60 mEq/L in childhood is consistent with the diagnosis of cystic fibrosis. It should be recognized that some normal adults may have values slightly above 60 mEq/L. Values between 45 and 60 mEq/L are considered borderline and are usually repeated. Reported cases of children with "positive" sweat tests, later proven to be normal, suggest that all positive tests should be confirmed at a later date unless clinical evidence for the presence of cystic fibrosis is strong. Repetition is often helpful in convincing family members that the diagnosis is correct.

False-positive results not related to technical error are infrequent, but they could occur with adrenal insufficiency and have been reported with a small number of other disease entities.

C. Sputum Collection and Evaluation

1. Purpose: Sputum, like other body fluids, may be studied by cytologic methods or culture and sensitivity techniques to clarify the cause of the patient's illness and dictate management.

2. Selection of Patients:

a. Indications: Sputum study is particularly advantageous in patients with chronic lower respiratory symptomatology such as cough or wheezing who may have asthma, cystic fibrosis, focal bronchiectasis, or other causes of excess secretion. The study of sputum is probably underused in office practice because it requires time to collect and prepare the specimen. In addition, many patients have either not mastered the technique of coughing and expectorating mucus or find the process distasteful enough that requests for specimens are not met.

When the history and physical examination indicate that endobronchial secretions are excessive in quantity, consider sputum study. There are numerous anecdotes that could illustrate how worthwhile sputum study is. Older, healthy appearing adolescents and adults have been proven by sweat testing to have cystic fibrosis with pulmonary manifestations after pseudomonas was detected in their sputum. Patients with prominent or nocturnal cough, but no audible wheezing by history, have been investigated more fully and treated for asthma after sputum showed significant eosinophilia. Many patients have previously received ineffective antibiotic or cough suppressant therapy before they were correctly diagnosed.

b. Contraindications and Precautions: There are virtually no contraindications to sputum study. Careful preparation often allows office sputum collections even in infants.

The most significant hazard involved in sputum collection is the associated vomiting of stomach contents from gagging that appears to occur, particularly in younger individuals. This risk can be diminished by withholding all oral intake from the patient before coming to the office. The mouth should not contain gum or food particles at the time of the collection in any case. Rinsing the mouth may be necessary.

3. Equipment and Supplies (See Appendix for equipment and supplies manufacturers and suppliers. Appendix is keyed to italicized words in the equipment and supplies lists):

- A sterile plastic *cup* with a tight lid
- Tongue *blades* (See Figure 9-20, page 97)
- Cotton-tipped *applicators* (See Figure 14-5, page 167)
- Aerobic and anaerobic bacterial culture media
- Hansel stain

4. Description of Procedure:

- The collection process is easy for the *older patient who expectorates* mucous from the lower respiratory tract into the collection cup after vigorous, deep coughing on command. Many of these patients are more at ease producing a specimen if provided privacy. Some are more successful if allowed to collect the specimen after the forced exhalation of spirometry or a session of chest physical therapy. Sputum induction with inhaled, nebulized sterile saline or a bronchodilator may be tried (See Emergency Management of Asthma, Acute Asthma Attack, page 249).

- *Younger patients* and those with very little sputum or a distaste for expectorating sputum require a different approach. Variously described as a "deep throat" or "gag" culture, the procedure is used to obtain a hypopharyngeal specimen that contains either fresh sputum or secretions that have been brought to this area by ciliary activity and previous coughing. A hypopharyngeal specimen is frequently small unless obtained while the child is coughing and does not lend itself to the usual screening procedures before culture. Most children resist this procedure, and the level of apprehension is high.

- The successful collection of a hypopharyngeal specimen by swabs requires patience, experience, and judgment and should be performed by the physician rather than by office staff trained in performing throat cultures for streptococci. Use two swabs. Preparation is a key element in successful hypopharyngeal collections. Parents are helpful in calming their young child, but are less helpful in restraining the child and anticipating quick body movements.

- The experienced office nurse is essential in stabilizing the young child's upper extremities and head to avoid those twisting motions that move the target area away from the physician's line of view. With the child recumbent, have the child's arms held extended next to the head, the assistant's hands compressing the arms and head together and retarding motions that interfere with

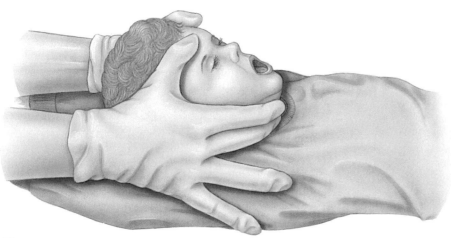

Figure 11-6.
Sputum collection and evaluation. Technique for restraint of patient for collection of sputum from the hypopharynx.

the collection (Figure 11-6). When needed, have the lower extremities and hips held by another assistant. Restrainers can be gentle initially, but should provide vigorous restraint while the swabs are in the throat.

• It is frequently necessary or even advantageous to allow an infant to cry while he is being restrained: the deep breathing that occurs with crying often promotes coughing and mobilizes sputum found in larger airways. Coughing after crying may be triggered also by depressing the tongue with a tongue blade and touching the pharyngeal wall with the swabs. Briefly retracting the swabs may result in coughing and significant sputum production. For sputum collection, listen for the sound of moving mucus and use a tongue blade and overhead lighting to watch the pharynx. By collecting the specimen at the optimal moment, you may prevent trauma or gagging from "hunting" for the specimen. If vomiting occurs, the value of an ongoing collection is questionable; usually the procedure must be terminated and tried at a later time.

• Note the characteristics of the sample at the time of collection. Sputum may be bloody, clear, colored yellow or green, relatively thin, or thick and tenacious. If possible, it is wise to inspect a questionable specimen microscopically to ascertain that true sputum is present. Each laboratory develops its own criteria for rejecting culture specimens they consider oral secretions rather than sputum. Clinical laboratories customarily screen specimens submitted as "sputum" with a Gram's stain to assure that the cellular content is predominantly leukocytes and that few squamous cells are seen. If flecks

of mucopurulent material are present in saliva, separation is necessary so that the mucopurulent material can be better studied. If the purpose for collection is cytologic study, confirmation of its origin is equally important. The Gram's stain also helps the technician identify the predominating organism and may help simplify the interpretation of the culture results.

• If a significant aliquot of sputum has been obtained, a portion may be separated first and saved on slides for bacterial stains, Hansel stain, or other cytologic study. If no identifiable sputum is present on the culture swabs, you will need to decide whether to proceed with the culture or not. It may be helpful in those with ongoing lower respiratory tract infections to know what organisms are present in the hypopharynx. The presence of a potential pathogen insensitive to a previously used or currently selected antibiotic may suggest that a different antimicrobial agent is necessary.

• Drying of a specimen may alter the culture result. If secretions are collected by swab, a holding medium may be needed for transportation of the specimen to the laboratory. An alternative is to have the necessary culture plates available in the examining room so that swabs used in the collection can be applied to the medium promptly for initial streaking. Cross-streaking with a sterile wire loop may then be accomplished when the plates reach the laboratory.

• The laboratory can be very helpful in selecting the proper culture plates to use. When multiple potential pathogens are possible, use a sheep blood agar (broad range of organisms), a mannitol salt agar (staphylococci), a MacConkey's agar (gram-negative rods), and a chocolate agar (*Haemophilus sp.*). When sputum is from a patient with cystic fibrosis, include a selective agar for *Pseudomonas cepacia*. You can have an impact on the results of sputum study by your personal involvement in the gross study of the specimen and communication with laboratory personnel.

5. Side Effects and Complications: There are no likely side effects except those already mentioned under Contraindications and Precautions.

6. Interpretation: On the day of the office visit, only results of simple sputum studies will be available. If a wet mount or Hansel stain of sputum reveals Charcot-Leyden crystals (elongated bodies from degeneration of eosinophils and coalescence of their granules), Curschmann's spirals (thin, long bronchial casts), or significant eosinophilia, asthma may emerge as a primary diagnosis. The Gram's stain may suggest

a predominant organism that antimicrobial therapy should cover while awaiting the final culture and sensitivity reports. This study, or the Hansel stain, may identify a heavy population of neutrophils and give support to an infectious cause. Sputum study can be a useful tool in initiating patient management as well as in adjustment of care when final reports and the patient's response to medications are known. The results of hypopharyngeal specimen cultures, however, do not correlate as well with the actual flora of the lower respiratory tract as do expectorated sputum cultures.

References

1. ATS Statement—Snowbird Workshop on Standardization of Spirometry. Am Rev Respir Dis 1979; 119:831.
2. Cystic Fibrosis Foundation, 6931 Arlington Road, Bethesda, MD 20814.

Chapter 12

Gastrointestinal Procedures

James L. Sutphen

I. Diagnostic Procedures

A. Rectal Examination

1. Purpose: A rectal examination is a valuable component of the physical examination of any child with a gastrointestinal complaint.

2. Selection of Patients:

a. Indications: This examination is particularly important in the child with abdominal pain, chronic diarrhea, constipation, or painful bowel movements.

b. Contraindications and Precautions: A relative contraindication to a rectal examination is extreme anxiety on the part of the child. Also, severe rectal fissures and fistulae may contraindicate a rectal examination because of the possibility of associated severe pain. In situations where the rectal examination is anxiety provoking or particularly painful, intramuscular analgesia with meperidine (Demerol) may be useful.

3. Equipment and Supplies (See Appendix for equipment and supplies manufacturers and suppliers. Appendix is keyed to italicized words in the equipment and supplies lists):

- Nonsterile *gloves*
- Lubricating *jelly*
- Occult blood detection *slide*
- Glass microscope *slide*
- Tissue paper

4. Description of Procedure:

- Because of the discomfort associated with a rectal examination, save this procedure until the end of the physical examination.
- Explain to the child that the examination is not painful, merely uncomfortable. Children less than 10 years of age rarely understand (or believe) this distinction. Therefore, a more graphic explanation is sometimes useful. This explanation of the procedure will often

evoke peals of laughter or frank stares of horror from siblings. Therefore, before performing a rectal examination, ask all siblings of the child to leave the room. If possible, invent a convenient excuse for them to be out of the room. If one asks a child's siblings to leave the room immediately before a painful procedure, it is virtually certain that the child will tense up and react with fear. It is essential for the child to relax as much as possible during the performance of the procedure.

· The preferred position for a rectal examination is to have the child lie on his left side with the right leg appropriately flexed at the hip (Figure 12-1).

· Don nonsterile gloves, and apply a generous amount of lubricating jelly to the tip of the index finger (for a procedure on children over 6 years of age) or small finger (for a procedure on children under 6 years of age).

· After lubricating the perianal area, examine it for skin tags, abscesses, or tears before inserting the finger. It is extremely painful to have a rectal examination done across a torn anal area. You also may have difficulty convincing the parent that the rectal examination did not cause the anal tear.

· Massage a small amount of lubricant into the distal anal canal and insert the tip of the finger. First insert the ball of the finger into the canal, followed by the upper or nail (cut short) portion of the finger.

· When your finger encounters the rectal sphincter (Figure 12-2), do not advance the finger quickly. Rapid advancement produces painful spasm of the sphincter. The rectal sphincter will relax as you very slowly advance the finger into the anal canal. To this end, have the patient open his mouth and take deep breaths in and out through the mouth while you advance the examining finger.

· After you advance the finger past the point of the sphincter, palpate the anterior rectal shelf in a sweeping fashion (Figure 12-2). Then turn the hand 180 degrees so that you can examine the posterior shelf. The sweeping action allows you to feel small polyps on the rectal mucosa.

· On withdrawing the finger from the rectal canal, it is prudent not to have your head or body in harm's way. This is especially true when examining a child who has Hirschsprung's disease, because on withdrawal of the examining finger, there is often an explosive watery stool.

· After your finger is withdrawn, rub the tip of the examining finger on an occult blood detection slide.

· Rub another surface of the tip of the finger on a microscope slide for later examination for leukocytes. Do this latter step even if stool is not visible on the finger.

· Wipe the jelly off the perianal area with tissue paper.

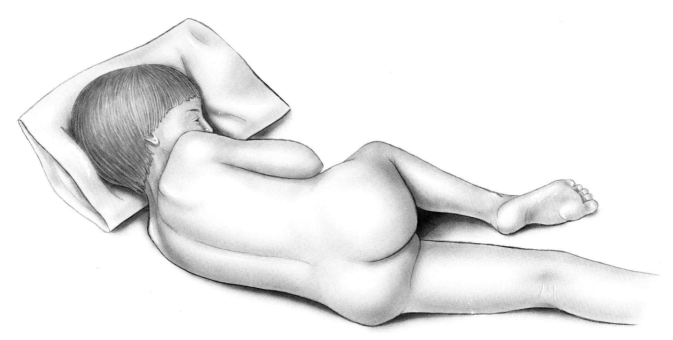

Figure 12-1.
Rectal examination. Proper positioning of patient.

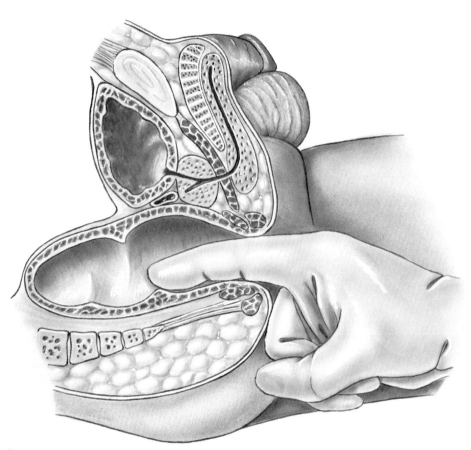

Figure 12-2.
Rectal examination. Technique.

· Suggest to the patient that he can use the bathroom to clean himself more thoroughly or to defecate.

5. Side Effects and Complications: In patients with significant fissures and fistulae, it is possible to irritate these areas with the examiner's finger. In patients with significant perianal inflammation, rectal examinations rarely induce bacteremia; therefore, routine rectal examinations are not considered an indication for antibiotics for bacterial endocarditis prevention.

B. Proctoscopy/Sigmoidoscopy

1. Purpose: The purpose of proctoscopy/sigmoidoscopy is to provide direct visualization of the rectum and distal colon.

2. Selection of Patients:

a. Indications: The indications for proctoscopy/sigmoidoscopy include undiagnosed rectal bleeding, chronic bloody or nonbloody diarrhea, and suspected rectal polyp(s).

b. Contraindications and Precautions: Proctoscopy/sigmoid-oscopy is relatively contraindicated in selected individuals who have severe fissures and fistulas or bleeding hemorrhoidal varices, or who are immunosuppressed. Insertion of the tip of a glass laboratory test tube to provide a direct view of the rectum is not recommended, because it provides limited visualization and can be hazardous.

3. Equipment and Supplies (See Appendix for equipment and supplies manufacturers and suppliers. Appendix is keyed to italicized words in the equipment and supplies lists):

· Saline *solution,* for irrigation

· Enema *bottle* (See Figure 12-14, page 139) or enema *bag*

· Tilt table

· *Sigmoidoscope,* rigid, with insufflating balloon—available in two pediatric sizes (Figure 12-3). In full-term infants and in children up to 6 to 7 years of age, the infant size sigmoidoscope is preferable. An intermediate size sigmoidoscope is available for younger school-age

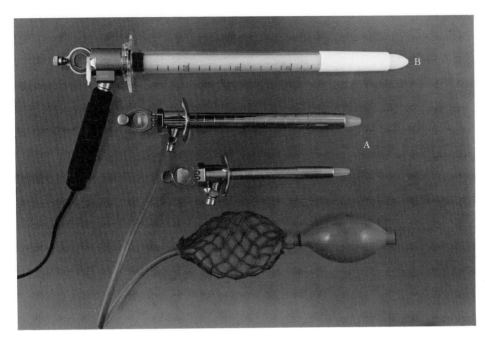

Figure 12-3.
Proctoscopy/sigmoidoscopy. Equipment and supplies: **A,** Sigmoidoscope, rigid (two pediatric sizes; one attached to insufflating balloon); **B,** Sigmoidoscope, flexible.

children. The standard adult size sigmoidoscope is used for teenagers.

· *Sigmoidoscope,* flexible (Figure 12-3)
· Lubricating *jelly* with lidocaine (2%)
· Lubricating *jelly*
· Sigmoidoscopic cotton-tipped *applicators*
· Rectal suction *catheter*
· Tissue paper

4. Description of Procedure:

· Examine an infant or toddler by having him lie with the left side down in a knee–chest position (See Figure 12-1, page 127). You can examine an older child in this position, but he is best examined through the use of a special tilt table designed for sigmoidoscopic examination. When using the tilt table, show the child how to position the knees close to the table on the knee supports. Explain to the child that he will be tilted head down in a somewhat unnatural position. Tell the child that he will not fall and position an assistant to prevent slipping. If a special table is not available, perform a sigmoidoscopy by asking the patient to kneel on the examining table on his knees, lie down on his forearms, and place his forehead on his forearms (See Figure 14-7, page 168).

· Do not perform a sigmoidoscopy without first per-

forming a rectal examination (See Rectal Examination, page 126). On the rectal examination, determine the amount of stool in the rectum.

· If significant stool is present, precede the sigmoidoscopic examination with an enema (See Enemas, page 138). Use a saline enema, because other enema solutions may induce subtle histologic changes that may confuse the microscopic interpretation of biopsy material.

· Attach the insufflating balloon to the sigmoidoscope before inserting the sigmoidoscope; the attachment of the balloon can be difficult after the sigmoidoscope has been inserted.

· Apply lidocaine anesthetic jelly through the anus with the oval applicator.

· Apply a generous amount of lubricating jelly to the sigmoidoscope, and slowly advance the tip into the anal canal.

· On encountering the sphincter, tell the child to "Push on the tube like you push when you are trying to have a bowel movement."

· After the sigmoidoscope has been advanced into the rectum, remove the obturator. Keep your head and body out of the direct line of fire during removal.

· With your left hand keep the sigmoidoscope in the

same relative position to the anus at all times by resting the side of the palm of the left hand on the buttock, using the fingers on the left hand to hold the scope in position (Figure 12-4). Do not pivot the sigmoidoscope in the anal canal without using the left hand as a fulcrum to stabilize its position.

· After inserting the sigmoidoscope, do not advance the tip of the tube without adequate visualization of the anal canal. To see the anal canal, you will usually have to insufflate the sigmoidoscope using the attached balloon. Insufflate only enough air into the anal canal to allow for adequate visualization of the lumen. If you are inexperienced, do not advance the tube beyond the most distal anal area.

· Pass a sigmoidoscopic swab through the tube to remove stool or adherent membranes and to assess the friability of the mucous membranes. Remove excessive soft or liquid stool through a suction catheter.

· As the sigmoidoscope is removed, rotate it in a 360-degree manner to allow visualization of all sides of the colon (Figure 12-5). This maneuver is best done on withdrawal of the sigmoidoscope, as it may be painful if it is done on insertion of the sigmoidoscope.

· Provide the patient with adequate tissue paper for cleaning lubricant from the perianal area.

5. Side Effects and Complications: Rectal perforation, tran-

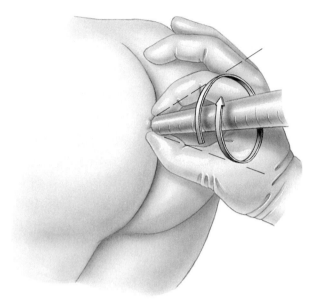

Figure 12-5.
Proctoscopy/sigmoidoscopy. Technique.

sient bacteremia, or anal tears may occur, but are unusual complications.

C. String Test

1. Purpose: The purpose of the enteral string test is to obtain a sample of small intestinal fluid for analysis for *Giardia lamblia*. It is also possible to use the string test to localize gastrointestinal bleeding by examining the withdrawn string for the location of blood.

2. Selection of Patients: Patients who are suitable candidates for the string test include older children who are able to swallow intact capsules and who can tolerate the somewhat nauseating feeling of having a string in the back of their throat.

a. Indications: In general, patients who have giardia infestations will manifest a chronic watery, often gassy, diarrhea. There may be a past history of contact with contaminated fresh water. The diarrhea tends to be worsened by the ingestion of lactose-containing foods.

b. Contraindications and Precautions: It is inadvisable to attempt to force an enteral capsule on a young child who cannot cooperate.

3. Equipment and Supplies (See Appendix for equipment and supplies manufacturers and suppliers. Appendix is keyed to italicized words in the equipment and supplies lists):

· Topical anesthetic *spray*
· Enteral *capsule* (Figure 12-6)
· Large glass of water
· Adhesive *tape*

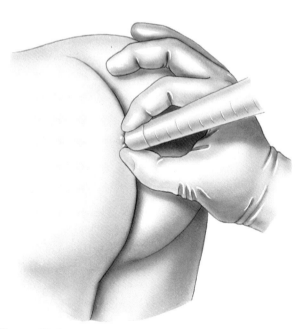

Figure 12-4.
Proctoscopy/sigmoidoscopy. Technique.

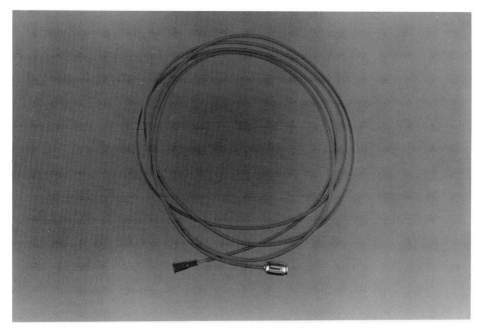

Figure 12-6.
String test. Equipment and supplies: **A,** Enteral capsule.

- Nonsterile *gloves*
- Petri *dish*
- Glass microscope *slides*
- Microscope
- pH *paper*

4. Description of Procedure:

- After the patient fasts overnight, anesthetize the posterior pharynx with a topical anesthetic spray.
- Pull a short length of cord from the capsule and hold it in your hand.
- Instruct the patient to swallow the capsule with a glass of water.
- Tape the proximal end of the cord to the patient's cheek and instruct him to drink water *ad libitum.*
- A major problem with children is that it requires 3 to 4 hours for the capsule to pass into the small intestine. During this time you must entertain most children. Also, they may begin to complain about the string in their mouth. Therefore, have available numerous diversions (toys, books, etc.) in the office to occupy the child's time. If at any point the child becomes nauseated, instruct him to breathe through his nose and put his chin to his chest.
- After a 3- to 4-hour period, instruct the patient to open the mouth. Then rapidly withdraw the string from the intestine.

- If significant resistance develops during withdrawal, cut the string and allow it to pass in the stool.
- Place the withdrawn string in a petri dish and squeeze duodenal fluid from the bile-stained segment of yarn.
- Check the pH of the yarn by touching it with pH paper at various locations to verify the position of the yarn in the gastrointestinal tract (acid pH indicates a gastric position; alkaline pH indicates an intestinal position).
- Place a sample of bile-stained duodenal fluid on a glass slide and examine under the microscope for the presence of active giardia organisms.

5. Side Effects and Complications: The most frequent side effect of this procedure is the nauseating feeling of the string in the posterior pharynx. If this problem persists, positioning of the head with the chin against the chest may be useful. Age-appropriate activities will provide diversions for the patient, which will facilitate cooperation. Instructing the patient to breathe through the nose instead of through the mouth when a gagging episode begins will help the patient abort the gagging episode. Repeat spraying of the posterior pharynx with topical anesthetic is sometimes useful. However, the mere act of spraying is sometimes enough to stimulate regurgitation once the string is in place. Occasionally the capsule does not exit the stomach and enter the duodenum, and the results are not useful.

6. Interpretation: The presence of giardia in the duodenal fluid in symptomatic individuals is suggestive of giardia-related diarrhea. If no giardia are found, the pH of the fluid should be carefully checked to make certain that the capsule was passed into the appropriate area.

D. Specimen Collection

Pinworm Collection—Scotch Tape Test

1. Purpose: The purpose of the scotch tape test is to detect the presence of pinworm eggs in the perianal area.

2. Selection of Patients:

a. Indications: Suitable candidates for this examination include patients who have perirectal itching.

b. Contraindications and Precautions: A rare allergy to the scotch tape adhesive is a contraindication.

3. Equipment and Supplies (See Appendix for equipment and supplies manufacturers and suppliers. Appendix is keyed to italicized words in the equipment and supplies lists):
  • Commercially available clear adhesive tape test *kits* are available with a microscope slide included. Alternatively, clear adhesive *tape* and a standard glass *slide* may be used.

4. Description of Procedure:
  • Expose the adhesive side of the scotch tape and gently apply to the perianal area several times.
  • Then apply the tape to a microscope slide and microscopically examine the slide for eggs.

5. Side Effects and Complications: None

6. Interpretation: If eggs are found, treatment of the infestation is indicated. If no eggs are found, infestation is not excluded and you must rely on your clinical judgment in deciding whether treatment is indicated.

Stool Specimen Collection for Examination for White Blood Cells or Ova and Parasites, for Detection of Rotavirus, or for Bacterial Culture

1. Purpose: The purpose of this examination is to find evidence of colitis (presence of white blood cells), parasitic infestation, viral infection, or bacterial infection.

2. Selection of Patients:

a. Indications: The indications for a stool examination for *white blood cells* include chronic diarrhea, rectal bleeding, suspicion of inflammatory bowel disease, or acute diarrhea with fever, blood, mucus, or abdominal cramping.

The indications for an examination for *ova and parasites* include a history of unidentified worms in a diaper or stool, chronic diarrhea, peripheral blood eosinophilia, unexplained bowel obstruction, rectal bleeding, or manifestations of possible extraintestinal parasitic infestation.

The indications for seeking evidence of rotavirus infection include significant and persistent vomiting associated with dehydration with or without diarrhea or fever, especially in younger children and infants. The manifestations can be especially severe and even life-threatening in the immunocompromised patient.

The indications for *bacterial culture* include the presence of white blood cells or blood in the stool of a patient with diarrhea or diarrhea with fever or abdominal cramping.

b. Contraindications and Precautions: None

3. Equipment and Supplies (See Appendix for equipment and supplies manufacturers and suppliers. Appendix is keyed to italicized words in the equipment and supplies lists):
  • Wooden applicator *stick*
  • Sterile *gloves*
  • Glass microscope *slides*
  • Methylene blue stain
  • Microscope
  • Bacterial culture media

4. Description of Procedure:

a. Examination for white blood cells:
  • From a *fresh* stool, obtain a very small specimen, using a wooden applicator stick, and smear the stool thinly on a microscope slide.
  • If stool samples are not available, or if an answer is needed rapidly, use stool that is obtained on rectal examination. In fact, even if no stool is visible on the examining finger, swab the mucus that is on the finger. This may not be visible on the glove, but is apparent when the finger is gently swabbed on a microscope slide. For patients with severe colitis, occasionally only mucus containing abundant polymorphonuclear leukocytes is available.
  • You need not decolorize or fix the stool on the microscope slide. Merely allow the stool to air dry.
  • Flood the slide with methylene blue stain and allow to stand for 1 or 2 seconds.
  • Rince with tap water and air dry.
  • Examine microscopically with a 10× lens to screen for white blood cells and, if necessary, with a 100× lens under oil immersion for verification of white blood cells.

b. Examination for ova and parasites, detection of rotavirus, or bacterial cultures:
  • The collection procedure is basically the same as for Examination for white blood cells. Many parasitic forms do not appear in fecal specimens in concentrated numbers on a daily basis; thus, collect specimens on separate days to yield a higher percentage of positive results. Examine these specimens within 1 hour of their collection or preserve them in fixatives such as PVA (polyvinyl alcohol) solution and formalin solution.
  • You should also obtain specimens for the detection of rotavirus or culture for bacteria; a fresh stool optimizes the yield. Alternatively, you can freeze the specimen and

store it at −20°C. Commercial immunoassay kits are available for the detection of rotaviruses and require a small sample of stool. For the growth and identification of bacteria, swab a small sample on to appropriate bacterial culture media.

5. Side Effects and Complications: None unless a specimen is obtained with a swab and some discomfort occurs.

6. Interpretation:

a. Examination for white blood cells:

Actual quantitative interpretation is problematic. Generally the results are classified into occasional (only one white blood cell in several high-power microscopic fields), scattered (several white blood cells in a high-power microscopic field), and diffuse or sheets (a confluent mass of white blood cells easily visible in many high-power microscopic fields). White blood cells may be seen in the stool of any patient with colonic inflammation. The most common cause of white blood cells in the stool in children is bacterial diarrhea with invasive organisms such as salmonella, shigella, and campylobacter. However, occasional cases of viral diarrhea, food protein sensitivity, hemolytic uremic syndrome, ulcerative colitis, Crohn's disease, rectal fissure, intussusception, hemorrhoids, diaper rashes, and inflammatory polyps may produce white blood cells in the stool.

Although the stool examination for white blood cells generally indicates inflammation in the colon, it does not always mean that there is colitis. Stool samples obtained from diapers in the presence of a diaper rash may show white blood cells from the inflamed perineal area. Stools obtained in the presence of a rectal fissure may demonstrate white blood cells as a result of local irritation from the fissure. Similarly, stools obtained in presence of an inflamed hemorrhoid or polyp may demonstrate white blood cells.

b. Examination for ova and parasites:

Identification of parasitic forms rests on well-established morphologic criteria that are dependent on correct collection and fixation techniques. Several microscopic examinations are generally used for identification of different parasitic form. Wet preparations made directly from the fecal specimen detect motile trophs. Wet preparations made from a fixative solution detect troph forms, Helminth eggs, larvae, and protozoan cysts. Permanent stain preparations such as Trichrome detect protozoan cysts and troph forms.

c. Rotavirus detection:

Rotavirus antigen can be detected in stool specimens using one of a number of immunoassay tests that have a sensitivity of 70% to 100% and a specificity of 50% to 100%.

d. Bacterial culture:

Gastrointestinal bacterial pathogens isolated on culture media are identified on the basis of growth characteristics, Gram staining properties, antigen–antibody reactions, and biochemical profiles.

E. Enteral Intubation

1. Purpose: These procedures have both diagnostic and therapeutic purposes. They can be used to obtain gastric or duodenal material for analysis, to provide decompression of the bowel, or to administer drugs or feedings.

2. Selection of Patients:

a. Indications: Patients with a surgical abdomen, patients with inability to tolerate oral feedings or medications, and patients with infectious or other digestive diseases requiring gastric or other fluid analyses are candidates for enteral intubation.

b. Contraindications and Precautions: Nasal obstruction and esophageal fragility from burns or collagen vascular disease are contraindications to this procedure.

3. Equipment and Supplies (See Appendix for equipment and supplies manufacturers and suppliers. Appendix is keyed to italicized words in the equipment and supplies lists):

- Appropriate size polyvinyl chloride, silastic, or polyurethane *tube* (size according to easy passage through the nasal passageway). Tubes should be weighted when used for transpyloric passage (Figure 12-7).
- Stiffening *wire* (Figure 12-7)
- Nonsterile *gloves*
- Nasal decongestant drop or spray (e.g., *phenylephrine hydrochloride*)
- Lubricating *jelly* with lidocaine (2%)
- Cotton-tipped *applicator* (See Figure 14-5, page 167) for application of lubricating jelly
- Restraint *board* (See Figure 13-20, page 159)
- Topical anesthetic *spray*
- Bite *block*
- Broad-range pH *paper*

4. Description of Procedure:

a. Nasogastric intubation:

- Passage of a nasogastric or orogastric tube inevitably requires considerable patient cooperation. It is uncommon to achieve good cooperation if the patient is less than 13 to 14 years of age; therefore, appropriate patient restraint is important. Calm discussion of the procedure before starting goes a long way toward achieving a more successful intubation.
- Approximate an end point for insertion by a single two-step process. First, holding the tip of the tube at the patient's earlobe, stretch a length of tube to the tip of the patient's nose (Figure 12-8A). Second, keeping the first measured length of tube below the xyphoid, stretch a second length between the xyphoid and the tip of the patient's nose (Figure 12-8B). Make a mental note of which mark on the premarked tube represents the proximal end of the second measured length. This mark should be passed to the point of entry into the nostril once the tube is inserted.
- Don gloves.

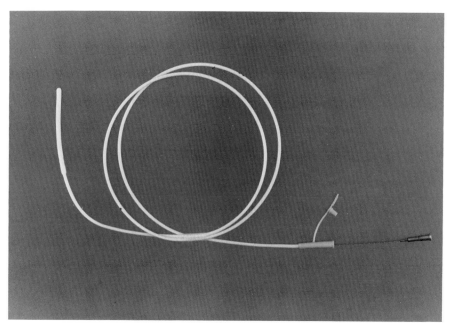

Figure 12-7.
Enteral intubation. Equipment and supplies: **A,** Enteral intubation tube with stiffening wire.

· Ascertain that the patient can breathe through both nostrils. Young infants are obligate nose breathers and will need to have both nasal passages open after the nasal tube has been passed. Any patient who is undergoing a procedure that involves stimulation of the gag reflex generally experiences less gagging if they can successfully breathe through their nose instead of their mouth. Both the nasal passage that is receiving the tube and the other nasal passage must be clear. Use a nasal decongestant drop immediately before nasal intubation.

· Determine which nasal passage is larger and begin anesthetizing this nasal passage with topical xylocaine jelly. Apply the xylocaine jelly to a nasal swab and progressively swab it down the passage. Have the patient lie on his back while the swab is gently and slowly inserted into the nasal passage. Alternatively, in an older, cooperative patient, have the patient sniff a small amount of lidocaine jelly into the nasal passage. For very uncooperative patients, preliminary topical anesthetics may not be tolerated and will simply prolong the procedure.

· After the initial topical sedation, apply a small amount of xylocaine jelly to the tube that is to be passed through the nasal passage.

· Only stiff tubes may be successfully passed through the nasal passage. You must reinforce very floppy tubes with a stiffening wire, which is often provided by the manufacturer with the tube. If the tube is to be passed for a short time, use the stiff polyvinyl chloride tube. For prolonged use, use silastic or polyurethane tubes, as they do not become stiff and brittle when exposed to gastric secretions. Bend the tip of the tube slightly in a curved position so that it may be directed down in the posterior nasopharynx rather than curling upward in a superior portion of the nasopharynx (Figure 12-9). Rotate the curved tube approximately 180 degrees after the tube has cleared the nasopharynx and is proceeding down the posterior pharynx (Figure 12-9). By doing this you direct the tip of the tube back toward the esophagus and away from the larynx, preventing insertion into the airway.

· After you have successfully passed the tube beyond the nasal passage and rotated it, subsequent manipulation will depend on the position of the patient.

· For infants and young children, you can best perform the procedure with the child restrained with a restraint board (Papoose Board) and lying on his side with the right side down.

(a) Gently press the head forward so that the chin touches the anterior chest. By doing this you decrease the gagging sensation and facilitate passage of the tube toward the esophagus and away from the larynx.

(b) Pass the tube into the stomach by feeding the

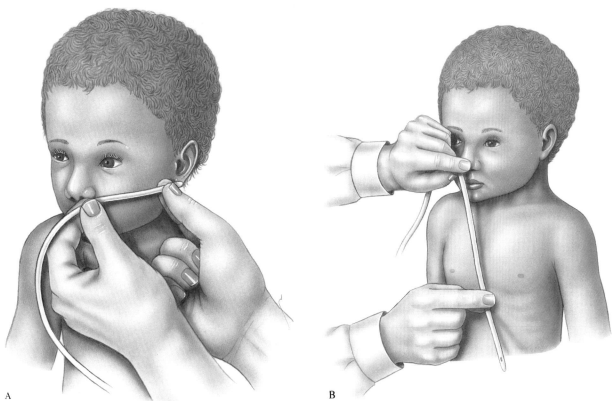

A   B

Figure 12-8.
Enteral intubation—Nasogastric intubation. Technique for estimation of appropriate
nasogastric tube length.

tube into the point where the predetermined mark
(See above) reaches the opening of the nostril.

(c) If severe coughing occurs or the patient is unable
to cry during the passage of the tube, immediately
withdraw the tube and reinsert it, as these signs generally indicate tracheal passage of the tube. Verify tube
position by aspirating gastric contents from the tube
or injecting air through the tube and auscultating over
the stomach to hear gastric bubbling. Alternatively,
you may hold the proximal end of the nasogastric
tube to your ear to detect breath sounds.

(d) After passage of the nasogastric tube and ascer-
tainment of its position in the stomach, securely tape
it along its track, beginning below the nose and extending out on the cheek (Figure 12-10).

· In an older, more cooperative patient, you can more
easily pass a nasogastric tube with the patient in a sitting
position. In these patients, you can further anesthetize
the posterior pharynx with topical spray anesthetics.

(a) The initial stages of intubation are identical for
the older patient who is to be intubated in a sitting
position. Once the tube has passed to the posterior
pharynx, instruct the patient to take several deep
breaths through the nose. Have the patients sit on
their own hands to provide a small amount of additional restraint that will prevent them from reaching
for the tube. You may find other distracting techniques such as instructing the patient to pull up on
his toes or pull back on his thumbs useful to decrease
the gag reflex.

(b) When the patient has calmed himself, offer a glass
of cold water with a straw. Instruct him to take several
rapid swallows with the straw. Lubricate the tube over
the entire length of passage. Quickly (but not forcefully) advance the tube in coordination with the patient's swallows.

(c) As in the younger uncooperative infant, have the
patient keep the chin down toward the chest.

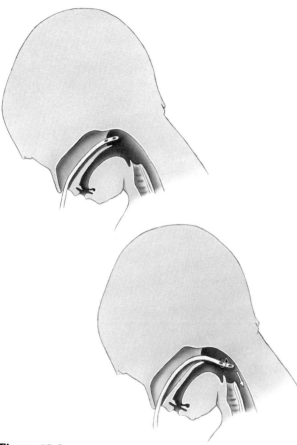

Figure 12-9.
Enteral intubation—Nasogastric intubation. Technique for insertion of the tube.

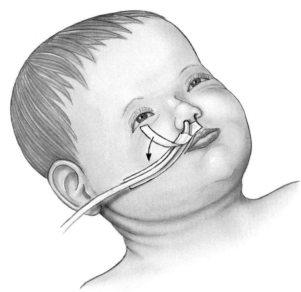

Figure 12-10.
Enteral intubation—Nasogastric intubation. Technique for securing the tube in an infant.

(d) Ascertain the tube's position as it is done in younger patients.

(e) After passing the nasogastric tube and confirming its position in the stomach, securely tape it to the nose and then tape it at a second point, either on the cheek or on the forehead (Figure 12-11).

b. Orogastric intubation:

• Larger caliber gastric tubes can be passed by the oral route, but can be left in place for only limited periods.

• If a gastric tube is to be passed through the mouth of a cooperative patient, first anesthetize the posterior pharynx with a topical spray. Further suppress the gag reflex by keeping the tube out of the midline during passage. Place your index finger in the mouth adjacent to the buccal mucosa but well outside the range of the teeth. Firmly hold the tube against the buccal mucosa, and pass it along the finger (Figure 12-12).

• In uncooperative patients, you may need to use a bite block to prevent the tube (and the examiner's finger) from being bitten (Figure 12-13).

• Immediately pass the tube into the posterior pharynx. During the swallow that follows the initial gagging, pass it down into the esophagus.

• When it it necessary to pass a tube forcefully, quickly pass the tube toward the lateral side of the mouth adjacent to the buccal mucosa immediately after successful passage into the esophagus.

• Remove the bite block and gently pass the tube as described above.

• If it is necessary to leave the tube in the mouth for a short time, keep the tube adjacent to the buccal mucosa with finger pressure. Orogastric tube passage is not suitable for prolonged intubation, because it is necessary to apply constant pressure. In a very young (preterm) infant, you can leave these tubes in successfully for the duration of a bolus feeding.

c. Small bowel intubation:

• If either a nasogastric or orogastric tube must be passed into the small intestine, pass an additional amount of tubing into the stomach to allow sufficient slack for passage of the tube into the duodenum. In general, you can more easily pass tubes with distal weights into the small bowel, as the weight provides a traction point for gastric peristalsis. You will need light anesthesia for small children.

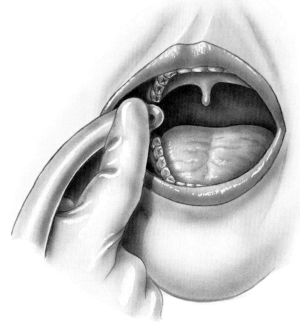

Figure 12-12.
Enteral intubation—Orogastric intubation. Technique for insertion using an index finger as a guide.

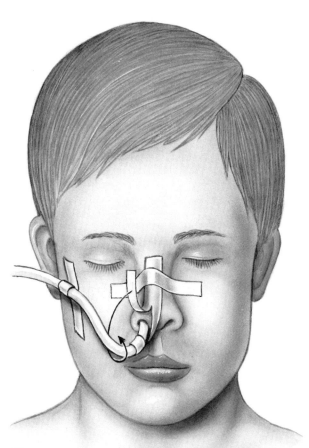

Figure 12-11.
Enteral intubation—Nasogastric intubation. Technique for securing the tube in a child.

· Facilitate passage of the tube into the small intestine by having the patient lie with the right side down. If it is possible to tilt the examining table, have the patient's head slightly lower than the feet. After entering the proximal duodenum, have the feet lowered to facilitate passage into the more distal duodenum.

· You may administer metaclopromide (Reglan) either intravenously or orally before passage of the tube unless this medication is contraindicated. Other maneuvers that may facilitate your passing the tube into the duodenum include having the child drink a small amount of warm liquid to facilitate gastric peristalsis. In cooperative older patients, suggest eating favorite foods to induce gastric peristalsis. Some children refuse to eat after the tube has been inserted.

· Check the position of the tube in the duodenum by determining, with pH paper, the pH of any aspirated

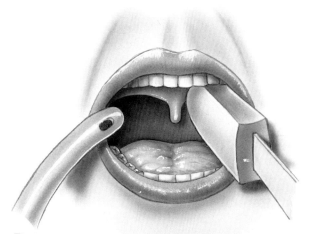

Figure 12-13.
Enteral intubation—Orogastric intubation. Technique for insertion using a bite block.

fluid. If you aspirate alkaline fluid, the tube has probably reached the duodenum. It is insufficient for you simply to note the color of the aspirate, because the gastric contents may occasionally appear yellow or even green to you. If fluoroscopy is available, examine the tube for the characteristic curve it assumes when properly positioned.

• If these simple techniques for passage of the tube are not successful, it may be necessary for you to use fluoroscopy to push the tube manually through the pylorus. You will need a relatively stiff tube. During fluoroscopy, position the patient with the right side down and pass the tube along the greater curve of the stomach under fluoroscopic guidance. When the tube is seen on fluoroscopy to be lying in the distal portion of the stomach and not curled back on itself, have the fluoroscope turned off and wait 5 minutes for the tube to pass. If the tube does not pass within 5 minutes, place the patient in the supine position, put on a radiopaque glove, and press your fingertips on the mid-abdomen immediately inferior to the curl of the tube. Apply a gentle caudal pressure with your fingers to press the curl of the tube into an anterior–posterior plane, as the pyloric outlet is slightly posterior in the stomach. Hold the tube in this position while you gently feed more tubing in through the nose or mouth. Take care not to induce into the stomach a large redundant curl that might absorb any forward pushing on the tube. When the tube has passed into the duodenum, it will assume a very characteristic turn as it proceeds through the first and second portion of the duodenum.

• Remove any enteral tube by a smooth rapid withdrawal.

5. Side Effects and Complications: The major complication of enteral intubation is aspiration of gastric contents. This risk can be lessened by having the patient receive no oral intake for at least 6 to 8 hours before tube passage (4 hours for young infants). Even in this situation, it is best to be prepared with adequate suction equipment and resuscitation equipment to deal with an aspiration episode. Other complications include inadvertent passage of the tube into the trachea and gastric perforation.

II. Therapeutic Procedures

A. Enemas

Enemas are often necessary for the removal of impacted fecal material. There are several commercial varieties available. In addition, there are numerous "home remedies." If an enema is being given before a rectal biopsy, it is important that the enema be only isotonic saline. All other enema solutions may induce subtle histologic changes that may confuse the microscopic interpretation of biopsy material. In addition to commercial products, tap water, soap suds, and milk and molasses (really) have been employed by grandmothers and clinicians for generations. The relative proportions and tolerance limits for detergents or milk and molasses have been inadequately investigated in children. These and other "exotic" enemas should be avoided. A commonly used and effective commercial enema is the sodium phosphate and biphosphate solution enema (Fleet's Enema). An oil retention enema also has been marketed by the Fleet company. The latter is useful as a nighttime enema for the removal of very firm fecal impactions. It is often combined with a cleansing phosphate enema on the following morning. The appropriate dosage of enema solution is poorly defined. In general, the adult size Fleet's enemas are reserved for older school-age children. However, the chronically constipated child may require a larger volume enema to produce results.

1. Purpose: The purpose of an enema is to remove impacted fecal material.

2. Selection of Patients:

a. Indications: The most common indication for an enema is constipation.

b. Contraindications and Precautions: Enemas are generally contraindicated in a patient who is immunosuppressed or believed to have a surgical abdomen. Also, in patients with calcium and phosphorus or electrolyte abnormalities, enema solutions may exacerbate the underlying abnormalities by absorption of enema components or by loss of fluid and electrolytes. Finally, patients with bleeding hemorrhoidal varicies, recent rectal biopsies, or recent rectal surgical procedures should not receive enemas.

3. Equipment and Supplies (See Appendix for equipment and supplies manufacturers and suppliers. Appendix is keyed to italicized words in the equipment and supplies lists):

• Disposable waterproof *pads*
• Nonsterile *gloves*
• Lubricating *jelly*
• Lubricating *jelly* with lidocaine (2%)
• Commercial enema *bottle* (Figure 12-14) or enema *bag* or *syringe* with feeding *tube* (Figure 12-14), for small infants
• Tissue paper

4. Description of Procedure:

• Carry out the procedure in close proximity to toilet facilities.

• Have all of the patient's clothing from the waist down removed before administering an enema. Use a sheet or towel to cover the child's buttocks so that some degree of modesty is maintained.

• Asminister an enema with the child lying on the left side with the right leg or both legs drawn up to the chest (See Figure 12-1, page 127). You may prefer to

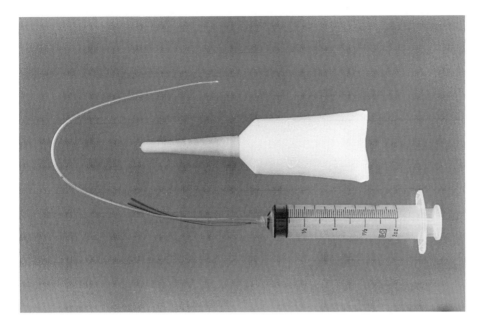

Figure 12-14.
Enemas. Equipment and supplies:
A. Commercial enema bottle;
B. Syringe with feeding tube.

allow infants to lie supine or prone with the legs gently flexed. You may restrain the patient for him to remain in the proper position. Older children may prefer to kneel down on their knees and rest their heads on their arms on the examining table (See Figure 14-7, page 168).
· Place disposable waterproof pads on the table below the patient's buttocks.
· Don nonsterile gloves and lubricate the tip of the enema catheter. If a rectal fissure is present, use a commercial lubricating jelly with lidocaine.
· Slowly advance the enema catheter past the anal sphincter.
· Then gently squeeze the enema bottle to deliver the solution slowly into the anal canal. If an enema bag is used, elevate the bag above the level of the rectum.
· After the enema has been instilled, have an assistant or parent hold the buttocks together to facilitate retention. In the uncooperative patient, enema solution will generally be expelled as soon as the tip of the catheter is withdrawn. The disposable pads directly under the patient are useful as barriers.
· If there is a large fecal impaction with fecal material easily palpable throughout the abdomen, you may find it necessary to use repeated enemas on several sequential days to remove the impaction.
5. Side Effects and Complications: Electrolyte imbalance, water intoxication, rectal perforation, and transient bacteremia are recognized unusual complications.

B. Disimpaction
Disimpaction of a severely constipated child is not pleasant for either the operator or the child. It is very useful to spend some time discussing the procedure with a frightened child. Light sedation may be very useful when manual disimpaction is being performed. In addition, the use of lidocaine jelly applied to the anus through a rectal applicating tube may make the procedure somewhat more acceptable.
1. Purpose: The purpose of a disimpaction procedure is to remove impacted fecal material from the rectum.
2. Selection of Patients:
a. Indications: Recurrent constipation unresponsive to repeated courses of laxatives or enemas, overflow diarrhea, and palpable firm fecal impactions are indications for the procedure.
b. Contraindications and Precautions: Contraindications include an acute surgical abdomen, evidence of toxic megacolon, or immunosuppression. Manual disimpaction should not be used before a trial of enema disimpaction (See Enemas, page 138).
3. Equipment and Supplies (See Appendix for equipment and supplies manufacturers and suppliers. Appendix is keyed to italicized words in the equipment and supplies lists):
· Waterproof *pads*
· Nonsterile *gloves*
· Lubricating *jelly*
· Commercial enema *bottle* (See Figure 12-13, page 137) or enema *bag* or *syringe* with feeding *tube* (See Figure 12-13, page 137), for small infants.

4. Description of Procedure:

· You can best perform simple manual disimpaction with a patient lying on water-impermeable pads with the left side down and facing away from the physician (See Figure 12-1, page 127). It is preferable for hygiene considerations to have the patient place *both* knees in a knee–chest position.

· Insert a gloved finger (well lubricated with lubricating jelly) into the anus and manually break hard impacted fecal material into smaller chunks that can be pulled across the anus with a curve finger. Often you may need to remove manually only a few large impacted masses.

Either the act of your removing these plugs or the dilation and stimulation of the anal area or both are sufficient to stimulate the passage of more stool.

· After manual disimpaction, begin a series of enemas to insure complete removal of more proximal fecal material. (See Enemas, page 138). The Fleet's mineral retention enema may be given initially at night and followed in the morning with the Fleet's cleansing enema.

5. Side Effects and Complications: Rectal perforation, anal tear, toxic megacolon, or transient bacteremia are unlikely occurrences.

Chapter 13

Urogenital Procedures

Jacob A. Lohr

Stuart S. Howards

Michael F. Rein

I. Diagnostic Procedures

A. Transillumination of the Scrotum

1. Purpose: The purpose of this procedure is to facilitate the diagnosis of scrotal masses.

2. Selection of Patients:

a. Indications: Transillumination of the scrotum is indicated in all patients with scrotal masses in whom there is any doubt about the diagnosis after a simple history and physical.

b. Contraindications and Precautions: None

3. Equipment and Supplies (See Appendix for equipment and supplies manufacturers and suppliers. Appendix is keyed to italicized words in the equipment and supplies lists):

· The procedure is done with a flashlight in a darkened room. It is preferable to have a flashlight with a small bright bulb at the end of a pencil-like projection to focus the light. A sinus *transilluminator* (Figure 13-1) is ideal.

4. Description of Procedure:

· After physical examination of the scrotum, turn off the light in the room and place the light source behind the scrotum (Figure 13-1). Take care not to use a light source that has become hot to touch.

· Then determine whether or not the scrotum transilluminates.

5. Side Effects and Complications: None other than discomfort or pain from a hot light source.

6. Interpretation: Transillumination through a significant portion of the scrotal mass suggests it is a fluid-filled mass. This is most consistent with a hydrocele. In a young infant, a scrotal hernia may also transilluminate. Because of the small size of the scrotum in the very young boy, a mass that is solid may be misinterpreted as transilluminating. However, in the older child transillumination is very useful in distinguishing between solid and fluid-filled scrotal masses.

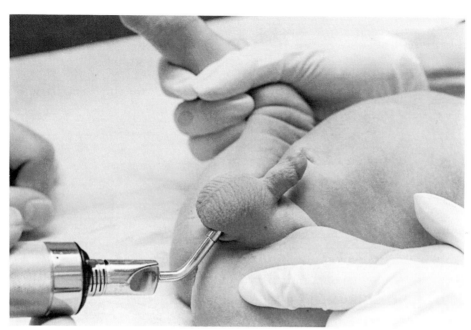

Figure 13-1.
Transillumination of the scrotum. Technique.

B. Specimen Collection—Urine for Urinalysis or Culture

1. Purpose: The purpose of this procedure is to collect a urine specimen for chemical or microscopic analysis or for bacteriologic culture.

2. Selection of Patients:

a. Indications: Collection of urine for chemical or microscopic analysis is indicated for a wide variety of patients believed to have primary renal disease or renal manifestations of other disease. Urine analysis is also occasionally performed as a screening procedure on healthy patients. Collection of urine for culture is indicated for patients with symptoms or signs of a urinary tract infection. Specific symptoms and signs include dysuria, increased frequency of urination, incontinence (including nocturia in a child previously dry at night), suprapubic pain, foul-smelling urine, macroscopic hematuria, suprapubic tenderness, and costovertebral angle tenderness. Suggestive findings include abdominal or flank pain, unexplained vomiting or diarrhea, and others.

b. Contraindications and Precautions: There are no contraindications for performing a urinalysis or urine culture. A urine specimen collected for microbiologic diagnosis must be collected with careful attention to the collection technique. The implications of a diagnosis of urinary tract infection (exposure to antimicrobial therapy, costly and invasive radiographic procedures, and costly long-term follow-up) mandate that an

accurate diagnosis be made. The diagnosis of a urinary tract infection can be suggested by certain chemical (nitrite and leukocyte esterase tests) and microscopic (presence of white cells, white cell casts, or bacteria) findings, but it is inappropriate for the diagnosis to be based on anything less than a quantitative culture of a urine obtained with a limited risk of microbial contamination. Contamination is minimized by selecting the most appropriate technique for the individual patient, by carefully performing the collection, and by using experienced personnel in the collection process. The methods of choice for urine collection for different age groups are shown in Table 13-1. On occasion, the likelihood of success in collecting a urine specimen is enhanced by offering the patient oral fluids; however, one must be mindful of the fact that the urine may be diluted by this process, thus decreasing the number of colony-forming units of an organism grown from a milliliter of urine.

(1) Urine bag collection: A urine bag collection is often suitable for routine analysis, but should not be used to diagnose a urinary tract infection, because the contamination rate is unacceptably high. One should use caution in applying a urinary bag to an infant with a diaper rash, because of the likelihood of producing additional irritation and discomfort.

(2) Voided midstream collection: This method is fraught with possibilities for contamination of the urine specimen

Table 13-1. Methods of Choice for Urine Specimen Collection for Microbiologic Analysis and Culture

Age Group	Gender	
	Males	Females
Neonates	Suprapubic aspiration	Suprapubic aspiration or urethral catheterization
Infants and incontinent children	Suprapubic aspiration	Urethral catheterization or suprapubic aspiration
Continent children	Midstream voided specimen collection	Midstream voided specimen collection, preferably times 2 or urethral catheterization

by skin, urethral, vaginal, or preputial flora; however, if proper technique is used, it can be the method of choice for continent (toilet-trained) children.

(3) Catheter collection: This method approaches the suprapubic aspirate in terms of low rates of contamination. The length and small caliber of the male urethra and the hazardous course of its posterior portion limit the use of this method in males.

(4) Suprapubic aspirate: This method remains the standard by which other methods are judged, because the rate of contamination is negligible. Its use is limited by the invasive nature of the procedure and by a low yield for obtaining urine if carelessly performed by an inexperienced practitioner. If properly performed, it is a safe procedure with a high success rate for obtaining urine. It is the procedure of choice in all neonates and in male infants and male non–toilet-trained children, and shares that distinction with catheter collections in female infants and female non–toilet-trained children. Although not the procedure of choice in continent children, it is safe and acceptable in this group. Because it provides a highly reliable specimen for culture, it is often used to obtain an early, accurate diagnosis in the more seriously ill patient.

3. Equipment and Supplies (See Appendix for equipment and supplies manufacturers and suppliers. Appendix is keyed to italicized words in the equipment and supplies lists):

a. Urine bag collection:

- 2 × 2 or 4 × 4 gauze *pads*
- Warm soapy water
- Warm water
- Sterile plastic urine collection *bag* with adhesive strips, newborn or pediatric size (Figure 13-2)
- Isopropyl alcohol (70%) *pad*
- 21-gauge *needle* (See Figure 20-7, page 262) on a 5-mL *syringe* (See Figure 20-7, page 262)

b. Voided midstream collection:
- Sterile *container* with a leak-proof screw cap (Figure 13-2)

c. Catheter collection:
- Povidone-iodone *solution* or *swabs*
- Sterile *gloves* for operator and assistant
- Cotton-tipped *applicator*
- Catheters
  - Feeding *tube,* for infants up to 1 year of age (Figure 13-3)
  - Urinary *catheters* (straight catheter or plastic catheter attached to a collection device), for older infants and children (Figure 13-3)
- Sterile bacteriostatic *lubricant*
- Sterile *container* with a leak-proof cap (Figure 13-2)

d. Suprapubic aspirate:
- High-intensity *transilluminator* (See Figure 9-14, page 94)
- Povidone-iodine *swabs*
- Isopropyl alcohol (70%) *pad*
- Sterile *gloves*
- *Lidocaine* (1%)
- 25-gauge *needle* (See Figure 20-7, page 262) on a 3-mL *syringe* (See Figure 20-7, page 262), for lidocaine injection
- 21- or 23-gauge, 1½-inch *needle* (See Figure 20-7, page 262) on a 10- to 12-mL *syringe* (See Figure 20-7, page 262), for urine aspiration. A 1.5- to 2.0-inch spinal *needle* (See Figure 17-3, page 212) may be needed in patients with a thick anterior abdominal wall.
- Sterile *container* with a leak-proof cap (See Figure 13-2, page 144)
- Sterile adhesive *bandage*

4. Description of Procedure:

a. Urine bag collection:
- Instruct the parent to hold the infant in a frog-leg position (Figure 13-4), which keeps a female's labia spread to decrease the likelihood of specimen contamination and makes attachment of the bag simpler in patients of either gender.
- Using a 2 × 2 or 4 × 4-inch gauze pad saturated with warm soapy water, cleanse the genitalia and an area that extends beyond the skin that will be exposed to the opening of the collection bag.

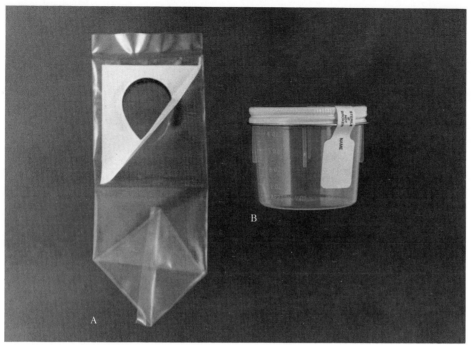

Figure 13-2.
Specimen collection—Urine for urinalysis or culture. Equipment and supplies:
A, Urine collection bag (with paper backing partially peeled from the bag's adhesive
surface); **B,** Sterile container.

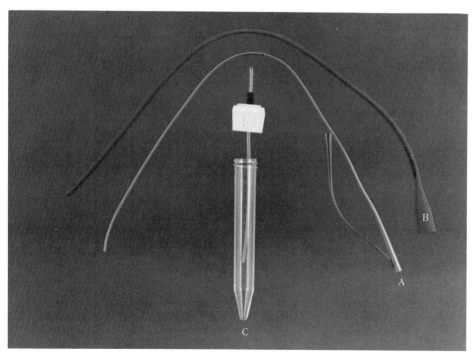

Figure 13-3.
Specimen collection—Urine for urinalysis or culture. Equipment and supplies:
Devices for catheterization—**A,** Feeding tube; **B,** Straight catheter; **C,** Plastic catheter
with a collection device.

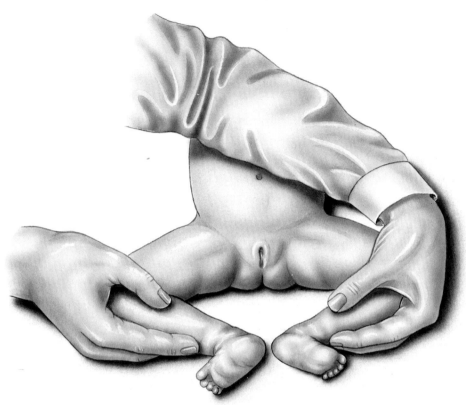

Figure 13-4.
Specimen collection—Urine for urinalysis or culture. Urine bag collection: frog-leg
position for attachment of urine collection bag.

• Rinse the soap off with warm water.
• Dry the cleansed area with a gauze pad to facilitate attachment of the bag.
• Peel off the paper backing on the bag, thus exposing the adhesive surface.
• For a girl, apply the adhesive so that the uretheral meatus is centered in the bag opening.
• For a boy, insert the penis (and the scrotum of a small infant) through the bag hole and apply the adhesive to the perineal skin.
• Make certain the adhesive is firmly attached around the bag opening.
• The patient may be diapered or covered with a blanket for comfort; but check the bag for urine every 10 minutes. Early detection of urine and prompt removal of the bag minimize the likelihood of contamination or loss of the specimen.
• Remove the bag by peeling off the adhesive surface from the skin.
• Take a specimen from the bag aseptically. The collec-

tion bag has a blue tab at the lower corner of the pouch that you can remove so that urine pours from the bag. However, we do not use this method for urine retrieval, because of concern about specimen contamination from the outside of the pouch and because the stream from the bag is often difficult to direct. We clean with isopropyl alcohol (70%) a small spot on the bag and insert into the bag a 21-gauge needle on a 5-mL syringe and withdraw a sample.
• Cap the needle and immediately transport the urine in the syringe to the laboratory for processing.

b. Voided midstream collection:
For the purpose of bacterial culture, the first voided morning urine is ideal. It is usually not possible to obtain such a urine specimen in the office, and collection of voided urine at home should be discouraged because proper technique may not be followed.

In the past, the midstream voided specimen collection was preceded by a laborious and time-consuming cleansing technique. Recent evidence indicates that the procedure can be greatly simplified,[1-3] and cleansing before the urine collection may be unnecessary.

(1) Boys

· Obtain a specimen by having the child urinate into a toilet. Then pass the mouth of a sterile container into the stream (midstream collection).

· Cap the container and transport the specimen to the laboratory.

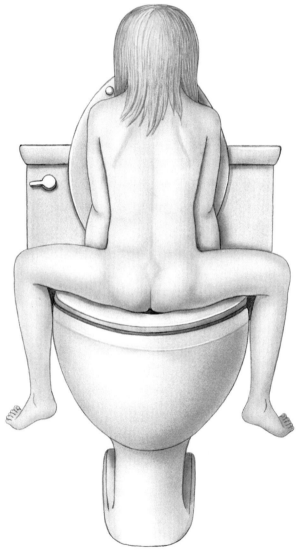

Figure 13-5.
Specimen collection—Urine for urinalysis or culture.
Midstream voided collection: position of a girl for urine collection.

(2) Girls

· The labia should be spread to expose the urethral opening before urinating. You can instruct an older child or adolescent to manually spread the labia, being careful not to touch the periurethral area. The younger child can sit in reverse position on a toilet seat (Figure 13-5). This position will spread the labia and expose the urethral opening (Figure 13-6), avoiding the necessity of touching the genital area by a medical assistant. In an era of "good touching" and "bad touching," avoiding unnecessary genital contact seems prudent. Some girls refuse to assume the reverse position. If such a girl sits in a forward position far enough back on the toilet seat, appropriate labial spreading will still be achieved.

· Have the girl maintain the proper position until she can urinate. Once the urine stream is initiated, pass the mouth of the sterile container into the stream (midstream collection).

· Cap the container and transport the specimen to the laboratory.

c. Catheter collection:

(1) Girls

· An experienced assistant is essential to you.

· You can often avoid restraint by gaining the confidence of the girl who is old enough to understand a careful explanation of the technique and a description of the minimal discomfort associated with the procedure.

· Have the girl lie on her back and assist her into a frog-

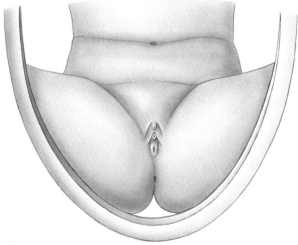

Figure 13-6.
Specimen collection—Urine for urinalysis or culture.
Midstream voided collection: exposure of a girl's urethra with proper patient positioning.

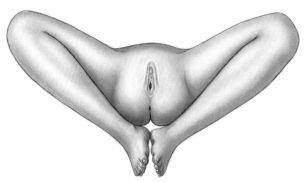

Figure 13-7.
Specimen collection—Urine for urinalysis or culture.
Catheter collection: position of a girl for urethral catheterization.

leg position, with the soles of the feet in apposition (Figure 13-7). When necessary, provide restraint by having the assistant lean across the child's body from above, restraining the child's trunk with her trunk. The assistant's elbows and arms are also used to restrain the child's body and arms, and the assistant's hands are used to hold the child's legs in the proper position.

· Carefully cleanse the periurethral area with povidone-iodone. Make circular motions with the povidone-iodine swab, starting at the urethral opening and extending out a few centimeters.

· Don gloves and gently retract the labia minora with the gloved fingertips of the left hand. You may prefer to have an assistant retract the labia (Figure 13-8).

· Occasionally the urethral opening is obscured by a fold of introital mucosa. If so, move the mucosal fold downward with a cotton-tipped applicator, exposing the urethral meatus (Figure 13-8). If this maneuver is necessary, an assistant will have to retract the girl's labia.

· Apply sterile bacteriostatic lubricant to the selected transparent feeding tube or urinary catheter.

· After verbally preparing the patient, gently insert the catheter a few centimeters or until urine flow is apparent.

· Discard the first few millimeters of urine, because of possible contamination by distal urethral organisms captured by the catheter at the time of insertion.

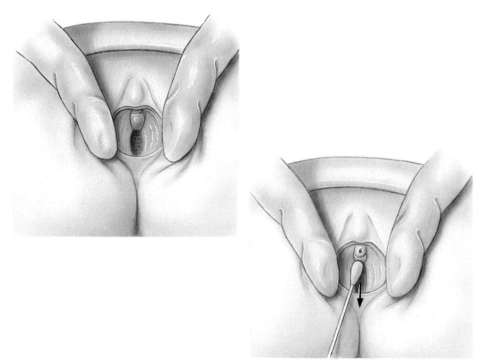

Figure 13-8.
Specimen collection—Urine for urinalysis or culture. Catheter collection: technique for a girl.

- Collect a specimen in a sterile container and immediately transport it to the laboratory for processing.

(2) Boys

  - An experienced assistant is essential to you.
  - Have the boy lie on his back, with his arms by his side and with his legs extended (Figure 13-9).
  - Restraint is virtually always required. Have an assistant lean across the boy's body from above, restraining the boy's trunk with his or her trunk (Figure 13-9). The assistant's elbows and arms are also used to restrain the boy's body and arms, and the assistant's hands are used to hold the boy's legs in the proper position.
  - Don gloves.
  - With the thumb and index finger of the left hand, without force retract the foreskin, if present, to reveal the meatus and glans. Carefully cleanse the glans with povidone-iodine. Make circular motions with the povidone-iodine swab, starting at the urethral meatus, extending out to cover as much of the glans as possible. Repeat the process with povidone-iodine and then repeat several times with isopropyl alcohol.
  - Apply sterile bacteriostatic lubricant to the selected transparent feeding tube or catheter.
  - After verbally preparing the patient, gently insert the catheter until urine flow is apparent (Figure 13-10). The length of the catheter to be inserted is a few centimeters more than the length of the shaft of the penis. Never force the catheter. When resistance is felt on insertion,

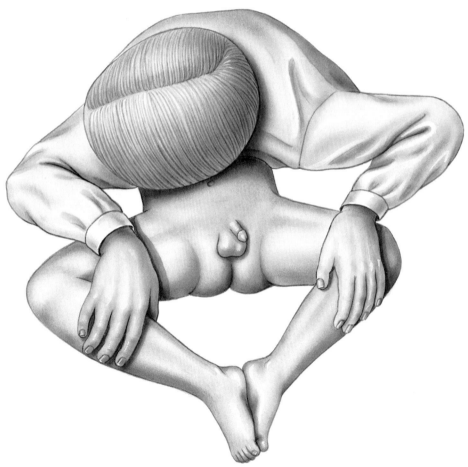

Figure 13-9.
Specimen collection—Urine for urinalysis or culture. Catheter collection: position and restraint of a boy for urethral catheterization.

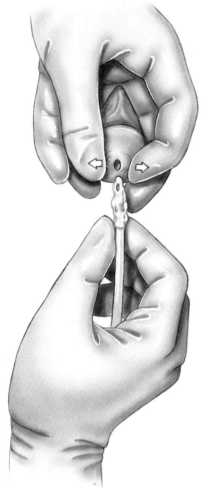

Figure 13-10.
Specimen collection—Urine for urinalysis or culture.
Catheter collection: technique for a boy.

withdraw the catheter slightly and gently reinsert. Discontinue the procedure if insertion is not successful after several attempts.

· Discard the first few milliliters of urine, because of possible contamination by distal urethral organisms captured by the catheter at the time of insertion.

· Collect a specimen in a sterile container and immediately transport it to the laboratory for processing.

d. Suprapubic aspirate:

The success rate for this technique is increased by assuring that the bladder is full. The presence of a full bladder also decreases the risk of missing the bladder with the needle and injuring the bowel or other organs.

· Wait at least 30 minutes and preferably 60 minutes after the last voiding before attempting the procedure.

· Handle an infant gently, not prompting urination.

· Have the patient lie flat on the examination table in a supine position with the legs extended.

· Ordinarily you will assess fullness of the bladder by palpation and percussion over the bladder. During these maneuvers (and during the cleansing and aspiration procedures), it is important that you have the urethral opening of an incontinent patient held closed by an assistant, because stimulation of the bladder by these maneuvers may lead to urination. (For male infants, it is useful to have a sterile container handy in case voiding occurs with stimulation. During the voiding, a midstream collection can be obtained.) In the neonate, infant, and small child, a thin abdominal wall may allow you to transilluminate a well-filled bladder with a high-intensity light source. Some have advocated the use of ultrasound to assess the fullness of the bladder, but expense and lack of availability in most outpatient settings make it an impractical adjunct.

· Cleanse with povidone-iodine the lower mid-portion of the abdomen down to slightly below the symphysis pubis. Apply the povidone-iodine in a circular motion, starting in the center of the lower abdomen. Increase the circles in diameter until the selected area is prepared.

· Repeat the same procedure.

· Allow the povidone-iodine applications to dry and then cleanse with isopropyl alcohol (70%) using the same circular motion. Be certain to remove any povidone-iodine that has accidentally run down the patient's flanks, because it may cause a chemical irritation if left on undiluted. Irritation or even a chemical burn is more likely if tincture of iodine is used.

· Don sterile gloves.

· Restrain the patient if necessary by gently immobilizing the arms and legs (See Figure 13-9, page 148). Continue to be aware that stimulation of the patient may led to urination.

· You may choose to use local anesthesia with lidocaine (1%). We recommend it for infants and find it is especially beneficial in an anxious older patient. Draw a milliliter of the anesthetic through a 25-gauge needle into a 3-mL syringe. Inject 0.5 mL into the skin and subcutaneous tissues at the site selected for the aspiration.

· Using a 21- or 23-gauge, 1½-inch needle attached to a 10- to 12-mL syringe, insert the needle into the skin 1 to 2 cm above the symphysis pubis in the midline (Figure 13-11). Keep the axis of the needle and syringe at a 0- to 20-degree angle from the perpendicular to the skin;

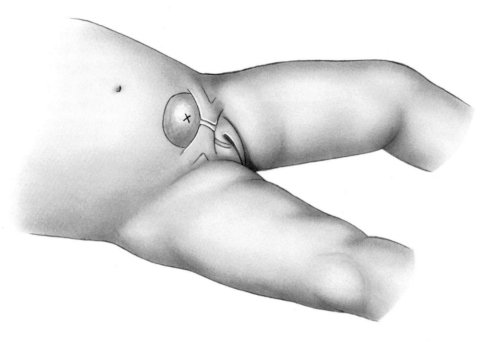

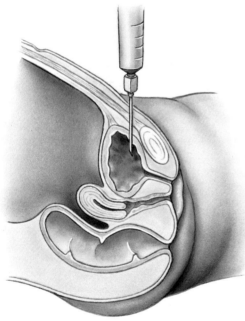

Figure 13-11.
Specimen collection—Urine
for urinalysis or culture.
Suprapubic aspirate: technique.

i.e., the top of the syringe should be angled slightly toward the patient's head. The angle used depends on the age of the patient, with the angle being decreased as the age of the patient increases, because the bladder sits more caudally in the younger patient.

· Insert the needle through the skin.
· With a smooth and moderately forceful motion, advance the needle through the bladder wall. Gently aspirate as the needle is advanced or as urine flows into the syringe as the bladder lumen is entered.

- Gently aspirate urine until the desired amount of urine (usually a milliliter is sufficient) is obtained. With forceful aspiration you may pull bladder mucosa into the needle.
- If no urine is obtained, rotate the needle to remove the bevel from a possible position against the bladder wall.
- If aspiration is still unsuccessful, return the needle tip to a position just below the skin, increase the angle of the needle slightly, and repeat the procedure.
- If two attempts are unsuccessful, make no further attempts until after allowing the bladder to fill more completely (30 to 60 minutes).
- After an adequate specimen is obtained, quickly withdraw the needle.
- Take the specimen to the laboratory in the syringe or place it in a sterile container for transportation.
- Apply a sterile adhesive bandage to the small wound.

5. Side Effects and Complications:

a. Urine bag collection: Skin irritation can occur and diaper rashes can be aggravated. The rate of contamination is significant.

b. Voided midstream collection: This procedure presents no hazard to the patient. The rate of contamination with urinary tract pathogens is low (slightly higher in uncircumcised males), but contamination with nonpathogenic vaginal and periurethral flora is high in girls.

c. Catheter collection: The most serious complication is damage to the urethra, which is most likely to occur in the posterior portion of a male's urethra. A potential risk for acquiring bacteriuria during the procedure exists. This risk in childhood is not well defined but is thought to be very low for in and out catheterization for specimen collection in otherwise healthy children.

d. Suprapubic aspiration: Although this procedure is invasive, significant complications are rarely seen. Postcatheterization hematuria is common, but is almost always minimal and resolves spontaneously. Hematomata can occur, but serious subcutaneous or visceral bleeding is rare. Needle entry into an intestine is a potential complication, especially when the bladder is not full or the bowels are distended. It is usually a benign occurrence, but significant perforation of the bowel has occurred. Vaginal entry, abdominal wall abscess, bacteremia, and pubic bone osteomyelitis have been reported as isolated complications.

6. Interpretation: It should be reemphasized that accurate interpretation of a urinalysis or urine culture depends on obtaining a urine specimen collected with careful attention to the collection technique.

A detailed discussion of the interpretation of all of the facets of a urinalysis is beyond the scope of this chapter. The normal values for a physiochemical (dipstick) analysis and for a microscopic examination of a urine specimen are shown in Tables 13-2 and 13-3, respectively. For additional information, the reader is referred to several excellent resources: Haber M. *Urinary Sediment: A Textbook Atlas.* American Society of Clinical Pathologists 1981, and Strasinger SK. *Urinal-*

Table 13-2. Urine Physiochemical Analysis Normal Values

Test	Normal Value
Appearance	Clear to hazy
Color	Yellow to amber
pH	5 to 8
Specific gravity	1.005 to 1.030
Protein	Negative*
Glucose†	Negative
Ketone	Negative
Blood	Negative
Bilirubin	Negative
Nitrite	Negative
Leukocyte esterase	Negative

* Any positive result should be confirmed by the sulfosalicylic acid test.

† To detect other reducing sugars (e.g., galactose) a Benedict's copper reduction reagent (Clinitest®) should be used.

Table 13-3. Urine Microscopic Examination Normal Findings

Entity	Normal Finding
White blood cells	
Males	0 to 1 per high-power field
Females	1 to 5 per high-power field
Red blood cells	0 to 2 per high-power field
Bacteria	0 per high-power field
Epithelial cells	0 to 2 per low-power field
Mucus	Small amount per low-power field
Casts	
Hyaline	0 to 1 per low-power field
Other	0 per low-power field
Nonpathologic crystals	
Acid urine pH	Amorphous urate, calcium oxalate, and uric acid
Alkaline urine pH	Amorphous phosphate, calcium oxalate, triple phosphate, calcium phosphate, calcium carbonate, and ammonium biurate

Table 13-4. Criteria for Diagnosis of Urinary Tract Infections[*]

Method of Collection	Colony Count (pure culture)	Probability of Infection (%)
Suprapubic aspiration	Gram-negative bacilli: any number	>99
	Gram-positive cocci: > than a few thousand	
Catheterization	$>10^5$	95
	10^4–10^5	Infection likely
	10^3–10^4	Suspicious; repeat
	$<10^3$	Infection unlikely
Clean-voided (male)	$>10^4$	Infection likely
Clean-voided (female)	3 specimens: $>10^5$	95
	2 specimens: $>10^5$	90
	1 specimen: $>10^5$	80
	5×10^4–10^5	Suspicious; repeat
	10^4–5×10^4	Symptomatic; suspicious; repeat
	10^4–5×10^4	Asymptomatic; infection unlikely
	$<10^4$	Infection unlikely

* Compiled from the data of many investigators including: Aronsonson AS, Gustafoson B, Svenningsen NW. Acta Paediatr Scand 1973;62:396. Boshell BR, Sanford JP. Ann Intern Med 1958;48:1040. Kass EH. Trans Assoc Am Physicians 1956;69:56. Kass EH. Arch Intern Med 1957;100:709. Pryles CV, Steg NL. Pediatrics 1959;23:441. Pryles CV, Atkin MD, Morse TS, et al. Pediatrics 1959;24:983. Pryles CV, Luders D, Alkan MK. Pediatrics 1961;27:17. Stamey TA. Urinary Tract Infections. Baltimore: The Williams & Wilkins Co., 1972, 1–29, with permission.

ysis and Body Fluids. Philadelphia, FA Davis Company, 1989. As stated previously, the urinalysis should not be used to rule in or rule out the clinical diagnosis of a urinary tract infection.

What specifically constitutes significant bacterial growth from a urine specimen culture is not known. It is widely held that growth of greater than 10^5 colony-forming units (CFU) per milliliter urine of a single organism documents the presence of a urinary tract infection. Recently it has been shown that growth of as few as 10^2 CFU/mL of voided urine may be associated with clinically significant urinary tract infections in women. Whether a single urine sample is adequate to document a urinary tract infection remains debatable. Most believe that the method of collection influences the need for obtaining more than one urine specimen for culture as well as the significance of various magnitudes of counts of CFU/mL urine. Hellerstein[4] has provided a table of guidelines for the interpretation of urine culture results (Table 13-4).

C. Examination of the Male Urethra

1. Purpose: The purpose of this procedure is to provide additional clinical evidence for the presence or absence of urethritis.

2. Selection of Patients:

a. Indications: Urethral evaluation is indicated for sexually active (or sexually abused) boys who complain of urethral discharge, urethral discomfort, or dysuria or for asymptomatic sexually active boys who require evaluation for sexually transmitted infections, or as a test of cure for boys after treatment for such infections.

b. Contraindications and Precautions: Dysuria in boys who are not sexually experienced is more likely due to urinary tract infection and should be evaluated as such. Although brief, urethral examination is uncomfortable, and genital examination *per se* is often frightening. The details of the procedure should be carefully explained to the child and when appropriate, to parents. Particular caution must be exercised when examining a child believed to have a urethral stricture.

3. Equipment and Supplies (See Appendix for equipment and supplies manufacturers and suppliers. Appendix is keyed to italicized words in the equipment and supplies lists):

- Examination *glove* (left hand for right-handed examiner)
- Calcium alginate or rayon *swabs* (Figure 13-12)
- Clean glass microscope *slides*
- *Cover slips* (if wet mount is to be performed)
- Alcohol *lamp* or 95% methanol
- Gram stain reagents
- Culture medium for *Neisseria gonorrhoeae*
- Transport medium for *Chlamydia trachomatis* or slide for direct fluorescent antibody staining for chlamydial antigens or tube for enzyme-linked immunosorbent assay (ELISA) or DNA hybridization
- Rarely, culture medium for genital mycoplasmas and *Ureaplasma urealyticum*
- Rarely, tube with 0.5 mL of 0.9% saline *solution* for wet mount or medium for culture of *Trichomonas vaginalis* or slide for direct fluorescent antibody staining
- Rarely, transport medium for herpes simplex virus

4. Decription of Procedure:

- Explain the procedure carefully to the child as appropriate to his level of understanding.
- Whereas you can evaluate older adolescents standing before the seated examiner, you can best examine younger children who are supine on an examining table to minimize inadvertent urethral trauma caused by avoidance behavior. Gentle restraint by sympathetic assistants is usually required with younger children (See Figure 13-9, page 148).
- Examine the patient as long after his last micturition as possible.

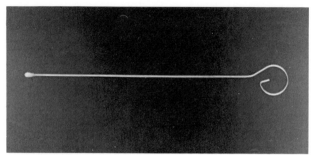

Figure 13-12.
Examination of the male urethra. Equipment and supplies:
Calcium alginate swab.

· Examine the entire genital area for lesions and adenopathy. Examine the meatus for erythema and discharge. Palpate the scrotal contents.

· Using the gloved hand, grasp the penis with the thumb gently compressing the urethra; move the hand distally to deliver any urethral discharge at the meatus (Figure 13-13). Collect the delivered discharge on a swab.

· If no discharge is delivered, hold the penis from above between the third and fourth gloved fingers with the palm facing the examiner (Figure 13-14). Gently spread the meatus with the gloved thumb and index finger to visualize the distal mucosa.

· Sequentially insert one or more swabs into the urethra with a straight movement of the ungloved hand. (Large [3-mm] cotton swabs on wooden shafts should not be inserted into the meatus. Cotton swabs and wooden

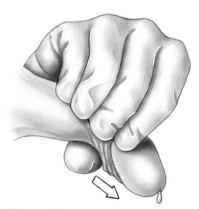

Figure 13-13.
Examination of the male urethra. Technique for delivering urethral discharge.

shafts may be toxic to some sexually transmitted organisms [chlamydia].) Insert each swab slightly deeper than the preceeding, with each swab reaching at least into the fossa navicularis (Figure 13-15). Remove each swab promptly while rotating the shaft.

· Immediately on obtaining the first specimen, rotate the swab against a clean glass slide to transfer a thin layer of material. You may then rotate the same swab against the surface of an agar selective for *N. gonorrhoeae*. Remember that Transgrow must be kept upright to preserve its CO_2 atmosphere.

· To evaluate the patient for chlamydial infection, one should obtain urethral cells, so you must insert a second swab into the urethra using the above technique. Do not use expressed discharge. The swab is rotated against a prepared slide for immunofluorescence or inserted in a carrier tube for ELISA or DNA hybridization, or the swab is broken off in a tube of transport medium for chlamydial cultures. Refrigerate the inoculated transport tube.

· Obtain a third swab for agitation in mycoplasma or ureaplasma transport medium or saline and trichomonas medium if indicated.

· Fix the first slide for examination by warming it briefly in the flame of an alcohol lamp or by flooding it briefly with 95% methanol. The slide is then Gram stained and examined microscopically using the oil-immersion objective and then with the substage condenser wide open and fully elevated.

· Prepare a wet mount by transferring a drop of material from the tube to a slide and applying a cover slip. The slide is examined microscopically using the high-dry objective with the substage condenser racked down and the substage diaphragm closed down to increase contrast. Phase contrast microscopy is used for this examination if it is available.

5. Side Effects and Complications: Urethral discomfort is universal. Urethral trauma may cause slight hemorrhage, which soon ceases. Gently compress the urethra laterally to speed hemostasis.

6. Intrepretation: Meatal erythema is nonspecific but suggests urethritis. Expressible urethral discharge signifies urethritis. The presence of even small numbers of polymorphonuclear neutrophils (PMN) diagnoses urethritis. The presence of gram-negative intracellular diplococci (GNID), shaped like kidney beans with their flat edges opposed, diagnoses gonorrhea, and the condition should be treated without awaiting the results of the culture. Other bacterial morphotypes, present in small numbers, may be disregarded. Polymorphonuclear neutrophils without GNID suggest nongonococcal urethritis, which should be treated immediately. One cannot use the gram-stained smear to diagnose coincident nongon-

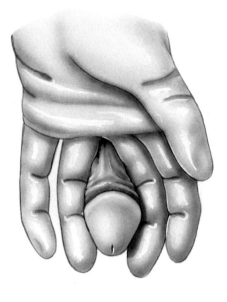

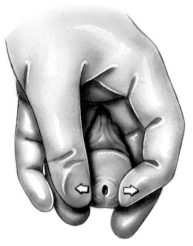

Figure 13-14.
Examination of the male urethra. Technique for spreading the meatus for insertion of a swab into the urethra.

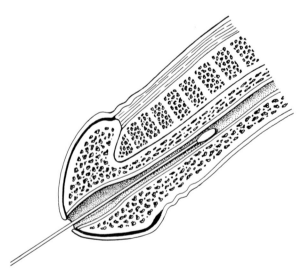

Figure 13-15.
Examination of the male urethra. Technique for inserting a swab into the urethra to collect a specimen.

ococcal urethritis in the presence of gonorrhea. The presence of motile flagellate protozoa (usually about $7 \times 10 \ \mu m$) diagnoses trichomoniasis, but the procedure is insensitive.

Direct immunofluorescence, ELISA, and DNA hybridization for chlamydia are highly specific but may be somewhat insensitive in the male urethra.

Do not overlook the implications of the presence of a sexually transmitted disease for the diagnosis of sexual abuse.

D. Examination of Male Genital Ulcerations—Darkfield Examination

1. Purpose: The purpose of this procedure is to provide additional information regarding the cause of genital ulcerations. Darkfield microscopy is used to identify *Treponema pallidum,* the cause of syphilis. History and physical examination are critical in the identification of suitable lesions.

2. Selection of Patients:

a. Indications: This evaluation is indicated for sexually active (or sexually abused) boys who present with or are found to have genital ulcerations on physical examination. Darkfield examination is usually performed on any genital ulcer for which a specific diagnosis is not strongly supported.

b. Contraindications and Precautions: Genital ulcerations in sexually inexperienced boys are most likely caused by trauma (e.g., zipper injury, vigorous masturbation) or nonsexually transmitted infections, some of which can be quite serious. Systemic antibiotics or topical therapies dramatically reduce the sensitivity of darkfield examination.

3. Equipment and Supplies (See Appendix for equipment and supplies manufacturers and suppliers. Appendix is keyed to italicized words in the equipment and supplies lists):

- Excellent light source
- Hand-held *magnifier* (See Figure 8-7, page 73)
- Examination *gloves*
- 2 × 2-inch or 4 × 4-inch gauze *pads*
- Clean glass microscope *slides*
- Clean glass (or less satisfactorily, plastic) *cover slips*

4. Description of Procedure:

- Explain the procedure carefully to the child as appropriate to his level of understanding.
- Lay out three gauze pads and several cover slips before gloving, then glove both hands.
- Isolate and support the genital ulcer by gently squeezing the surrounding skin (Figure 13-16).
- Rub the surface of the ulcer with a gauze pad to remove debris and purulent material.
- Lightly abrade the ulcer base with a clean gauze pad until a small amount of bleeding occurs.
- Using a third gauze pad, repeatedly blot the ulcer base until bleeding has largely ceased.
- Squeeze the sides of the ulcer gently but firmly until some serous (or slightly serosanguinous) fluid is expressed.
- Grasping a cover slip by the edges, pick up a drop of fluid by touching the surface of the cover slip to the lesion (Figure 13-16). Place the cover slip fluid side down on a glass side. The drop will spread out over the central portion of the cover slip. Take care to avoid contaminating the cover slip or slide with starch grains from the gloves.
- It is usually advisable to make several preparations. This is particularly important if the initial specimen is visibly red-tinged, for excessive blood in the specimen interferes with microscopy. Prepare additional specimens, beginning by blotting the ulcer base. Additional abrasion, often uncomfortable, is generally not required.

5. Side Effects and Complications: Local discomfort is the only complication.

6. Interpretation: Preparation and interpretation of darkfield examinations is highly dependent on practice, and consultation with an experienced colleague is strongly advised.

Insure by careful history that the patient has received

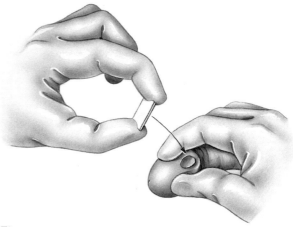

Figure 13-16.
Examination of male genital ulcerations—Darkfield examination. Technique for specimen collection.

neither oral nor parenteral antibiotics and has not treated the lesion with topical antibiotic or antiseptic preparations. These could eliminate spirochetes, rendering a negative darkfield examination uninterpretable.

An adequate darkfield has a black background and is spectacularly filled with bright objects. Small granules jerking about from Brownian movement *must* be seen in an adequate preparation. Erythrocytes appear as circles, and PMNs are brightly filled objects in which individual granules can be seen in motion. Bacteria are often seen in outline.

A positive test results from observing even a single organism morphologically identified as *Treponema pallidum.* Look for a pale spiral organism about 0.3 μm × 7 to 15 μm with well-maintained curves. The organisms may be observed to rotate about their long axes, move back and forth along that axis, and sometimes flex in the middle.

A positive test is diagnostic of syphilis.

The specimen is infectious and slides must be disposed of in a contaminated material container.

The presence of a sexually transmitted disease should raise the question of sexual abuse.

E. Examination of Male Genital Ulcerations—Culture for *Haemophilus ducreyi*

1. Purpose: The purpose of the procedure is to provide additional information regarding the cause of genital ulcerations, in particular, to confirm a diagnosis of chancroid.

2. Selection of Patients:

a. Indications: This procedure is indicated for sexually active (or sexually abused) boys who present with or are found to have single or multiple, ragged appearing, tender, genital ulcers accompanied by tender, inguinal adenopathy.

The sensitivity and specificity of the Gram stain for the diagnosis of chancroid are very low. Culture for *Haemophilus ducreyi* is preferred for diagnosis.

b. Contraindications and Precautions: Chancroid is not found in sexually inexperienced children. In this setting consider trauma or nonsexually transmitted infections (e.g., ulceroglandular tularemia), some of which can be quite serious.

3. Equipment and Supplies (See Appendix for equipment and supplies manufacturers and suppliers. Appendix is keyed to italicized words in the equipment and supplies lists):

- Cotton or other *swabs*
- Examination *glove* (left hand for right-handed examiners)
- Plates containing Muller-Hinton chocolate agar or gonoccal base supplemented with 2% bovine hemoglobin and 5% fetal calf serum are probably the best culture media, but others can be used.

4. Description of Procedure:

- Explain the procedure and the possibility of brief discomfort to the patient and parent.
- Grasp the lesion with the gloved hand (See Figure 13-16, page 155). Vigorously swab the base of the lesion and transfer material to the culture medium by rolling the swab on its surface.

5. Side Effects and Complications: Minimal, brief, local discomfort.

6. Interpretation: Identification of *Haemophilus ducreyi* makes the diagnosis of chancroid. Unfortunately the culture is only 80% sensitive.

F. Examination of Genital Ulcerations— Tzanck Smear and Culture for Herpes Simplex

1. Purpose: The purpose of these procedures is to provide additional evidence for the diagnosis of genital herpes simplex infection.

2. Selection of Patients:

a. Indications: The tests can be performed on sexually active (or sexually abused) males or on infants who present with or are discovered to have genital ulcerations on physical examination.

b. Contraindications and Precautions: Explain to the patient or parent that brief discomfort may result.

3. Equipment and Supplies (See Appendix for equipment and supplies manufacturers and suppliers. Appendix is keyed to italicized words in the equipment and supplies lists):

- These are described in Chapter 7: Skin Procedures.

4. Description of Procedure:

- This is described in Chapter 7: Skin Procedures.

5. Side Effects and Complications: Brief, local discomfort can occur during and after the procedure.

6. Interpretation: The presence of multinucleated giant cells on a Tzanck smear strongly supports a diagnosis of infection with a herpes group virus (*Herpes simplex, Herpes zoster,* rarely cytomegalovirus). The sensitivity of the test is about 90% on intact vesicles, but it is no greater than 30% on the ulcers remaining after vesicles have spontaneously ruptured. On these lesions, culture for *Herpes simplex* is preferred.

II. Therapeutic Procedures

A. Newborn Circumcision

In the past this procedure was usually performed during a male infant's nursery stay. With early discharge of mother and infant being the standard of practice, circumcision is now frequently an outpatient procedure.

1. Purpose: The purpose of this procedure is to remove the foreskin.

2. Selection of Patients:

a. Indications: In the view of the authors, the primary indication for newborn circumcision is the desire of the family to have this procedure done for social or religious reasons. There is considerable controversy over whether or not newborn circumcision should be performed routinely. The authors think that there is no overwhelmingly convincing medical evidence either for or against the procedure. Opponents of circumcision cite the possibility of surgical complications, the increased incidence of meatitis, and possible meatal stenosis in circumcised boys, the virtual absence of penile cancer in individuals with proper hygiene, and the cost of the procedure. The proponents of circumcision cite an apparent increased incidence of urinary tract infections in uncircumcised boys, the possible complications of being uncircumcised during an entire lifetime such as phimosis, balanitis, etc., the potential to develop penile cancer, and finally, the increased costs of the circumcision after the newborn period.

b. Contraindications and Precautions: Contraindications to newborn circumcision include the presence of hypospadias, bleeding dyscrasias, and significant systemic illnesses. Newborn circumcision should certainly be done in an appropriate setting with sterile technique and by experienced individuals. We believe electrocautery should not be used, as this can result in serious burns. Local anesthesia adds an element of risk to the procedure. Circumferential anesthesia may be additionally hazardous. More data are needed to define the degree of risk when local anesthesia is used with this procedure.

3. Equipment and Supplies (See Appendix for equipment and supplies manufacturers and suppliers. Appendix is keyed to italicized words in the equipment and supplies lists):
- Restraint *board* (See Figure 13-20, page 159)
- Povidone-iodine *solution*
- "Circumcision drape" (Figure 13-17)
- 25-gauge *needle* (See Figure 20-7, page 262) on a 3-mL *syringe* (See Figure 20-7, page 262), for lidocaine injection
- *Lidocaine* (0.5%–1.0%) without epinephrine
- Probe (Figure 13-18)
- Curved mosquito *clamps* (Figure 13-18)
- One pair of toothed forceps (Figure 13-18)
- Small *scissors* (Figure 13-18)
- Needle holder (Figure 13-18)
- Two packages of 3–0 chromic *suture* material
- Large suture *scissors* (Figure 13-18)
- Three straight mosquito *clamps* (Figure 13-18)
- Set of circumcision *clamps* ranging in size from 1.1 to 2.1 cm (Figure 13-19). A complete set includes five such clamps sized 1.1, 1.3, 1.45, 1.6, and 2.1 cm. Two of the intermediate sizes could be eliminated.
- No. 15 scalpel *blade* (Figure 13-18)
- Scalpel *handle* (Figure 13-18)
- 4 × 4 gauze *pads* (6)
- *Bacitracin* or similar antibacterial ointment
- Petroleum jelly *gauze*
- Finger roll *gauze*

4. Description of Procedure:
- You should fully inform the parents of the possible benefits and potential risks of the procedure.
- Place the patient on a restraint board or table and wrap him so that movement of the legs and arms is eliminated (Figure 13-20).
- Prepare the penis with povidone-iodine and drape the area as a sterile field.
- Draw lidocaine (1%) into a 3-mL syringe attached to a 25-gauge needle. Insert the needle on the dorsum at the base of the penis down through Bucks fascia to the tunica albuginea to block the dorsal nerve of the penis (Figure 13-21). This requires 0.5 to 1.0 mL of lidocaine. If the block appears inadequate, inject additional lidocaine at the operative site. We recognize that circumferential anesthesia of the skin is considered hazardous by some, but we have used this additional local anesthesia without incident.

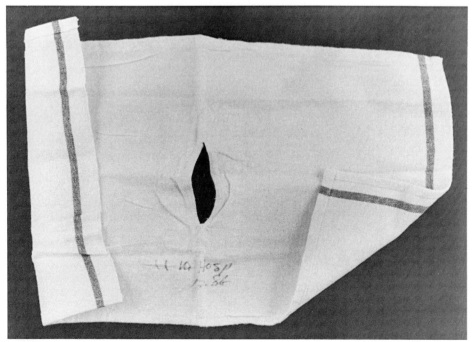

Figure 13-17.
Newborn circumcision. Equipment and supplies: Circumcision drape.

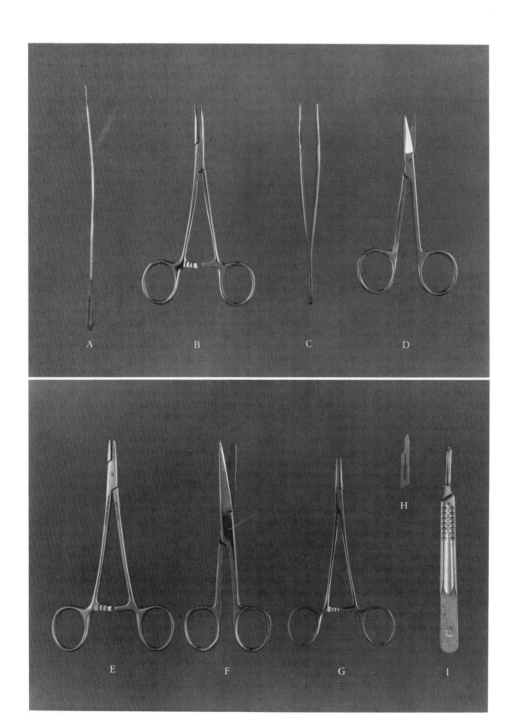

Figure 13-18.
Newborn circumcision. Equipment and supplies: **A,** Probe; **B,** Curved mosquito clamp; **C,** Toothed forceps; **D,** Small scissors; **E,** Needle holder; **F,** Large scissors; **G,** Straight mosquito clamp; **H,** No. 15 scalpel blade; **I,** Scalpel handle.

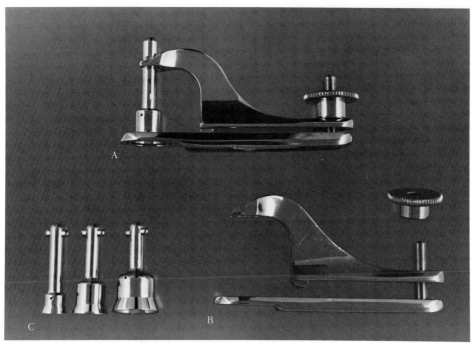

Figure 13-19.
Newborn circumcision. Equipment and supplies: Circumcision clamps (**A,** Assembled clamp; **B,** Disassembled clamp; **C,** Cones of various sizes)

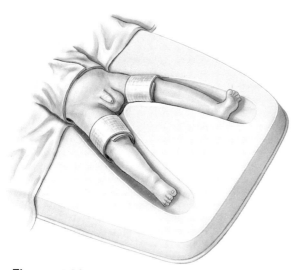

Figure 13-20.
Newborn circumcision. Restraint of patient.

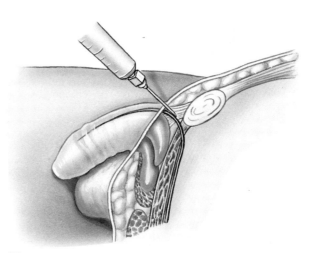

Figure 13-21.
Newborn circumcision. Technique for local anesthesia.

· Lyse the adhesions of the foreskin to the glans with a flexible probe or with a small curved mosquito clamp, and clearly identify the meatus (Figure 13-22). It may be necessary for you to hold the foreskin with toothed forceps and slit with small scissors the dorsal aspect of the foreskin to approximately the mid glans to accomplish this step. Importantly, be certain all of the adhesions are lysed so that the foreskin can be retracted and the coronal sulcus clearly visualized circumferentially. This does not take great force, but incomplete separation is common if care is not taken to divide all of the adhesions.

· Place three 3–0 chromic holding sutures in the foreskin equidistant from each other (Figure 13-23A). Cut off the needle with large suture scissors and apply a straight mosquito clamp to each holding suture.

· Place an appropriate size bell from the bell clamp set over the glans penis and pull the foreskin through the open ring in the bell clamp (Figure 13-23B). Apply the curved portion of the clamp in place and tighten the screw (Figure 13-23C). Leave in place for 5 minutes. The procedure can also be done with a Plastibell™.

· After 5 minutes, cut off the foreskin with a no. 15 scalpel blade and remove the clamp (Figure 13-24). If there is bleeding, stop it with pressure using 4 × 4 gauze pads.

· Apply bacitracin or a similar antibacterial ointment.

· Place a petroleum jelly gauze and a roller gauze around the incision.

· Instruct the parents to call you if fever, bleeding, or evidence of infection occurs.

· Instruct the parents to put petroleum jelly and clean gauze over the surgical site if the dressing falls off (which it usually does). Usually no dressing is required after 3 to 5 days following surgery.

5. Side Effects and Complications: The principal side effect of circumcision in the newborn period is discomfort, which is difficult to quantitate and lasts 24 to 48 hours.

Complications of a newborn circumcision occur in less than 1% of patients. The major complications include:

1. Severe damage to the penile shaft and urethra if electrocautery if used with a metal clamp
2. Wound infection
3. Bleeding
4. Excessive skin removal necessitating a prolonged healing period or, on rare occasions, a skin graft
5. Insufficient skin removal, necessitating a repeat circumcision
6. Meatitis
7. Systemic response to lidocaine injection

B. Foreskin Adhesion Release

1. Purpose: The purpose of releasing adhesions of the foreskin is to allow normal voiding and cleansing of the penis.

2. Selection of Patients:

a. Indications: The only indications we believe that are valid for release of foreskin adhesions in the uncircumcised boy

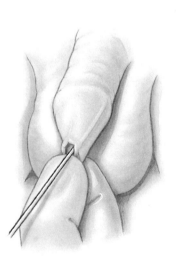
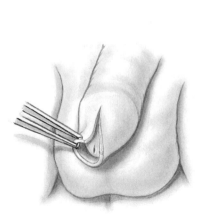
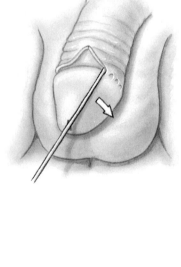

Figure 13-22.
Newborn circumcision. Technique.

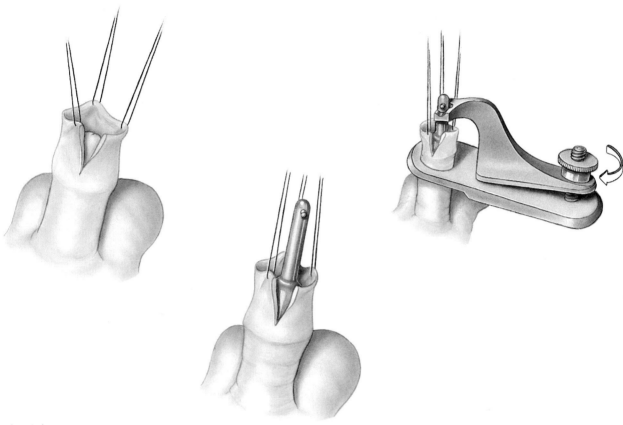

Figure 13-23.
Newborn circumcision. Technique.

are painful urination or significant ballooning of the foreskin during urination. Conversely, if a boy has been previously circumcised and there are adhesions to the glans penis, these adhesions should be released.

b. Contraindications and Precautions: There are no contraindications to releasing adhesions except contraindications to general anesthesia when this is required. It should be re-emphasized, however, that releasing the adhesions in an uncircumcised boy is not necessary unless he is symptomatic from the adhesions.

3. Equipment and Supplies (See Appendix for equipment and supplies manufacturers and suppliers. Appendix is keyed to italicized words in the equipment and supplies lists):

· Povidone-iodine *ointment*
· 23-gauge *needle* (See Figure 20-7, page 262) attached to a 3- or 5-mL *syringe* (See Figure 20-7, page 262)
· *Lidocaine* (1%) without epinephrine
· One pair of toothed *forceps* (See Figure 13-18, page 158)

· *Probe* (See Figure 13-18, page 158)
· Two curved mosquito *clamps* (See Figure 13-18, page 158)
· Small *scissors* (See Figure 13-18, page 158)
· Needle *holder* (See Figure 13-18, page 158)
· 5–0 chromic *suture* material (See Table 18-3, page 221)
· Petroleum jelly *gauze*
· Roller *gauze*
· Nonallergenic *tape*

4. Description of Procedure:

a. The simplest way for you to release adhesions is merely to retract the foreskin. This procedure requires no equipment or supplies. In many instances, however, it is too painful to be done without anesthesia.

b. In instances in which local anesthesia is required, do the following:

· Prepare the penis with povidone-iodine.
· Provide a circumferential penile block using the li-

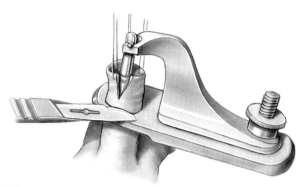

Figure 13-24.
Newborn circumcision. Technique.

docaine at the base of the penis (See Figure 13-21, page 159).

• After 3 minutes, retract the foreskin as far as possible and hold it with toothed forceps as you lyse the adhesions with a probe, clamp, or scissors, if necessary (See Figure 13-22, page 160).

• If a significant defect is created by the lysis of the adhesions, close the defect with 5–0 or 6–0 chromic suture material.

• Apply bacitracin or another appropriate antibiotic ointment.

• Apply petroleum jelly, roller gauze, and tape as a dressing.

5. Side Effects and Complications: The major side effect of this procedure is minor pain. The major complication of the procedure is wound infection. It should be added that in many instances the procedure is too traumatic to be done in the office and should be done under general anesthesia. The decision to not do the procedure in the office depends on the extent of the adhesions, the age of the patient, and the skill of the physician.

References

1. Lohr JA, Donowitz LG, Dudley SM. Bacterial contamination rates for non–clean-catch and clean-catch midstream urine collections in boys. J Pediatr 1986; 109:659–60.
2. Saez-Llorens X, Umana MA, Odio CM, Lohr JA. Bacterial contamination rates for non–clean-catch and clean-catch midstream urine collections in uncircumcised boys. J Pediatr 1989; 114:93–5.
3. Lohr JA, Donowitz LG, Dudley SM. Bacterial contamination rates in voided urine collections in girls. J Pediatr 1989; 114:91–3.
4. Hellerstein S. Recurrent urinary tract infections in children. Pediatr Infect Dis J 1982; 1:271–81.

Chapter 14

Gynecologic Procedures

Deborah E. Smith

Gynecologic examinations and procedures in the young child or adolescent provide information about genital anatomy and pathology and allow specific testing. Examinations and procedures must be performed gently and without haste. The mother may stay with the very young girl, but older children and adolescents can usually be examined better alone. Fears must be allayed (Was there a previous painful experience?) and care is needed to protect the adolescent's heightened sense of privacy by using gowns and sheets. The examiner must be familiar with normal genital anatomy (Figures 14-1 and 14-2). Procedures associated with the evaluation of suspected sexual abuse are described elsewhere (Sexual Abuse Evaluation Procedures, page 177).

I. Screening Procedures

A. Pelvic Examination

1. Purpose: The purpose of the examination is to assess the anatomy of the external genitalia and pelvic organs and to screen for sexually transmitted diseases (STDs) or changes associated with cervical cancer.

2. Selection of Patients:

a. Indications: All prepubertal girls should have an examination of their external genitalia at least once during childhood (and perhaps as a regular part of the annual well child visit) to ascertain normal anatomy. Additional examinations will be indicated by related history and symptoms. After puberty, the first full pelvic examination is done when sexual activity is initiated, or during late adolescence if the girl is not already sexually active. Subsequent screening is done annually in sexually active adolescents. More frequent pelvic examinations with STD screening are needed with changes in sexual partners, and depending on the local community STD prevalence. A pelvic examination also is needed in pa-

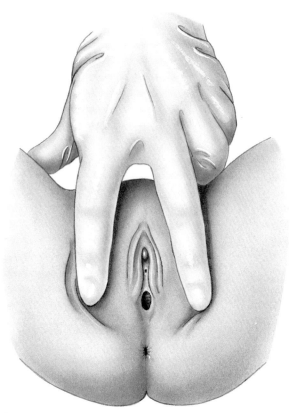

Figure 14-1.
Normal genital anatomy. Prepubertal girl.

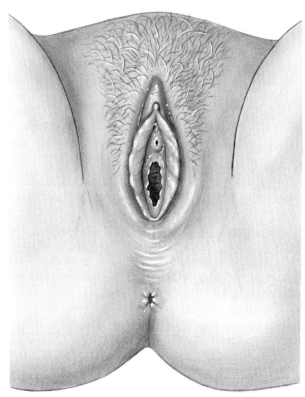

Figure 14-2.
Normal genital anatomy. Adolescent girl.

tients symptomatic with abdominal pain, amenorrhea, vaginal discharge, or dysfunctional uterine bleeding. It is also indicated before starting birth control pills or before hormone therapy is used to treat severe dysmenorrhea. In addition, girls exposed to diethylstilbestrol *in utero* need careful pelvic examinations (See Papanicolaou Smear, page 170). An examination including specimen collection is needed in patients in whom sexual abuse is suspected.

b. Contraindications and Precautions: In the absence of symptoms, the young adolescent girl does not need to have a pelvic examination until she expects to initiate sexual activity. The exceptions are the diethylstilbestrol-exposed girl (See Papanicolaou Smear, page 170) and a suggestive history such as of alleged sexual abuse.

3. Equipment and Supplies (See Appendix for equipment and supplies manufacturers and suppliers. Appendix is keyed to italicized words in the equipment and supplies lists):

· Source of direct lighting (e.g., goose-neck light). A pediatric *otoscope* (Figure 14-3) may also be used and provides low-power magnification.

· Standard gynecology examining table with adjustable stirrups. Such tables are necessary for adolescents and useful but not essential for younger patients.

· Examining *gloves*

· Specula

· Veterinary otoscope *specula* may be useful for girls over 3 to 4 years of age and can be attached to a standard pediatric *otoscope* head. There are three speculum sizes (5.5 cm × 4.0 mm; 6.5 cm × 5.0 mm; and 7.0 cm × 7.0 mm), obtainable as a set (Figure 14-3).

· Vaginal specula of various shapes and sizes are available. It is necesary to have one standard size speculum, for example, a Pederson *speculum* (11.5 cm × 2.6 cm (Figure 14-4), to examine sexually active adolescents.

· The Huffman-Graves *speculum* (11.0 cm × 1.5 cm) (Figure 14-4) is most useful for young adolescents who are not sexually experienced.

· Lubrication *jelly*. This can *not* be used if a Papanicolaou smear is to be done (See Papanicolaou Smear, page 170).

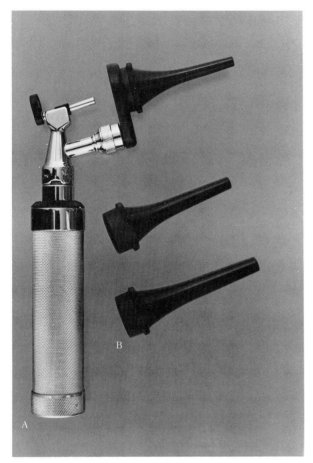

Figure 14-3.
Pelvic examination. Equipment and supplies: **A,** Otoscope with operating head; **B,** Veterinary specula.

- Large cotton-tipped *applicators* (Figure 14-5)
- Small cotton- or dacron-tipped *applicators* (Figure 14-5)
- *Non*bacteriostatic saline *solution*
- Glass or plastic eye *dropper* (Figure 14-5)
- Cytology *brushes* (See Figure 14-13, above)
- Glass microscope *slides* and *cover slips*
- *Fixative* for Papanicolaou smears. This may be isopropyl *alcohol* (95%) or an aerosol formula
- Normal saline *solution* and potassium hydroxide *solution* (KOH) (10%)
- Microscope
- Culture media such as Martin-Lewis agar plate for the isolation of *Neisseria gonorrhoeae*
- Test kit for diagnosing *Chlamydia trachomatis.* Cultures are expensive and not widely used. More available

are fluorescent antibody tests such as the Syva Micro-Trak. Most recently, kits for DNA probe testing have become available. These provide very accurate results.

- Viral culture media for isolation of *Herpes simplex* (See Skin Procedures, Vesicopustule Evaluation, page 62).
- Wright's stain for quick diagnosis of *Herpes simplex*

4. Description of Procedure:

a. Positioning:

(1) Frog-leg position (Figure 14-6): This position is most appropriate for genital examination when vaginal instrumentation is not required.

- Instruct the child to lie on her back with her knees flexed.
- Tell her to place her ankles or the soles of her feet together and let her knees fall out to the side as far as possible.
- Ask her to assist by holding her labia apart.
- As she coughs, or takes in a deep breath, the vaginal introitus should gape open, allowing a good view of the vagina.
- You may improve visualization by gently pulling the labia downward and laterally.

(2) Knee–chest position (Figure 14-7): This position is useful for the prepubertal girl who is over 2 years old.

- Instruct the child to kneel. Then tell her to lie forward onto her chest and folded arms with her head to one side, while keeping her botom up. An assistant may help by holding the buttocks up and apart.
- When a deep breath is taken, the vaginal orifice opens. In up to 90% of prepubertal girls, the cervix may be visualized.

(3) Lithotomy position: The conventional position for gynecologic evaluations is most useful for older children and adolescents, particularly if instrumentation is necessary. Adjustable stirrups are essential to accommodate different leg lengths.

b. Insertion of the speculum: This is ordinarily done with the patient in the *lithotomy position only.*

- In the *preadolescent child,* the vaginal examination is almost always satisfactory without a speculum. On *rare* occasions for improved visualization, e.g., before foreign body removal, or for multiple specimen collection, a veterinary otoscopy speculum may be useful (See Figure 14-3, this page), particularly in older children.
- To prepare the child for the speculum, consider preceding insertion of the instrument with a gentle single-digit vaginal examination, if this is possible.

Encourage the child to feel the speculum after it has been warmed in water.

- Then place the speculum on the child's thigh, and on the labia, explaining that this may feel "strange," "cold," "funny," etc.

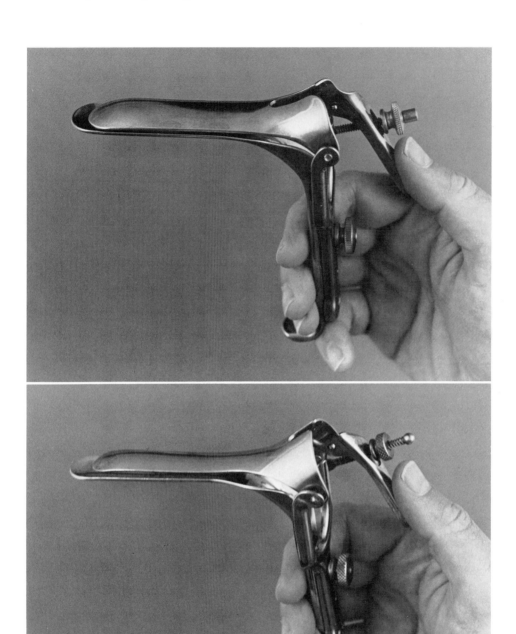

Figure 14-4.
Pelvic examination. Equipment and supplies: Vaginal specula (**A**, Pederson; **B**, Huffman-Graves).

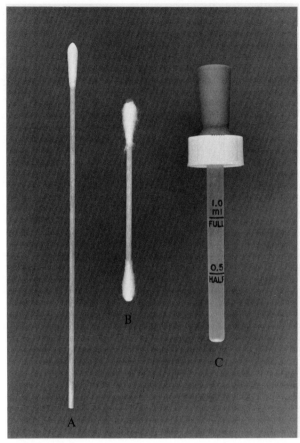

Figure 14-5.
Pelvic examination. Equipment and supplies: **A,** Large cotton-tipped applicator; **B,** Small cotton- or dacron-tipped applicator; **C,** Glass or plastic eye dropper.

· After application of a small amount of lubricant jelly, very gently and carefully insert the speculum while engaging the child with appropriate conversation.

· When the examination and any procedures are completed, carefully remove the speculum.

· In *adolescents,* the procedure is similar and should be equally unhurried and gentle.

· You can lubricate the vaginal speculum with warm water, or with jelly if a Papanicolaou smear is not needed.

· Before insertion of the speculum, perform a single-digit vaginal examination to prepare the patient for the speculum and to locate the cervix.

· Insert the speculum with the blades closed. Some people recomend inserting the speculum over the internal finger, which acts as a guide. In examining the young sexually inexperienced teenager, you may find it easier to insert the speculum blades at an angle, and then rotate the speculum once it has been inserted. Open the blades carefully in the horizontal position (Figure 14-8), allowing good visualization of the cervix and of the vagina (Figure 14-9).

· Before speculum removal, close the blades, being careful not to pinch any vaginal tissue.

c. Bimanual examination: This procedure involves placing the left hand on the lower abdomen and inserting the index finger or the index and middle fingers of the right hand into the vagina. In the prepubertal girl, one finger of the right hand may be placed in the rectum instead of the vagina. The pelvic area may then be examined with simultaneous palpation externally and internally. The position and size of the pelvic organs may be identified, and an assessment may be made of any abnormalities of these organs, the presence of

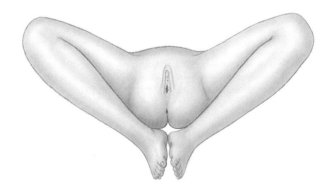

Figure 14-6.
Pelvic examination. Frog-leg position.

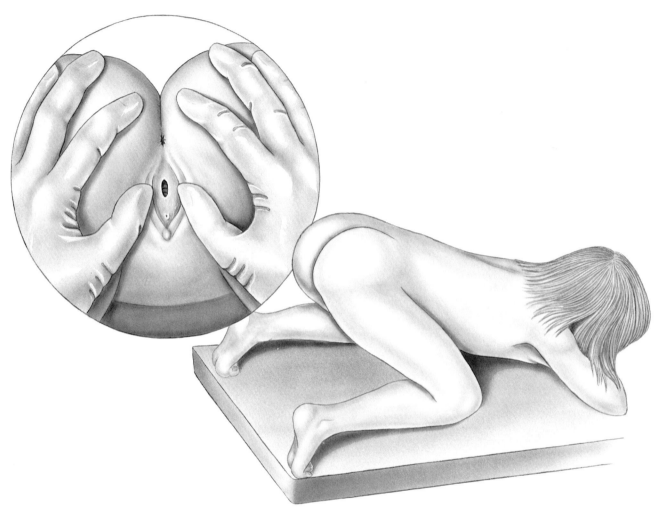

Figure 14-7.
Pelvic examination. Knee–chest position.

extra masses, and any areas of tenderness. The procedure is performed on all adolescents having a pelvic examination. The patient should be warned that she may feel as if she "needs to use the bathroom" and reassured that incontinence is most unlikely.

· Using lubrication, gently insert the index finger or the index and middle fingers of the right hand into the vagina, while placing the left hand on the abdomen just above the pubis. A single-digit vaginal examination is appropriate if the hymenal opening is small, and particularly in the pre-sexually active adolescent.

· You will feel the cervix internally and feel the uterus by pushing up on the cervix with the right hand and down on the abdomen with the left hand (Figure 14-

10). You will appreciate an anteverted uterus between your hands. The nulliparous uterus is normally the size of a small pear. Similarly, the adnexal areas are examined with the right hand palpating upwards lateral to the cervix and the left hand pressing down on the lower quadrants of the abdomen (Figure 14-11). The ovaries themselves may not be felt unless they are pathologically enlarged.

· You can best palpate an axial or retroverted uterus with a rectal-vaginal-abdominal examination (Figure 14-12). Insert the index finger of the right hand in the vagina, and place the middle finger of the same hand in the rectum. Use the left hand for the abdominal palpation as previously. Use the vaginal digit to palpate the

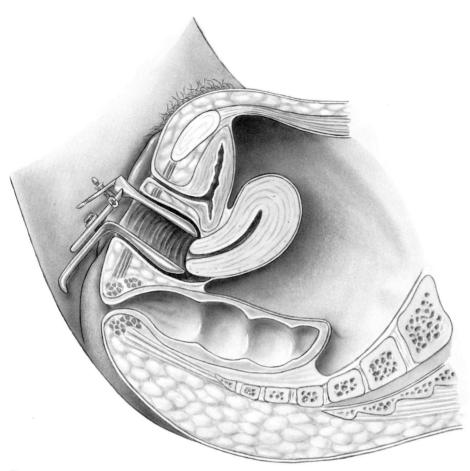

Figure 14-8.
Pelvic examination. Technique for visualization of the cervix and the vagina through a speculum.

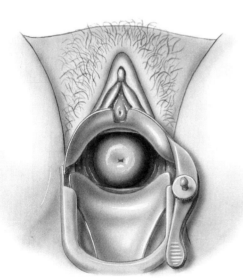

Figure 14-9.
Pelvic examination. Technique for visualization of the cervix and the vagina through a speculum.

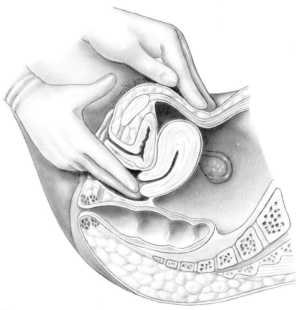

Figure 14-10.
Pelvic examination. Technique for palpation of the uterus.

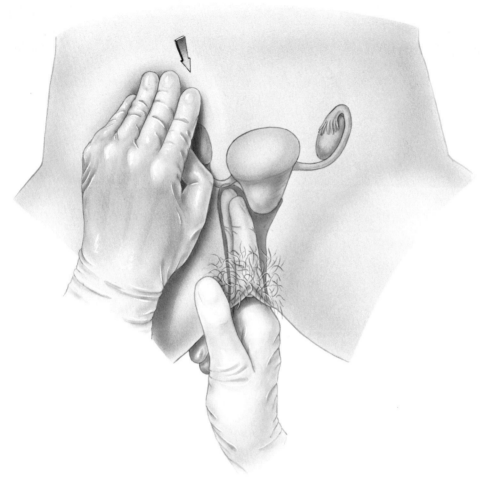

Figure 14-11.
Pelvic examination. Technique for palpation of the adnexal areas.

cervix, and with simultaneous abdominal pressure, feel the retroverted or axial uterus with the rectal digit. With the right hand in this rectal–vaginal position, palpate the uterosacral ligaments between the index and middle fingers. Painful nodules in this region are suggestive of endometriosis.

d. Specimen collection:
  • Moisten a small cotton applicator with *non*bacteriostatic saline for the collection of vaginal specimens in the young child.
  • If a copious discharge is present, or several samples are needed, aspirate vaginal secretions using a glass or plastic eye dropper. For the adolescent patient, details of specific procedures are described below.

5. Side Effects and Complications: In the adequately prepared patient, the gynecologic examination should be well tolerated. If, however, the patient cannot cooperate or if there are evi-

dent genital anomalies requiring further assessment, an examination under sedation or under anesthesia may be required. In such circumstances, referral to a gynecologist is appropriate. In severely obese patients, bimanual examinations may provide limited information. A pelvic ultrasound may be necessary to evaluate pelvic anatomy.

II. Diagnostic Procedures

A. Papanicolaou Smear

1. Purpose: The Papanicolaou (Pap) smear is used to detect changes in cervical cytology that indicate inflammation, dysplasia, or the presence of premalignant or malignant cells.
2. Selection of Patients:
a. Indications: A Papanicolaou smear is done at least annually after the onset of sexually activity and more frequently if there is a history of abnormal cervical cytology. It is particularly

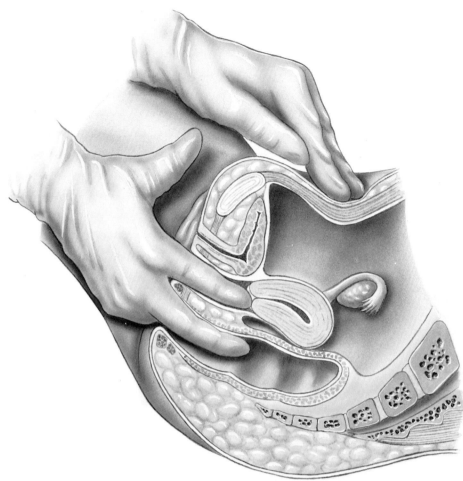

Figure 14-12.
Pelvic examination. Technique for palpation of an axial or retroverted uterus.

important in patients with condyloma acuminata. In girls exposed to diethylstilbestrol *in utero,* a Papanicolaou smear and careful vaginal examination are recommended shortly after menarche or by 14 years of age, because of an increased incidence of cervical and vaginal pathology in these young women. In addition, these patients should be referred for a full assessment including colposcopy.

b. Contraindications and Precautions: Lubricant should not be used, as it will interfere with the interpretation of the pathology specimen.

3. Equipment and Supplies (See Appendix for equipment and supplies manufacturers and suppliers. Appendix is keyed to italicized words in the equipment and supplies lists):

- Vaginal *speculum* (See Figure 14-4, page 166).
- Wooden *spatula* (Figure 14-13)
- Cytology *brushes* (Figure 14-13)

- Glass microscope *slides*
- Fixative: isopropyl *alcohol* (95%) or an aerosol formula

4. Description of Procedure:

- Insert the speculum using warm water for lubrication if needed (See Pelvic Examination, page 163).
- Visualize the cervix through the open speculum (See Figure 14-8, page 169).
- Scrape a wooden spatula around the whole exocervix with a circular sweep using moderate pressure. Smear the scrapings onto a slide.
- Insert a cytology brush 1 cm into the endocervical canal, rotate it, remove it, and then smear any collected material onto a second slide.
- Fix the two smears within a few seconds to prevent drying artefact.

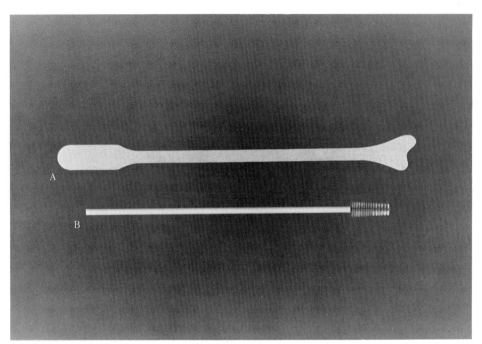

Figure 14-13.
Papanicolaou smear. Equipment and supplies: **A,** Wooden cytology spatula; **B,** Cytology brush.

5. Side Effects and Complications: Usually there are no side effects or complications. However, the patient should be forewarned that she may experience cramping while the cytology brush is manipulated in the endocervix.
6. Interpretation: Papanicolaou smears are usually classified as follows:
   · *Class I:* Normal
   · *Class II:* Atypical cells that may be inflammatory, e.g., secondary to chlamydia infection. The Papanicolaou smear is repeated after appropriate treatment.
   · *Class III:* Dysplastic cells are present.
   · *Class IV:* Carcinoma *in situ*
   · *Class V:* Invasive carcinoma
   Referral for colposcopy and treatment is appropriate for patients with class III, IV, or V Papanicolaou smears. Papanicolaou smears may also show trichomonads. Antibiotic treatment with metronidazole is then indicated; sexual contacts also should be treated.

B. Assessment of Cervical Mucus
1. Purpose: The estrogen status of a patient can be assessed by examining the cervical mucus.
2. Selection of Patients:
a. Indications: An estimation of estrogenization can be useful in evaluating patients with primary or secondary menorrhea.
b. Contraindications and Precautions: None
3. Equipment and Supplies (See Appendix for equipment and supplies manufacturers and suppliers. Appendix is keyed to italicized words in the equipment and supplies lists):
   · Vaginal *specula* (See Figure 14-4, page 166)
   · Lubrication *jelly*
   · Large cotton-tipped *applicator* (See Figure 14-5, page 167)
   · Small cotton- or dacron-tipped *applicator* (See Figure 14-5, page 167)
   · Saline *solution*
   · Glass microscope *slide*
   · Microscope
4. Description of Procedure:
   · Place the patient in the lithotomy position and insert the speculum (See Pelvic Examination, page 163).
   · Swab excess cervical secretions with the large cotton applicator.
   · Use a saline-moistened small cotton applicator to obtain a sample of endocervical mucus.
   · Smear the mucus onto a slide and allow to air-dry.
   · Examine the sample using the microscope.

5. Side Effects and Complications: None

6. Interpretation: Cervical mucus changes during the menstrual cycle. In the proliferative phase, which occurs in the beginning of the menstrual cycle, it is watery and scanty. At midcycle, it becomes profuse and is clear and string-like. During the secretory phase that follows, cervical mucus is thick and sticky. Microscopic examination of a dry smear will show "ferning" during the proliferative and midcycle phases, indicating estrogen action. Ferning is not seen when there is inadequate estrogen, or when progesterone levels are raised; for example, during the secretory phase of the menstrual cycle.

C. Wet Preparations

1. Purpose: In patients presenting with a vaginal discharge, direct microscopic evaluation of wet preparations of the discharge is useful in establishing a diagnosis, particularly in adolescents.

2. Selection of Patients:

a. Indications: Wet preparations should be examined on all patients with a vaginal discharge.

b. Contraindications and Precautions: None

3. Equipment and Supplies (See Appendix for equipment and supplies manufacturers and suppliers. Appendix is keyed to italicized words in the equipment and supplies lists):

- Vaginal *specula* (See Figure 14-4, page 166).
- Lubrication *jelly*
- Small cotton- or dacron-tipped *applicators* (See Figure 14-5, page 167)
- Glass microscope *slides* and *cover slips*
- Potassium hydroxide *solution* (10%) (KOH)
- Normal saline *solution*

4. Description of Procedure:

- Position the patient for specimen collection as previously described (See Pelvic Examination, page xxxx). Use a speculum in evaluating adolescents or if multiple specimens are to be collected (See Pelvic Examination, page 163).
- Take samples of the vaginal secretions using a small cotton or dacron applicator (See Pelvic Examination, page 163).
- Smear the secretions onto two different slides.
- Add a drop of potassium hydroxide to the specimen on one slide, and note any amine-like odor, i.e., "whiff test." Add a drop of normal saline to the specimen on the second slide, and place a coverslip over each slide.
- Examine the specimens directly under the microscope using both low- and high-power magnification, and with phase contrast, if available.

5. Side Effects and Complications: None

6. Interpretation: A positive "whiff test" is diagnostic of *Gardnerella vaginalis* infection.

When examined under the microscope, the potassium hydroxide preparation may show yeast or budding hyphae typical of *Candida albicans*.

The saline slide may show flagellated trichomonads dancing under the cover slip. Epithelial cells and leukocytes also will be seen. Epithelial cells that contain light-refractile bacteria are known as "clue cells" or "glitter cells." They are considered to be diagnostic of *Gardnerella vaginalis* infection. The finding of no leukocytes and only abundant epithelial cells is typical of a physiologic leukorrhea.

In the prepubertal girl, it is rare to diagnose a specific infectious cause for a vaginal discharge. If a child does have evidence of infection with *Candida albicans* or *Gardnerella vaginalis,* this does not constitute substantive evidence of sexual abuse. Similarly, the presence of these infections in an adolescent girl does not necessarily imply sexual transmission. By contrast, evidence of *Trichomonas vaginalis* generally implies sexual transmission; partners also should be treated. Treatment of sexual contacts of patients with *Gardnerella vaginitis* remains controversial.

D. Diagnosis of Chlamydia and Gonorrhea

1. Purpose: Genital infection with chlamydia or with gonorrhea may give rise to a mucopurulent discharge. Of note, these infections also may be asymptomatic. Chlamydial and gonorrheal infections are associated with cervicitis, endometritis, and salpingitis and are major causes of infertility. Early diagnosis and appropriate treatment is thus extremely important. In sexually active patients, screening is also necessary to diagnose asymptomatic infections, allowing appropriate treatment.

2. Selection of Patients:

a. Indications: Chlamydial and gonorrheal infections must be considered in all patients presenting with a vaginal discharge. In the prepubertal girl, screening is necessary if there is a history of alleged sexual abuse even without symptoms or if a purulent discharge is present even without a history of sexual abuse. The presence of either of these organisms is paramount to proof of sexual abuse. In the adolescent who has initiated sexual activity, screening for asymptomatic infections is appropriate at least annually and perhaps every 6 months if the local prevalence is high or when sexual partners are changed.

b. Contraindications and Precautions: None

3. Equipment and Supplies (See Appendix for equipment and supplies manufacturers and suppliers. Appendix is keyed to italicized words in the equipment and supplies lists):

- Vaginal *speculum* (See Figure 14-4, page 166)
- Lubrication *jelly*
- Small cotton- or dacron-tipped *applicators* (See Figure 14-5, page 167)

· Gonorrhea culture medium (e.g., Martin-Lewis agar plate)

· Chlamydia DNA probe test kit, including a very small dacron applicator

4. Description of Procedure:

a. Prepubertal patient:

· The frog-leg position (See Figure 14-6, page 167) is preferable for specimen collection in this age group.

· Vaginal specimens are adequate. Gonococcal organisms invade the vaginal mucosa in this age group. Chlamydia can also be isolated from vaginal specimens.

· A vaginal speculum may be used if multiple specimens are needed.

· Collect specimens using a very small dacron applicator premoistened with *non*bacteriostatic saline, taking care not to touch hymenal membrane.

· Smear the specimen directly onto the gonorrhea culture medium; and follow directions for the chlamydia kit.

b. Adolescent patient:

· Specimens must be cervical and should be collected with a small cottom or dacron applicator in the same way as the endocervical Papanicolaou smear (See Papanicolaou Smear, page 170).

· For the chlamydia test, obtain specimens with a small dacron applicator. Insert the applicator and rotate in the endocervix for 5 to 10 seconds.

· Process specimens as above.

5. Side Effects and Complications: Specimen collection from the endocervix may cause cramping or minor bleeding, particularly if the mucosa is friable.

6. Interpretation: Positive gonorrhea cultures indicate infection that should be treated appropriately. All sexual contacts also require treatment. Positive chlamydia DNA probe tests are diagnostic of infection; patients should be treated. Positive chlamydia antibody tests on cervical samples also are diagnostic of infection. However, the antibody test may be falsely positive on a vaginal sample, particularly if there is contamination with fecal flora. Positive antibody tests on vaginal samples must be followed up with a chlamydia culture before a definitive diagnosis is made and treatment initiated. The sexual partners of girls with genital chlamydia must also be treated.

E. Diagnosis of Herpes Genitalis

1. Purpose: Genital *Herpes simplex* is an acute and often recurrent disease that can be associated with significant pain and localized symptoms such as dysuria and urinary retention. It also may be asymptomatic. It is associated with considerable psychosocial dysfunction and can cause life-threatening illness in the newborn delivered vaginally to a woman with active infection (symptomatic or asymptomatic). Therefore, accurate diagnosis is important.

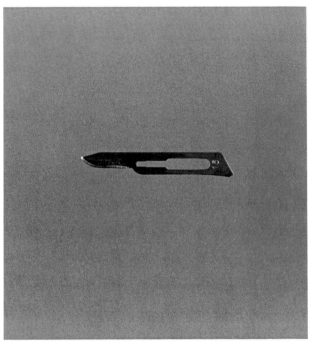

Figure 14-14.
Diagnosis of herpes genitalis. Equipment and supplies: No. 15 scalpel blade.

2. Selection of Patients:

a. Indications: Those patients who have undiagnosed genital ulceration should be cultured for *Herpes simplex*. Simultaneous counseling is also recommended.

b. Contraindications and Precautions: None

3. Equipment and Supplies (See Appendix for equipment and supplies manufacturers and suppliers. Appendix is keyed to italicized words in the equipment and supplies lists):

· No. 15 scalpel *blade* (Figure 14-14)

· Dacron-tipped *applicator* (See Figure 14-5, page 167)

· Viral culture medium

· Glass microscope *slide*

· Wright's stain

4. Description of Procedure:

· Inspect the external genitalia carefully.

· De-roof an intact blister using a broken-off applicator stick or a sharp blade.

· The Tzank smear is a useful quick diagnostic test. Obtain a specimen by firmly scraping the base of a lesion with a dacron-tipped applicator. Smear the specimen onto a slide, air-dry, and stain with Wright's stain.

· Obtain a specimen for culture from a second blister base using another dacron-tipped applicator. If there are no intact blisters, take a specimen for culture from an open lesion.

5. Side Effects and Complications: None

6. Intrepretation: The presence of multinucleated giant cells with inclusion bodies on Wright's stain is diagnostic of herpes infection. A positive culture then confirms the diagnosis. The patient needs counseling about the disease and how she should take care of herself to minimize symptoms and to prevent transmission to others. As yet there is no curative treatment.

III. Therapeutic Procedures

A. Release of Labial Adhesions

Labial adhesions are seen in young children, usually between the ages of 6 months and 6 years. Resolution usually occurs spontaneously within months, or at the latest by puberty in association with increasing estrogen levels.

1. Purpose: In certain cases, division of adhesions may be necessary.

2. Selection of Patients:

a. Indications: Treatment is needed for symptoms related to occlusion of the urethral meatus, such as dysuria or pooling of urine causing dribbling incontinence. In addition, the vaginal introitus may be obscured, giving rise to impaired drainage of vaginal secretions and causing considerable parental anxiety over the child's genital anatomy.

b. Contraindications and Precautions: Adhesions are partial in 20% to 50% of cases. The majority are asymptomatic and do not require treatment.

3. Equipment and Supplies (See Appendix for equipment and supplies manufacturers and suppliers. Appendix is keyed to italicized words in the equipment and supplies lists):
- Estrogen-containing *cream*
- Bland *ointment*

4. Description of Procedure:
- Place the child in the frog-leg position (See Figure 14-6, page 167).
- In mild cases only, separate adhesions by gentle bilateral traction of the labia (Figure 14-15) if this is not traumatic to the child.
- In more extensive cases, rub an estrogen-containing cream into the adhered area with gentle simultaneous bilateral traction of the labia (as above). A parent can do this twice daily for 2 weeks and then at bedtime only, if needed, for up to 2 more weeks, by which time the labia should have separated.
- After separation, continue a nighttime application of a bland ointment for several months or longer to prevent recurrences.
- Follow-up care includes good perineal hygiene with wiping from front-to-back, daily bathing, wearing white cotton underpants, and avoiding tight-fitting clothing.

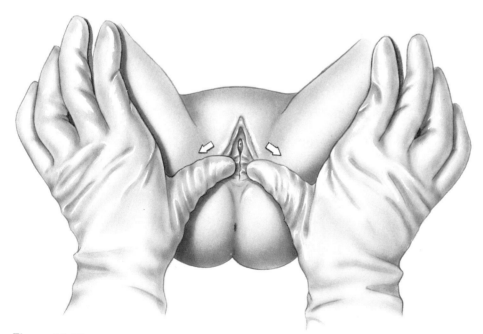

Figure 14-15.
Release of labial adhesions. Technique.

5. Side Effects and Complications: Side effects of topical estrogen treatment include breast development and tenderness. These breast changes reverse when the estrogen is stopped. Vulvar hyperpigmentation is a permanent side effect of topical estrogen-containing creams. Side effects secondary to topical estrogens are minimized if treatment is limited as described above.

The most frequent complication in the treatment of labial adhesions is recurrence of the adhesions. Treatment is as described above with prolonged use of a bland ointment at nighttime for up to 1 year if needed.

B. Foreign Body Removal

Foreign bodies such as wads of toilet tissue may be found in the vagina, particularly in the 3- to 8-year age group.

1. Purpose: The purpose of this procedure is to remove a vaginal foreign body.

2. Selection of Patients:

a. Indications: The presence of a foreign body in the vagina is suggested by the history of a bloody foul-smelling vaginal discharge confirmed by examination.

b. Contraindications and Precautions: None

3. Equipment and Supplies (See Appendix for equipment and supplies manufacturers and suppliers. Appendix is keyed to italicized words in the equipment and supplies lists):

· Veterinary otoscope *specula* (See Figure 14-3, page 165)
· Lubrication *jelly*

· Small cotton- or dacron-tipped *applicator* (See Figure 14-5, page 167)
· Saline *solution*
· Alligator *forceps* (See Figure 9-28, page 102)

4. Description of Procedure:

· You may occasionally find sedation (See Table 18-2, page 219) to be necessary, particularly if the child has had a previous traumatic experience with a similar procedure.
· Place the patient in the position that provides optimal visualization of the vagina (frog-leg position or the knee–chest position [See Figures 14-6 and 14-7, pages 167 and 168]).
· You will find instrumentation unnecessary in the majority of patients. Use a veterinary otoscope speculum if needed for better visualization (See Pelvic Examination, page 163).
· Manipulate the foreign body out with a saline moistened, cotton-tipped applicator or grasp it with alligator forceps.
· Send the foreign body for histologic examination.
· Irrigate the vagina with warm water.
· Instruct the patient to use twice-daily sitz baths until symptoms have resolved.

5. Side Effects and Complications: There are usually no problems associated with the removal of foreign objects from the vagina. In rare cases, sedation or even general anesthesia may be needed if the child cannot tolerate the procedure or if the foreign material is extensive.

Chapter 15

Sexual Abuse Evaluation Procedures

Frank T. Saulsbury

I. Diagnostic Procedures

A. Sexual Abuse Evaluation

1. Purpose: Sexually abused children require a medical evaluation for two reasons:

a. To diagnose and treat physical and psychological problems stemming from the sexual abuse.

b. To collect, under some circumstances, evidence for forensic analysis.

2. Selection of Patients: Dr. C. Henry Kempe defined sexual abuse of children as, "the involvement of dependent, developmentally immature children and adolescents in sexual activities that they do not fully comprehend, to which they are unable to give informed consent, or that violate social taboos of family roles." Although the legal definition of sexual abuse of children varies from state to state, any child subjected to sexual abuse, as defined above, should have a medical evaluation. This evaluation should take place regardless of the type of sexual abuse or the time elapsed since the last episode of abuse.

Recognition of the sexually abused child is the vital first step in conducting an evaluation and providing proper care.

A detailed discussion of the behavioral, psychological, and medical indicators of child sexual abuse is beyond the scope of this chapter. Suffice to say that children rarely, if ever, fabricate detailed stories of sexual activity. In addition, disclosure of sexual abuse by children is often delayed. Thus, a child who says he has been sexually abused should be believed and examined even if the alleged abuse occurred weeks or months before disclosure.

3. Equipment and Supplies (See Appendix for equipment and supplies manufacturers and suppliers. Appendix is keyed to italicized words in the equipment and supplies lists):

- Examining *gloves*
- Sheet

- *Lubricant*
- Vaginal *speculum* (See Figure 14-4, page 166)
- Cotton-tipped *applicators* (See Figure 14-5, page 167)
- Glass microscope *slides* and *cover slips*
- Potassium hydroxide *solution* (10%)
- *Scraper*
- Fingernail *clipper* or iris *scissors* (See Figure 18-2, page 220)
- Specimen containers (depending on the diagnostic tests used)
- Wood's *Lamp* (See Figure 7-1, page 59)
- Test *tubes*
- Sterile nonbacteriostatic saline *solution*
- Camera
- Gram stain materials

4. Description of Procedure:

a. History: A critical aspect of the evaluation of a sexually abused child is a careful, detailed history to establish an accurate database. This information will be pivotal in tailoring the extent of the physical examination as well as treatment and follow-up. For example, different measures would be taken in the following cases:

Example: A 12-year-old girl has been involved for 3 years in an incestuous relationship involving vaginal intercourse with her stepfather. The last episode of intercourse was 3 months before being seen by a physician.

Example: A 14-year-old girl was beaten and raped by a total stranger 1 hour before presenting to an emergency room for treatment.

Example: A 4-year-old boy was fondled in the genital area by a babysitter 1 week before being seen by a physician.

The following historical information should be collected:

(1) Type of abuse: This information should be as specific and detailed as possible. Drawings or dolls can be useful adjuncts in determining the nature of the abuse. In addition, record the activities, using the child's terms for various genital organs. However, establish that the child's terms correspond to the more traditional nomenclature (i.e., "worm" = penis, "kitty" = vagina, "where I poop" = anus).

(2) Identity of the perpetrator: Identify the perpetrator and determine any relationship to the child. Also, locate witnesses that may identify the perpetrator and corroborate the child's story. Finally, consider the possibility of other victims.

(3) Chronology of events: Determine the time and date of the abuse. Define whether the episode was an isolated event or one in a series of episodes. Equally importantly, determine when the last episode occurred.

(4) Threat of retaliation: Determine if a threat of retaliation for reporting the episode has occurred and define the specifics of the threat.

(5) Activities since last episode: Note whether the patient has carried out any of the following activities since the last episode of sexual abuse: bathing, douching, changing clothes, defecating, or brushing the teeth.

(6) Gynecologic history: Record the details regarding menarche, the last menstrual period, a current or past pregnancy, and the use of birth control pills.

(7) Signs or symptoms stemming from abuse: Describe in detail any of the following:

(a) Dysuria

(b) Vaginal discharge or bleeding

(c) Rectal pain or bleeding

(d) Sore throat

(e) Genital ulcers

(f) Behavioral and emotional changes (i.e., enuresis, insomnia, separation anxiety, withdrawal)

b. Physical examination: In preparing for the physical examination, the examiner must be sensitive to issues of privacy, confidentiality, and control. Before focusing on the genital exam, perform a complete, routine physical examination for signs of trauma. This approach helps desensitize the child to examination of the perineum.

The examination for sexual abuse addresses not only the genitalia, but also the breasts, the rectum, and the mouth. Again, a genital exam is warranted regardless of the amount of time elapsed since the last sexual encounter. The majority of sexually abused children will have no positive findings on physical examination. When positive findings are present, however, they are important for two reasons. First, they may require treatment, and second, they are important objective corroboration of the child's story.

Because the vast majority of sexually abused children are girls, the remainder of the discussion will focus on the examination of girls. Young children are often most successfully examined in the frog-leg position while in their mother's lap (Figure 15-1). Older children may be adequately examined on their back with their hips and knees flexed and legs abducted (Figure 15-2). It is controversial whether the knee–chest position (See Figure 14-7, page 168) is appropriate for the child who has been sexually abused. Adolescents may have a traditional pelvic examination, as described in Gynecologic Procedures. Throughout the examination, the presence and stage of development of anatomic structures should be noted.

Carefully inspect the genitourinary system, the perineum, and the anus for signs of trauma or infection. On occasion, photographic documentation of the findings is useful.

c. Laboratory specimens: The child's history and the findings on physical examination will dictate the type of laboratory

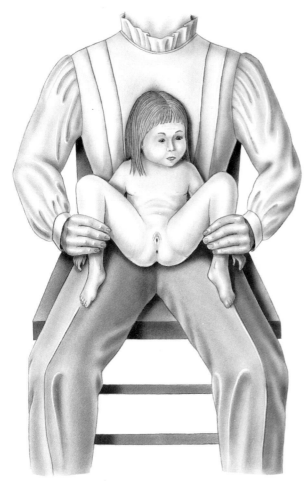

Figure 15-1.
Sexual abuse evaluation. Position for the physical examination of the young child.

specimens, if any, to be obtained. Many children will require the following specimens:

(1) Culture of appropriate sites (throat, rectum, vagina) or other laboratory tests for the following venereal infections (See Gynecologic Procedures, pages 163–176):

(a) Gonorrhea
(b) Chlamydia
(c) Herpes
(d) Syphilis
(e) Trichomonas

(2) Wet mount of vaginal, oral, and rectal secretions for identification of spermatozoa (See Gynecologic Procedures, page 163).

(3) Potassium hydroxide preparation of vaginal secretions

for identification of monilial infection (See Gynecologic Procedures, page 163).

(4) Urinalysis with emphasis on the presence of blood, white blood cells, or spermatozoa (See Urogenital Procedures, page 141).

(5) Pregnancy test

d. Evidence collection: The collection of evidence for forensic analysis is appropriate in some instances of sexual abuse. Such evidence may be helpful in corroborating the child's testimony concerning sexual abuse, and occasionally it may help to identify the perpetrator. In most circumstances, evidence collection is useful when the sexual assault has occurred within 24 hours of the examination, and may be useful within a longer period. Label all specimens to indicate the source of the specimen, the date and time of collection, and the signature of the physician who collected the specimen. To preserve the chain of evidence, you must maintain constant and sole possession of the specimens until a law enforcement officer personally collects and signs for the specimens. Collect the following specimens:

(1) Clothing: Have the child disrobe on a sheet and save all clothing.

(2) Fingernails: Scrape any material from beneath the fingernails or clip the fingernails and place the specimens in a container.

(3) Pubic hair: Collect suspicious, loose hairs and note where they were found. Pluck scalp and pubic hair from the victim and save them for comparison.

(4) Wood's lamp: Examine the body and clothes with a Wood's lamp (See Skin Procedures: Wood's Lamp Examination, page 58). Semen will fluoresce with a dark green color. Record the locations of fluorescence. Cut and label any scalp hair, pubic hair, or clothing that shows fluorescence.

(5) Semen identification: Swab the vaginal mucosa and each suspicious area with two swabs. Smear one swab onto a microscope slide and air dry, and place the other swab in a test tube. These specimens may be sent to a forensic laboratory for sperm identification and ABO semen typing. In addition, a wet mount of the vaginal fluid should be examined immediately for motile sperm.

(6) Acid phosphatase: Swab suspicious areas, air dry, and place in a test tube. Instill 1 or 2 mL of sterile saline into the vagina, aspirate, and place the fluid in a test tube for acid phosphatase determination.

(7) ABO Typing: Collect blood and saliva for determination of ABO blood type and secretor status. It is important to know the ABO and secretor status of the victim to intrepret the results of ABO semen typing.

(8) Photography: Photograph all visible evidence of trauma, both genital and nongenital.

e. Reporting: Child abuse is a crime. All 50 states require

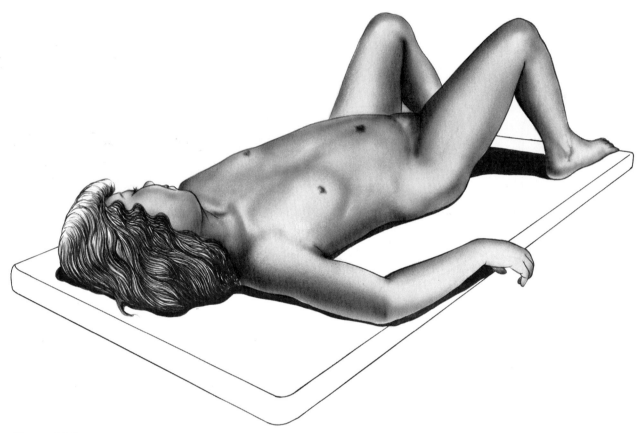

Figure 15-2.
Sexual abuse evaluation. Position for the physical examination of the older child.

physicians to report patients who have been sexually abused. The agency mandated to receive such reports varies from state to state, but in most instances, it is the Department of Social Services or the police. All states have criminal or civil penalties for willful failure to report the sexual abuse of children. Thus, the physician should report all suspicious cases to the legally mandated agencies.

5. Side Effects and Complications: There are very few, if any, complications of a properly performed sexual abuse evaluation.

Chapter 16

Musculoskeletal Procedures

Mary Williams Clark

Musculoskeletal complaints can be the presenting problem in up to three fourths of the visits to primary physicians. The procedures described in this chapter frequently will be useful in a pediatric or family medicine practice. Some techniques of physical examination are included because they are simple and useful but little known to most nonorthopedists.

I. Screening Procedures

A. Scoliosis Screening[1]

Minor body asymmetries occur in many children and may be physiologic but could also represent pathology. Asymmetry in a patient with growth remaining may be potentially progressive, and progressive asymmetry clearly requires further investigation. As most significant lateral spinal curvatures involve some vertebral rotation, an asymmetric thoracic prominence can indicate scoliosis. William Adams described the ''forward-bend'' test in 1865.

1. Purpose: The purpose of this test is to detect potentially progressive scoliosis.

2. Selection of Patients:

a. Indications: Girls 10 to 14 years of age and boys 10 to 16 years of age should be screened.

b. Contraindications and Precautions: None

3. Equipment and Supplies (See Appendix for equipment and supplies manufacturers and suppliers. Appendix is keyed to italicized words in the equipment and supplies lists):

- Equipment is not essential, but the Scoliometer, an *inclinometer* for measurement of degree of trunk rotation, is useful[2] (Figure 16-1).

4. Description of Procedure:

- Have the patient stand in shorts or swimsuit, with her back to the examiner, feet together, and knees straight.
- Look for asymmetry in shoulder height, scapular

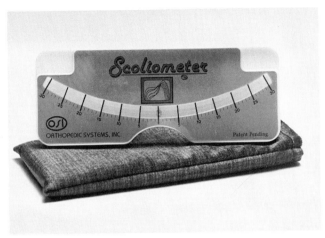

Figure 16-1.
Scoliosis screening. Equipment and supplies: Inclinometer.

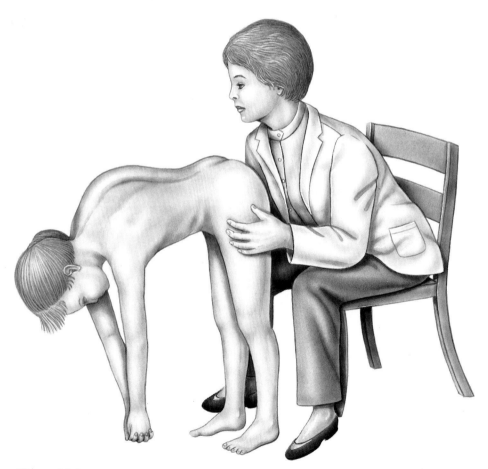

Figure 16-2.
Scoliosis screening. Technique.

prominence, distance of arm from flank, and hip height (See Leg Length Difference, page 186). If a leg length discrepancy is present, level the patient's pelvis and proceed with the Adams test.

· The patient bends forward with head down, arms dependent, and hands clasped.

· Look at the back with your eyes at the level of the mid-back. Observe the thoracic spine for asymmetry with the patient at a 45-degree angle forward, the thoracolumbar junction with the patient leaning farther forward, and the lumbosacral spine with the patient at 90 degree or maximum bend (Figure 16-2).

· An inclinometer is useful for quantifying any prominence seen on the Adams test. With the patient in the forward-bend position, place the device transversely on the back at the level of maximum asymmetry, with the zero mark directly over the tip of the spinous process at that level (Figure 16-3). Do not press down, as that may affect the reading. Read the angle of inclination directly from the scale, at the point where the indicator ball rests in the fluid.

5. Side Effects and Complications: None

6. Interpretation: Suspect scoliosis if asymmetries are present, and refer to an orthopedist who will provide an experienced second screen. The diagnosis of scoliosis is made roentgenographically, but unnecessary x-ray exposure may be avoided by referring to an orthopedist first. The orthopedist may follow the patient without taking any radiographs. Conversely, most orthopedists have available facilities for taking long-film views that show the entire spine and iliac crests (for evaluation of skeletal maturity) on a single film. If you obtain other films, they may have to be repeated.

The scoliometer provides a simple means to "second screen" at the primary level and an easy way to follow a minor asymmetry. An angle of rotation of 5 degrees or more indicates referral to an orthopedist. Smaller angles require reevaluation in 6 to 12 months, and an increasing angle requires referral.

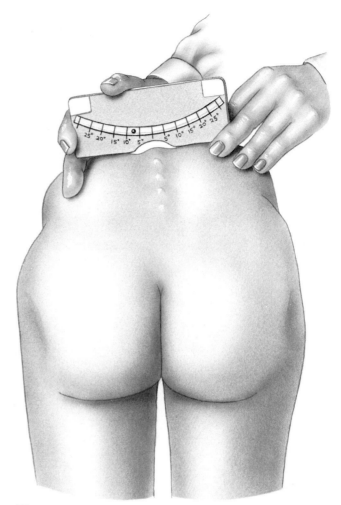

Figure 16-3.
Scoliosis screening. Technique using inclinometer.

B. Examination for Hip Flexion Contracture (Thomas Test)

This maneuver was described by Hugh Owen Thomas in 1876 for the detection of pathology in or about the hip joint.[3] It detects limited range of extension of the joint and can thus screen for many hip disorders, including transient synovitis, Legg-Calvé-Perthes disease, and septic arthritis.

1. Purpose: The purpose of the procedure is to test for the presence of a flexion contracture of the hip joint.

2. Selection of Patients:

a. Indications: All patients with symptoms in the abdomen, back, hip, or knee should be evaluated.

b. Contraindications and Precautions: The procedure should not be performed on patients with a suspected fracture of the femur or pelvis.

3. Equipment and Supplies:

· A firm examining table or surface

4. Description of Procedure:

· Have the patient lie supine on a firm surface, wearing only underwear or loose shorts.

· Flex both lower limbs onto the abdomen, flattening the lumbar spine against the table. Feel beneath the lumbar spine with your hand to ascertain if the spine is flattened optimally.

· Hold the asymptomatic leg in place, or have the patient do so ("Hug your knee to your chest.") (Figure 16-4).

· Extend the other leg toward the table; a normal leg comes easily to full extension and lies flat on the table.

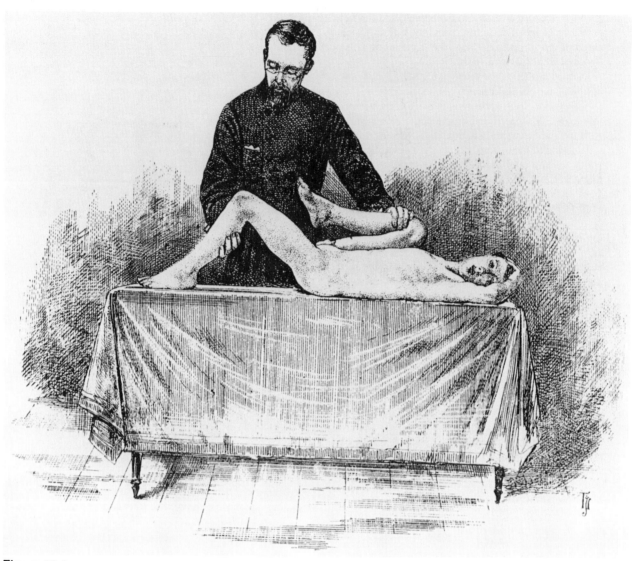

Figure 16-4.
Examination for hip flexion contracture (Thomas test). Technique.

- Contracture of the hip prevents full extension, and the extent of contracture is the angle the thigh forms with the table (e.g., "a flexion contracture of 15 degrees") (Figure 16-4).

5. Side Effects and Complications: None

6. Interpretation: Any measurable contracture in a child older than 6 months (normal neonatal contractures of the hip can take up to 6 months to resolve[4]) indicates pathology in or about the hip joint, and referral to or consultation with an orthopedist is appropriate.

C. Examination for Hip Abductor Weakness (Trendelenburg Test)

The peculiar gait of a person with an untreated dislocated hip was thought to be due to the uncovered head of the femur sliding proximally on the iliac wing when the patient places weight on that leg, until Friedrich Trendelenburg pointed out in 1897 that careful observation shows the pelvis moving downward on the side *opposite* the abnormal hip, not the same side.[5] This movement is due to weakness of the hip abductors, which normally stabilize the pelvis on the weight-bearing femur. A "Trendelenburg gait" is also known as a "gluteus medius lurch" and results from the trunk shifting toward the side of the abnormal hip when the patient's weight is on that leg. The trunk shifts to balance the drop of the pelvis in the opposite direction. The Trendelenburg test itself is done standing, and details of the procedure were clarified recently by Hardcastle and Nade.[6]

1. Purpose: The purpose of this procedure is to detect hip abductor weakness of various causes.

2. Selection of Patients:

a. Indications: All patients older than 4 years with a limp or symptoms at the back, hip, or knee should be evaluated. Patients younger than 4 years of age cannot consistently perform the test.

b. Contraindications and Precautions: None

3. Equipment and Supplies: None

4. Description of Procedure:

· Have the patient stand, wearing only underwear, facing away from the examiner.

· Observe the relationship between the pelvis (a line joining iliac crests or the posterior sacral dimples) and the ground.

· Have the patient stand on one leg (the side being tested), and raise the other leg, flexing the hip until the foot clears the ground (Figure 16-5A). Balance may be assisted by supporting *only* the hand on the stance side. Supporting the non-stance arm or hand will allow the trunk muscles to produce a false-negative test.

· Have the patient now raise the non-stance side of the pelvis as high as possible (Figure 16-5B). If the patient leans far over the supporting leg (another way to produce a false-negative test), correct by gently moving the shoulders until the base of the neck (C7 vertebra) is approximately over the hip and the weight-bearing foot.

· Have the patient maintain this position for 30 seconds.

· Observe the pelvis and record the time (if less than 30 seconds) at which the pelvis drops.

5. Side Effects and Complications: None

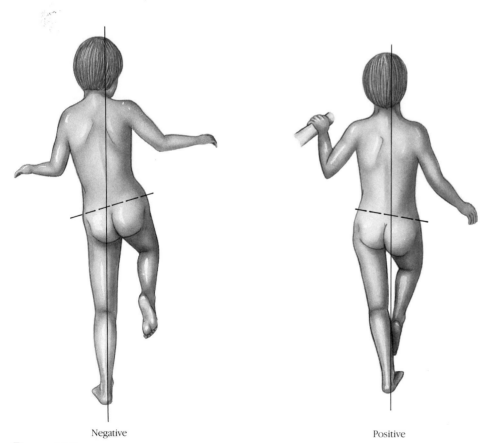

Negative   Positive

Figure 16-5.
Examination for hip abductor weakness (Trendelenburg test). Technique.

6. Interpretation: A normal patient can lift the pelvis as high as hip abduction on the stance side will allow and maintain it there for 30 seconds (negative test). A positive test is one in which the pelvis drops toward the floor on the unsupported side, either initially or during the 30 seconds (as the muscle fatigues). A positive test indicates significant weakness of the hip abductor muscles on the stance side, which could be caused by a hip disorder (subluxation, dislocation, Legg-Calvé-Perthes, etc.) creating altered mechanics, or by various disorders causing muscle weakness, including dystrophies or intraspinal pathology. The subluxated variety of "dislocated" hips, particularly those with an otherwise full range of motion, a negative Thomas test, full abduction, and only a minimal limp, can often be detected *only* in this way. Consultation with an orthopedist is indicated.

II. Diagnostic Tests

A. Girth Measurements

1. Purpose: The purpose of this procedure is to determine difference in limb girth or to follow results of a muscle-strengthening program. It is most often used for evaluating lower limbs; it can be done in the upper arm or the forearm as described for the calf.

2. Selection of Patients:

a. Indications: All patients with weakness or prolonged immobilization should be evaluated.

b. Contraindications and Precautions: Mid-shaft (diaphyseal) fractures (healing or healed) may lead to a misinterpretation (false-negative test), as callus of fracture healing can increase limb girth and obscure the amount of muscle atrophy.

3. Equipment and Supplies (See Appendix for equipment and supplies manufacturers and suppliers. Appendix is keyed to italicized words in the equipment and supplies lists):

> • Tape *measure:* preferably narrow ¼-inch cloth tape, marked in inches and centimeters. Metal tapes are cold and edges can hurt children. Paper tapes wrinkle and tear easily. Wide tape (½-inch or more) is difficult to handle and impairs accuracy.
> • Pen

4. Description of Procedure:

a. *Thigh girth measurement:*

> • Have the patient lie supine and relaxed, with legs unclothed.
> • Identify the medial joint line of the knee, palpable as a vertical depression (perpendicular to the table) on the medial side of the knee, just proximal to the level of the distal pole of the patella (Figure 16-6). If it is difficult to identify, ask the patient to extend and bend the knee slightly. (Note: the patella is an unreliable landmark. Though it is recommended as a landmark in some texts,

it is movable by a tense quadriceps muscle in a patient who is anxious, cold, or in pain.)

> • Measure the girth proximal to the joint line at a distance far enough to be above the suprapatella pouch of the knee joint, (at least 4 inches in a toddler, 6 or 7 inches in an adolescent) (Figure 16-6). Measurement at this distance avoids artifact if a joint effusion is present.
> • Mark the joint line and the point of measurement with a pen. Repeat the measurement, using your thumb to mark the point. (After 30 to 50 measurements, your intra-observer reliability should be sufficient to omit marking with a pen.)
> • Have the patient relax, and carefully measure the circumference transverse to the longitudinal axis of the thigh.
> • Record the measurements *or* the difference *and* the site (e.g., "Left thigh 1 inch smaller than right at 5 inches above the medial joint line").

b. *Calf girth measurement:*

> • Have the patient sit relaxed with her legs hanging over the edge of an examination table.
> • Measure the circumference of each calf at what appears to be the maximum calf bulk, carefully keeping the tape perpendicular to the long axis of the leg.
> • Measure again ¼-inch proximal and then ¼-inch distal to each original calf measurement, and record the maximum circumference of each calf. The gastrocnemius heads make the maximum circumference more proximal than it usually appears.

5. Side Effects and Complications: None

6. Interpretation: A difference in calf measurements of more than ½ inch in a child or adolescent (or ¼ inch in a small child) may be significant. Muscular atrophy on the smaller side is the most common cause of a difference; however, the differential diagnosis includes swelling, mass, or hemihypertrophy on the larger side.

B. Leg Length Difference

Leg-length differences are measured indirectly, as there are no specific external landmarks for the top of the femoral head. Measuring with the patient supine (anterior superior spine to malleolus) does not take into account the foot and ankle; measuring with the patient standing does.

Apparent leg length difference can be caused by pelvic obliquity, fixed deformities at hip or knee, or asymmetric positioning. Apparent leg lengths can be measured from the xiphoid or umbilicus to malleolus; orthopedists rarely find this information useful and rarely document it. The procedures defined here will describe accurate reflections of *true* leg lengths *if* hip and knee ranges of motion are full and there is no fixed pelvic obliquity (i.e., a line drawn from one

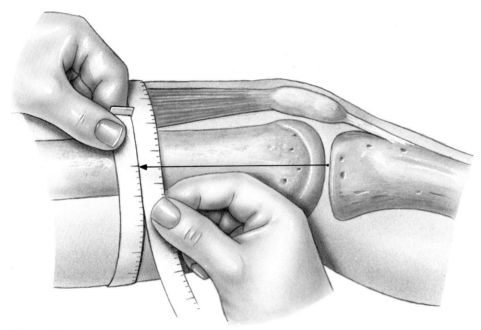

Figure 16-6.
Girth measurements—Thigh girth. Technique.

iliac crest to the other iliac crest is transverse to the spine in the coronal plane).

1. Purpose: The purpose of this procedure is to measure differences in leg lengths.

2. Selection of Patients:

a. Indications: All patients having an apparent leg-length difference, a limp, or scoliosis should be evaluated.

b. Contraindications and Precautions: None

3. Equipment and Supplies (See Appendix for equipment and supplies manufacturers and suppliers. Appendix is keyed to italicized words in the equipment and supplies lists):

· For supine measurement: ¼-inch cloth tape *measure* (See Girth Measurements, Equipment and Supplies, page 186)

· For standing measurement: Boards of varying thicknesses large enough to stand on. The ideal surface dimensions are 5 inches × 10 inches, in thicknesses of ⅛ inch, ¼ inch, ½ inch, ¾ inch, and 1 inch. If these are not available, firm books of varying thicknesses can be used.

4. Description of Procedure:

a. Supine measurement:

· Have the patient lie supine, in underwear, on a firm table. Have the legs aligned longitudinally with the trunk and pelvis level with the examination table.

· Identify the anterior superior spine of the ilium by

palpating the iliac crest and following it anteriorly; just inferior to the "lip" of the spine anteriorly there is a slight indentation, at the attachment of the sartorius and tensor fascia lata tendons to the iliac spine (Figure 16-7). Align the "0" mark of the tape with this indentation to allow best accuracy and reproducibility.

· Measure to the distal tip of the lateral malleolus (Figure 16-7). The distal tip is a more precise point than the greatest lateral prominence of the malleolus. Measuring to the lateral malleolus is more accurate than measuring to the medial malleolus in cases where thigh bulk is asymmetric.[7]

· Measure both legs and record the absolute measurements *or* the difference, and the points of measurements (i.e., "left leg shorter than right leg with ¾-inch difference, anterior superior spine to lateral malleolus").

b. Standing measurement:

· Have the patient stand in underwear facing away from the examiner. Have your eyes at the level of the patient's hips (Figure 16-8).

· Identify the iliac crests (by palpation) and observe the posterior superior iliac spines (the dimples) (Figure 16-8). If the crests or spines are not level, have the patient stand on the various boards, singly or combined until the pelvis levels.

· Record the amount of lift that levels the pelvis.

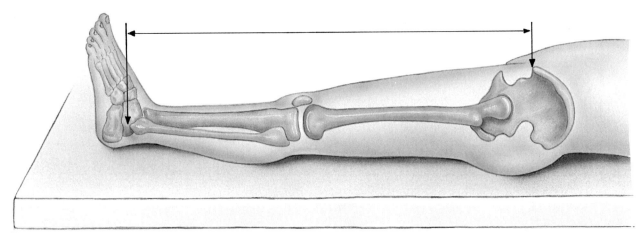

Figure 16-7.
Leg length difference—Supine measurement. Technique.

· Alternatively, have the patient face you and identify the crests and observe the anterior superior spines.

5. Side Effects and Complications: None

6. Interpretation: Leg length differences of more than ½ inch are worth following with serial measurements every 6 months; progressive differences indicate consultation with an orthopedist. Differences up to 1 inch are usually tolerated very well, although some children with such discrepancies have a smoother gait or are more comfortable with a heel lift. One-quarter to three-eighth-inch lifts of felt can be placed inside the shoe, in the heel only (under the insole); larger lifts keep the shoe from fitting well on the heel. The lifts flatten considerably with wear and should be replaced about every 3 months. Larger lifts should be attached to the sole of the shoe by a shoemaker or orthotist. The larger lifts should be added to *both* heel and sole, with the depth of the lift tapered to the toe.

Differences greater than 1 inch can be most accurately documented by scanograms or orthoroentgenograms. Orthopedists use these studies (with a radiographically determined bone age) to chart progressive differences and make estimations of differences likely at skeletal maturity.

C. Aspiration of Knee Joint

Aspiration or "tapping" of a knee joint is very useful in evaluating the cause of a swollen knee; and when done for significant hemarthrosis or for septic arthritis, it can be therapeutic as well as diagnostic. In many circumstances it is a procedure that can be appropriately done by nonorthopedists.

1. Purpose: The purpose of the procedure is to obtain fluid from a swollen knee joint for analysis and to decompress the joint for pain relief in some cases.

2. Selection of Patients:

a. Indications: Patients with suspected arthritis, bleeding into the knee, a traumatic effusion, or infection may benefit. The effusion usually obscures the hollows medial and lateral to the patella.

b. Contraindications and Precautions: Do *not* tap the knee joint through an area of inflammation or cellulitis, to avoid spreading infection into the joint.

If the history is compatible with a diagnosis of hemophilia, the patient should have the clotting abnormality corrected before the joint aspiration is attempted.

Do *not* tap the knee joint if the swelling is *pre*patellar and the peripatellar hollows are visible, because the joint is probably not involved. The bursa itself can be aspirated (See Aspiration of Bursas, page 190).

While the aspirating needle is in the joint, be careful not to gouge the articular cartilage with it.

3. Equipment and Supplies (See Appendix for equipment and supplies manufacturers and suppliers. Appendix is keyed to italicized words in the equipment and supplies lists):

· Disposable waterproof *pads*

· Povidone-iodine *solution* or povidone-iodine scrub *solution*

· 4 × 4-inch sterile gauze *pads* (4–6)

· Sterile towels

· Sterile *gloves*

· 2- to 5-mL *syringe* (See Figure 20-7, page 262)

· 10-mL *syringe* (See Figure 20-7, page 262)

· 25-gauge *needle* (See Figure 20-7, page 262)

· 18- to 20-gauge *needle* (See Figure 20-7, page 262)

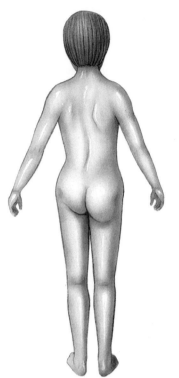 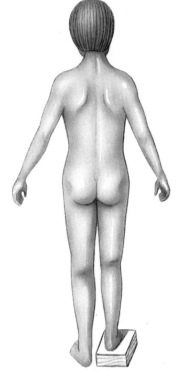

Figure 16-8.
Leg length difference—Standing measurement. Technique.

• 15-gauge *needle* (See Figure 20-7, page 262); if aspiration of blood is a possibility
• *Lidocaine* (1% or 2%), with or without epinephrine
• Sterile saline *solution*
• Culture *tubes* (aerobic, anerobic, fungal, and acid-fast bacillus)
• Collection *tubes* (See Figure 20-7, page 262), for cell count, glucose, and protein determinations
• Sterile adhesive bandage *strip*

4. Description of Procedure:
• Have the patient lie supine and relaxed.
• If the child is young or very anxious, have an assistant hold the leg at the ankle, and another gently hold the hands and talk to the patient.
• STERILE TECHNIQUE IS VERY IMPORTANT—DO NOT BE CASUAL ABOUT PREVENTION OF INFECTION.
• Place an impervious pad beneath the knee.
• If the knee is grossly dirty, clean with scrub solution first, but rinse with saline before using the prep solution, as the soap in scrub solutions can be toxic to deep tissues.
• Using 4-inch × 4-inch sterile gauze pads, prepare

the skin with povidone-iodine solution over an area extending at least 8 inches above and below the knee and to the posterior aspect of the knee medially and laterally.
• Drape with sterile towels above and below and on the sides (one towel should cover the *other* knee in a small child).
• Don sterile gloves.
• Draw up 1 to 2 mL of lidocaine (depending on size of child) in a small (2- to 5-mL) syringe.
• Your best approach is lateral to the patella, to avoid the intra-articular medial fat pad. If another approach is necessary because of inflammation, you can use the superior, inferior, or medial approaches.
• Using a 25-gauge needle, inject an intradermal bleb of anesthetic approximately 1 cm from the patella at your chosen site of entry. Slowly infiltrate the deeper tissues, advancing the needle toward the joint just beneath the patella. Withdraw the needle.
• Aim just beneath (posterior to) the patella, which will be anterior to the femoral condyles (not the tibia). *Do not* attempt to enter the femoral–tibial space, where the

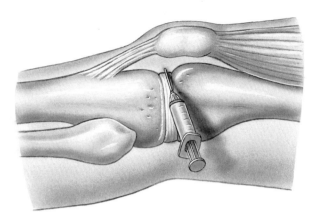

Figure 16-9.
Aspiration of knee joint. Technique.

meniscus can block your needle and the articular carti-lage will be at greater risk.

· Displace the patella laterally toward you with a finger and maintain it in that position. Advance an 18- to 20-gauge needle on a 10-mL syringe through the anesthe-tised track into the joint (Figure 16-9).

· There is usually a "popping" sensation as you move the needle through the capsule into the joint.

· Pull back on the plunger of the syringe. If there is no fluid, advance the needle farther, carefully avoiding dam-aging the articular cartilage. Rotate the needle to clear the bevel. If necessary, inject a small amount (0.5 to 1.0 mL) of sterile saline to clear the needle.

· Withdraw sufficient fluid for analysis—usually 2 to 5 mL. If the effusion or hemarthrosis is large enough to be tense and very uncomfortable, withdraw as much fluid as possible to decompress the joint. Palpation above the patella and from the side opposite the needle can "milk" fluid toward the needle and help you clear synovium that could block the needle.

· Withdraw the needle, using compression with a sterile sponge for hemostasis, and apply a sterile adhesive bandage strip.

· Place the fluid in appropriate tubes. Send the fluid for Gram stain, culture (for aerobes, anerobes, fungi, and acid-fast bacilli) and sensitivities, cell count, and glucose and protein if indicated.

· Record the amount and character of the removed fluid.

5. Side Effects and Complications: Possible complications in-clude allergic reaction to the local anesthetic, hematoma at the needle track site, and infection of a previously uninfected joint.

6. Interpretation: See Table 16-1.

D. Aspiration of Joints Other Than the Knee

The *hip* is a very difficult joint to tap, especially in a small child, and we strongly recommend that the aspiration be done by an orthopedist. This joint aspiration should always be done in the radiology department so that if no fluid is obtained, renografin can be injected and a radiograph or fluoroscopic examination can be done to document that the needle is in the joint.

Elbow, ankle, and *shoulder* joints rarely need aspiration. If they do, an orthopedic consult is appropriate.

E. Aspiration of Bursas

Swollen olecranon and prepatellar bursas (Figure 16-10) oc-cur frequently and may need aspiration to determine if they are infected. Trochanteric bursas at the hip occur but, being deep, are rarely infected and, therefore, rarely need aspira-tion.

1. Purpose: The purposes of the procedure are to determine if a swollen, tender bursa is infected and to relieve pain.

2. Selection of Patients:

a. Indications: Patients with a fluctuant, tender swelling over a bony prominence should be evaluated.

b. Contraindications and Precautions: A *pulsatile* mass, which could be a vascular entity, should not be aspirated; seek a pediatric surgical consult. Differentiate a swollen prepatellar bursa (Figure 16-10), which usually has a definite border, from a knee effusion, in which fluid can be moved from one side of the knee to the other. In addition, if a knee effusion is moderate in size, the fluid will obliterate the normal per-ipatellar hollows. Be very careful not to enter bone or a joint space when aspirating a bursa, so as to avoid spreading a possible infection.

Approach an olecranon bursa from the lateral side to avoid possible injury to the ulnar nerve.

3. Equipment and Supplies (See Appendix for equipment and supplies manufacturers and suppliers. Appendix is keyed to italicized words in the equipment and supplies lists):

· Disposable waterproof *pads*
· Povidone-iodine *solution* or povidone-iodine scrub *solution*
· 4 × 4-inch sterile gauze *pads* (4 to 6)
· Sterile towels
· Sterile *gloves*
· 2-mL *syringe* (See Figure 20-7, page 262)
· 5-mL *syringe* (See Figure 20-7, page 262)
· 25-gauge *needle* (See Figure 20-7, page 262)
· 18- to 20-gauge *needle* (See Figure 20-7, page 262)
· 15-gauge *needle* (See Figure 20-7, page 262), if aspi-ration of blood is a possibility
· *Lidocaine* (1% or 2%), without epinephrine

Table 16-1. Usual Synovial Fluid Findings

	Appearance	Leukocytes Per mm³ (range)	Leukocytes Per mm³ (usual)	Neutrophils Percent (usual)
Normal	Clear, yellow	10–200	<200	<25
Traumatic arthritis	Pink, bloody	2,000–5,000	2,000	<25
Septic arthritis	Turbid	10,000–200,000	75,000	>75
Tuberculous arthritis	Cloudy	2,000–136,000	20,000	<60
Rheumatic fever	Slightly cloudy	1,000–60,000	10,000	<50
Rheumatoid arthritis	Slightly cloudy	5,000–30,000	20,000	<75
Reiters syndrome	Cloudy	2,000–50,000	18,000	>60
Systemic lupus erythematosus	Slightly cloudy	2,000–24,000	3,000	<50
Lyme arthritis	Cloudy	500–76,000	9,000	>75
Kawaski syndrome	Cloudy	20,000–200,000	—	>75

Table prepared by Richard W. Kesler, MD.

- Sterile saline *solution*
- Collection *tubes* (See Figure 20-7, page 262), for cell count, glucose, and protein determinations
- Culture *tubes* (aerobic and anaerobic bacterial, fungal, and acid-fast bacillus)
- Sterile adhesive bandage *strip*

4. Description of Procedure:
- Have the patient lie in an appropriate position (supine for a bursa about the knee, prone with the affected arm overhead or supine with the affected arm across the chest for a bursa about the elbow).
- If the child is young or very anxious, have an assistant hold the leg at the ankle, or the arm at the wrist, and another gently hold the hands and talk to the patient.
- Carefully observe sterile technique.

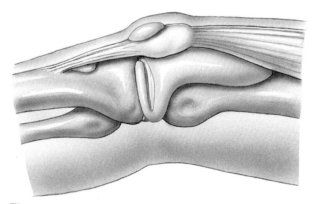

Figure 16-10.
Aspiration of bursa. Anatomy of swollen knee joint and prepatellar bursa.

- Place an impervious pad beneath the limb.
- If the skin is grossly dirty, clean with soap or a scrub solution, then rinse before using prep solution.
- Using 4 × 4 sterile gauze pads, prepare the skin with povidone-iodine solution, extending at least 4 inches around the area to be aspirated.
- Drape with sterile towels around the area.
- Don sterile gloves.
- Draw up approximately 1 mL of lidocaine in a small 2-mL syringe.
- Using the 25-gauge needle, infiltrate intradermally with anesthetic, creating a bleb in the skin over the bursa to be aspirated, injecting very slowly to decrease the pain and maintain a calmer child.
- Insert a 15- to 18-gauge needle attached to a 5-mL syringe into the bursa, and aspirate the contents of the bursa; rotating the needle may clear the bevel of obstructing tissue.
- Withdraw the needle.
- Apply compression with a sterile sponge for hemostasis.
- Then apply a sterile adhesive bandage strip.
- Obtain a Gram stain and culture. A cell count, which helps differentiate infection from rheumatoid arthritis in a joint, is not always necessary for bursa fluid.

5. Side Effects and Complications: Possible complications include formation of a hematoma, infection of a previously sterile bursa, and an allergic reaction to the local anesthetic.

6. Interpretation: The aspiration of purulent material from a bursa may indicate surgical incision and drainage, especially if the pus is thick and can not be fully aspirated.

Clear fluid may represent a sterile bursitis, but fluid culture is still indicated. Treatment of a sterile bursitis includes short-term immobilization and anti-inflammatory medication.

F. Ganglion Aspiration

Symptomatic ganglion cysts can sometimes be aspirated to produce relief of symptoms. Aspiration can be difficult, as the material inside is jelly-like. The relief is often temporary; splinting or surgical resection may be necessary.

1. Purpose: The purpose of the procedure is to provide symptomatic relief and, occasionally, to confirm a clinical diagnosis of ganglion.

2. Selection of Patients:

a. Indications: Patients with a smooth, noninflamed but symptomatic (tender or painful) or enlarging mass, over a tendon or joint, on the dorsum of the wrist or foot may require aspiration of a probable ganglion.

b. Contraindications and Precautions: We recommend against attempting to aspirate volar wrist ganglia—they can be too close to the median nerve. In addition, dorsal ganglia on the radial side may be close to the radial artery, and dorsal ganglia on the proximal foot may be close to the neurovascular bundle (between the anterior tibialis and long extensor tendons).

3. Equipment and Supplies (See Appendix for equipment and supplies manufacturers and suppliers. Appendix is keyed to italicized words in the equipment and supplies lists):

- Disposable waterproof *pads*
- Povidone-iodine *solution* or povidone-iodine scrub *solution*
- 4 × 4-inch sterile gauze *pads* (4 to 6)
- Sterile towels
- Sterile *gloves*
- 2- to 5-mL *syringe* (See Figure 20-7, page 262)
- 10-mL *syringe* (See Figure 20-7, page 262)
- 25-gauge *needle* (See Figure 20-7, page 262)
- 18- to 20-gauge *needle* (See Figure 20-7, page 262)
- 15-gauge *needle* (See Figure 20-7, page 262), if aspiration of blood is a possibility
- *Lidocaine* (1% or 2%), without epinephrine
- Sterile saline *solution*
- Culture *tubes* (aerobic, anerobic, fungal, and acid-fast bacillus)
- Collection *tubes* (See Figure 20-7, page 262), for cell count, glucose, and protein determinations
- Sterile adhesive bandage *strip*

4. Description of Procedure:

- Have the patient lie supine and relaxed.
- If the patient is young or anxious, have an assistant hold the leg at the ankle, and the foot or the forearm above the wrist and the hand, and another hold the other hand(s) gently and talk to the patient.
- STERILE TECHNIQUE IS VERY IMPORTANT; MANY GANGLIA COMMUNICATE DIRECTLY WITH JOINTS; DO NOT BE CASUAL ABOUT PREVENTION OF INFECTION.
- Place an impervious pad beneath the foot or hand.
- If the skin is grossly dirty, clean with soap or a scrub solution; rinse with water or saline before using prep solution.
- Using 4 × 4-inch sterile gauze pads, prepare the skin with povidone-iodine solution, extending at least 4 inches (radius) around the area to be aspirated.
- Drape sterile towels around the area.
- Don sterile gloves.
- Draw up approximately 1 mL of lidocaine in a small 1- to 2-mL syringe.
- Using a 25-gauge needle, infiltrate intradermally, creating a small bleb in the skin over the ganglion.
- Aspirate before injection of anesthetic, to rule out the possibility of intravascular injection. Very slow injection can decrease the painfulness of infiltration and help maintain a calmer child. Infiltrate the skin (and subcutaneous tissue if it is thick) only.
- Using a larger (18- or 20-gauge) needle on a 2- to 5-mL empty syringe, advance the needle through the anesthetized track into the ganglion and aspirate (Figure 16-11).
- After aspiration, withdraw the needle and apply pressure with a dry sterile pad for 1 to 2 minutes for hemostasis.
- Apply a sterile adhesive bandage strip.

5. Side Effects and Complications: Possible complications include allergic reaction to the local anesthesia, hematoma formation, infection, nerve or blood vessel injury, and intravascular injection of local anesthesia with resultant systemic effects or local ischemia.

6. Interpretation: Ganglions are filled with clear jelly-like material that usually has no color. Any material that does not look clear and jelly-like should be submitted to the pathology laboratory for microscopic examination, and a biopsy probably should be done on the mass.

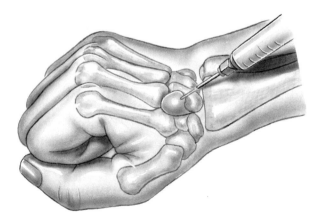

Figure 16-11.
Aspiration of ganglion. Technique.

III. Therapeutic Procedures

First Aid

1. Remember "RICE": **R**est, **I**ce, **C**ompression, **E**levation.

The procedure is applicable to *all* injuries immediately and over the first 24 hours, to keep bleeding and swelling to a minimum.

Rest means limited activity and in the case of lower extremity injuries includes no weight-bearing. Rest can result in decreased bleeding and swelling, less instability of an injured joint, and shorter duration of the recovery period.

"**Ice**" can be a commercial coldpack, ice cubes (mixed with a small amount of water to keep the temperature at approximately 0–4°C and prevent skin freezing), or a bulk pack (bag) of frozen vegetables(!) if nothing else is available. Use "ice" 10 to 20 minutes at a time and repeat as often as every 1 to 2 hours.

Compression is best maintained with an elastic bandage, wrapped figure-of-eight fashion (avoid direct circumferential wraps), with more tension at the end of the limb and less toward the hip or shoulder. *Don't* pull the bandage to maximum stretch; about one quarter (less tension) to one half (more tension) of the available stretch will do. Rewrap every several hours.

Elevation of the injured part above the *heart* is best. An injured ankle should be on several pillows, above the knee, which should be above the hip with the individual supine. An injured elbow should be above the shoulder. An individual with an injured shoulder should be sitting, or semisitting, or reclining on the unaffected side. Proper positioning minimizes swelling.

2. Heat: Application of heat to an injured area increases local circulation, and if the injury is recent (less than 24–48 hours) local heat increases swelling. Heat therefore should *not* be used to treat acute injuries.

After 48 hours, heat treatment can aid in mobilizing edema and speed local healing by increasing metabolism. "Moist" and "dry" heat are equally effective.

The combination of *ice* massage followed by *stretching* and exercise is more effective in decreasing swelling and restoring function than dependent soaking in warm water, and the therapeutic use of heat will be most effective *if* delayed until the *rice* approach has achieved full range of motion and no further swelling is occurring.[8]

A. Crutch Fitting and Use

Fitting of crutches and training in their use is most frequently done by a physical therapist, but in many physicians' offices and emergency rooms, physical therapists are not immediately available. The procedure detailed here can guide your initial instructions in such a situation. If the patient appears insecure or there is no time to instruct them in use of the crutches on ramps, steps, (both up and down), and over rugs, a follow-up appointment with a physical therapist is recommended.

1. Purpose: The purpose of this procedure is to enable a patient to walk with partial weight or no weight on an injured limb.

2. Selection of Patients:

a. Indications: All children aged 3 years or older who require protection of a lower limb from full weight-bearing are candidates. Two-year-olds, and some 3- and 4-year-olds, have difficulty with crutches, but may be able to handle a pick-up walker.

b. Contraindications and Precautions: Crutches may be contraindicated in children under 3 years of age or in children who are otherwise unreliable, and in children not able to demonstrate the ability to use the crutches on all surfaces.

If in doubt about the patient's stability, arrange for wheelchair use or assess the parents' ability to carry the younger child.

We do not recommend that you teach single-crutch use, which is appropriate in only a few cases and should be taught by a therapist.

3. Equipment and Supplies (See Appendix for equipment and supplies manufacturers and suppliers. Appendix is keyed to italicized words in the equipment and supplies lists):

· Adjustable wooden or aluminum axillary *crutches*, with adjustable handles.
· Rubber *tips* for bottom ends of crutches
· Rubber *pads* for tops of crutches (optional)
· Rubber *pads* for hand grips of crutches (optional)

4. Description of Procedure:

a. Fitting:

(1) With the patient standing and the crutch tip placed 5 to 6 inches lateral and 5 to 6 inches anterior to the patient's foot (the "starting position"), have the upper edge of the crutch three fingerbreadths beneath the axilla, leaning against the patient's lateral chest wall (Figure 16-12).

(2) Be sure both crutches are adjusted to the same height.

(3) Adjust the handle of the crutch so that when the hand is on the crutch in the above-described "starting" position, the elbow is flexed at approximately 10 to 15 degrees.

b. Gait:

There are many varieties of crutch gaits. The most basic of the gaits for patients who can bear full weight on one lower limb is the "three-point non–weight-bearing gait." It is

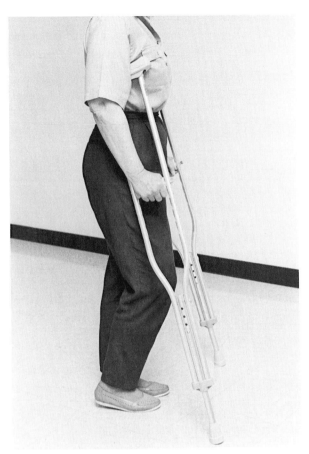

Figure 16-12.
Crutch fitting and use. Fitting technique.

the easiest to teach, but it has the disadvantages of instability, fatigue of muscles holding up the protected or "storked" leg, and promotion of atrophy and contractures on the non–weight-bearing side. Two alternatives are a "touchdown–non–weight-bearing" ("heel–toe non–weight-bearing gait"), and a "three-point partial–weight-bearing gait." Both of these are useful only in reliable children older than approximately 8 years. The latter gait is useful only for those patients who can safely put some weight on their limb. A "four-point partial–weight-bearing gait" can be used by patients who can not take full weight on either lower limb.

The three-point non–weight-bearing gait:

· Have a patient, standing on the sound leg, put both properly fitted crutches forward 8 to 12 inches, depending on the patient's height (Figure 16-13A).
· Have the patient place weight onto his or her hands by extending the elbows, pick up and swing forward the

sound leg, and land with the sound leg *in front of* the crutches (Figure 16-13B). The crutch tips and the sound foot should form a triangle on the floor at the beginning and the end of the step to provide anteroposterior stability. (If the sound leg and crutch tips form a straight line, the patient can fall forward or backward.) (Figure 16-13C).

· The tops of the crutches are held against the chest wall with no leaning (no weight taken in the axilla), and the arms are kept as straight as possible while weight is on them.
· Have the patient practice several steps in one direction, turn around, and take several steps in the opposite direction. Have her take steps on smooth and carpeted surfaces if possible.
· Have the patient also practice sitting down (approach the chair closely [Figure 16-14A], pivot around on the normal foot, take the crutches from under the arms, move one crutch to the other hand and hold both together, reach for the chair arm with the free hand [Figure 16-14B], and sit [Figure 16-14C]) and standing up again (reverse the procedure).
· Alternative gaits should be taught by a physical therapist or physical therapy aide.

B. Slings

Basic Sling

1. Purpose: The purpose of the basic sling is to contribute to the support and immobilization of an injured arm, to take the weight of the arm off an injured or painful shoulder, or to decrease the dependent edema in an injured forearm or hand.

2. Selection of Patients:

a. Indications: Patients with injury to the shoulder, arm, or hand may benefit.

b. Contraindications and Precautions: None

3. Equipment and Supplies (See Appendix for equipment and supplies manufacturers and suppliers. Appendix is keyed to italicized words in the equipment and supplies lists):

· The best *slings* currently available are commercially made. They are much more comfortable than the alternative "old-fashioned" triangle-bandage sling, are relatively inexpensive, and are available in various sizes. They come with "package directions" for application and adjustment.
· An alternative is the muslin *bandage,* triangular, 24 inches in its longest dimension.

4. Description of Procedure: If the commercial sling is not available, use the triangle sling.

· Place the long side of the bandage vertically along the anterior midline of the patient, with the point of the

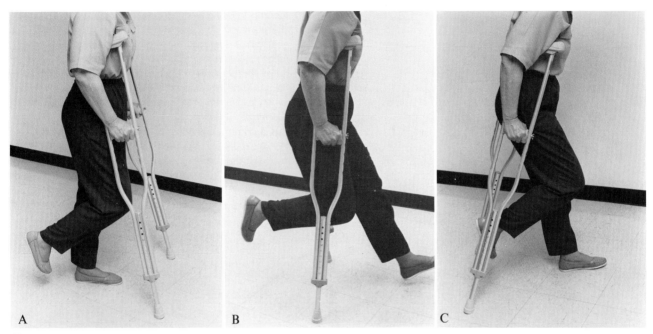

Figure 16-13.
Crutch fitting and use—The three-point non–weight-bearing gait. Technique.

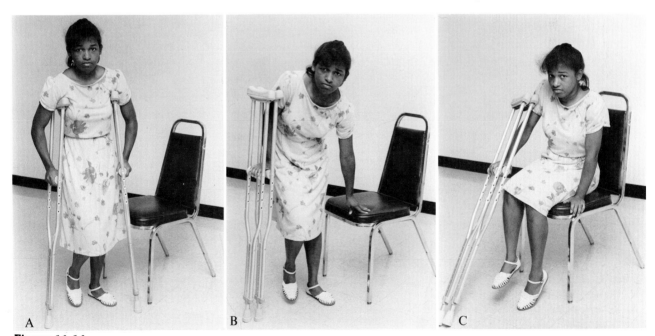

Figure 16-14.
Crutch fitting and use—Sitting. Technique.

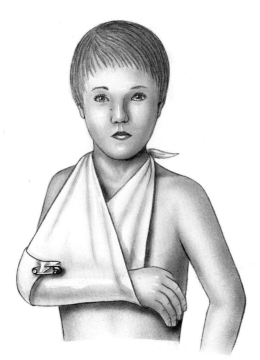

Figure 16-15.
Basic sling. Technique.

triangle beneath the elbow of the injured arm and the upper "tail" of the bandage over one shoulder (Figure 16-15).

· Bend the patient's elbow to 90 degrees and bring the lower "tail" of the bandage over the other shoulder. Be sure the edge of the sling is at the distal metacarpal level of the hand, to support the wrist. If this part of the sling is too short, the hand can "droop" over the edge and become swollen in an inactive patient.

· Tie the tails in a square knot behind the neck.

· Fold the point of the bandage behind the elbow and pin to the sling.

5. Side Effects and Complications: Complications include discomfort and skin pressure problems beneath the knot.

Sling and Swathe

1. Purpose: The purpose of the "swathe," an addition to a sling, is to secure the supported arm to the body, limiting rotation at the shoulder.

2. Selection of Patients:

a. Indications: All patients for whom shoulder rotation or elevation would be painful or harmful (e.g., a patient with a humeral fracture) might benefit.

b. Contraindications and Precautions: None

3. Equipment and Supplies (See Appendix for equipment and supplies manufacturers and suppliers. Appendix is keyed to italicized words in the equipment and supplies lists):

· The best sling and swathe are commercially available. Instructions are included in the package.

· An alternative is a muslin triangle sling plus a 3- or 4-inch elastic *bandage, or* a 4-inch sterile gauze *bandage, or* an additional muslin bandage, *or* a tube stockinette.

4. Description of Procedure:

Using a commercial sling and swathe, do the following:

· Place the sling over the injured arm, allowing the hand to extend at the buckle end of the sling (Figure 16-16). Attach the shoulder strap to the buckle at the top of the sling. Then bring the swathe strap (attached to the elbow end of the sling) around the child's body and

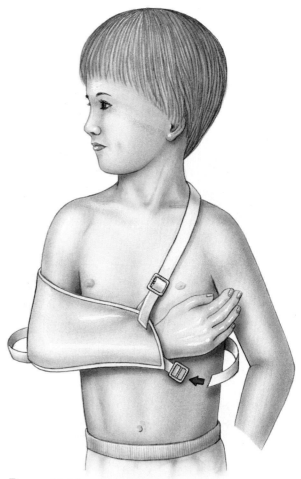

Figure 16-16.
Sling and swathe. Technique with commercially available equipment.

buckle the strap to the lower buckle (at the hand).
· If a commercial sling and swathe are not available, do the following:

After the basic sling is applied, wrap the arm to the trunk with the elastic bandage (pulling only approximately one third of the available stretch in the bandage, i.e., not too tightly) or with gauze, or fold the muslin bandage to approximately a 4- to 5-inch width and tie around the arm and trunk (Figure 16-17).

5. Side Effects and Complications: Maceration of the skin where skin touches skin, e.g., in the axilla, can occur if the swathe remains damp from perspiration or bath water. The maceration can be avoided by using an absorbent pad in the axilla if necessary or by daily damp sponging of the skin followed by careful drying.

Stockinette Sling and Swathe

1. Purpose: The purpose of the stockinette sling and swathe is to secure the supported arm to the body. In addition, it is difficult for an active child to wiggle out of this sling and swathe.
2. Selection of Patients: (See Basic Sling, page 194)
3. Equipment and Supplies (See Appendix for equipment and supplies manufacturers and suppliers. Appendix is keyed to italicized words in the equipment and supplies lists):
· Cotton tube *stockinette:* 2- to 3-yard length; 2-inch

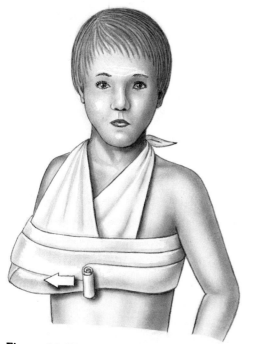

Figure 16-17.
Sling and swathe. Technique.

width for toddlers, 3-inch width for most children, 4-inch width for large adolescents
· Bandage *scissors*
· Large safety *pins,* at least 21

4. Description of Procedure:
· Cut a 3- to 5-inch longitudinal slit in the stockinette at a location about one third of the way from one end.
· Place the stockinette on the injured arm like a long glove, putting the hand through the slit in the direction of the longest end of the stockinette (Figure 16-18). The slit should end up at the shoulder.
· Place the short upper end of the stockinette around behind the neck and down the front of the chest.
· Cut a slit at the wrist in the "glove" portion, to allow the hand out.
· Bend the elbow to 90 degrees and support the wrist with the end of the stockinette on the chest (Figure 16-18). Bring the end of the stockinette around the wrist and pin it to itself to provide support.
· Bring the "hand" end of the stockinette around the trunk, between the elbow and the trunk, and around the arm just above the elbow, and pin it to itself.
· The stockinette will stretch; instruct the family in unpinning, taking up any slack gently, and repinning.

5. Side Effects and Complications: Maceration of the skin where skin touches skin, e.g., in the axilla, can occur if the stockinette remains damp from perspiration or bath water. The maceration can be avoided by using an absorbent pad between the stockinette and the skin if necessary or by daily damp sponging of the skin followed by careful drying. Possible neurovascular compromise at the wrist or elbow can occur if the wrap is too tight.

Figure-Eight Dressing, for Clavicle Fractures

1. Purpose: The purpose of the procedure is to reduce and hold clavicle fractures.
2. Selection of Patients:
a. Indications: Most patients with a minimally displaced clavicle fracture are more comfortable in a sling and swathe, but if there is significant over-riding of fracture ends and some reduction is desired, a figure-eight dressing is appropriate.
b. Contraindications and Precautions: A figure-eight dressing is not usually necessary in infants because of their significant remodeling potential; a stockinette sling and swathe or pinning the sleeve to the front of the garment works well.
3. Equipment and Supplies (See Appendix for equipment and supplies manufacturers and suppliers. Appendix is keyed to italicized words in the equipment and supplies lists):
· Figure-eight *dressing*—commercially available or
· 3- or 4-inch tube *stockinette*
· ½-inch-thick orthopedic *felt*
· Bandage *scissors* (See Figure xx-xx, page xxxx)
· Safety *pins*

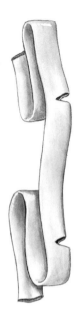
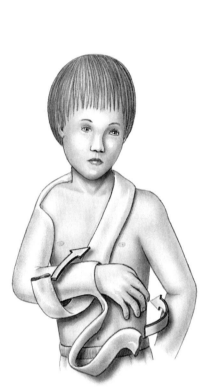
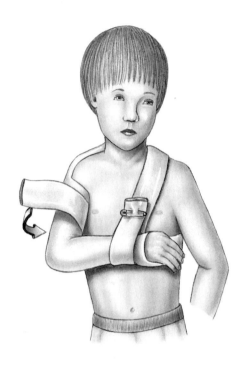

Figure 16-18.
Stockinette sling and swathe. Technique.

4. Description of Procedure:
Using a commercial figure-eight splint, do the following:
• Place the unbuckled splint between the patient's scapulae, and bring each strap over the proper shoulder, beneath the axilla from the front, and back to the midline, where it is buckled (Figure 16-19).
• Adjust the buckling to allow a finger to fit comfortably beneath the splint.
If a commercial dressing is not available, do the following:
• Cut two strips of felt (1 to 3 inches wide and 5 to 8 inches long) to fit from in front of to under or in back of the axilla.
• Cut a length of stockinette to go around both shoulders and to overlap in the back (Figure 16-20).
• Place one strip of felt into each end of the stockinette so that the center ends of the felt are 3 to 8 inches apart (depending on the size of the patient) (Figure 16-20). Have the patient bring the shoulders back as far as possible.

• Position the bandage around the shoulders and through the axilla, meeting between the scapulae. The enclosed felt strips should be positioned anteriorly and rest over the anterior axillary folds.
• Pin the ends of the stockinette to the middle of the stockinette.
5. Side Effects and Complications: Possible complications include neurovascular compromise from excessive pressure. Skin rashes or maceration can occur.

C. Compression Wrapping
1. Purpose: The purposes of compression wrapping are to decrease edema in an injured limb and to secure splints or dressings on an injured limb.
2. Selection of Patients:
a. Indications: The procedure is indicated for patients with an injury to a limb.
b. Contraindications and Precautions: The procedure cannot

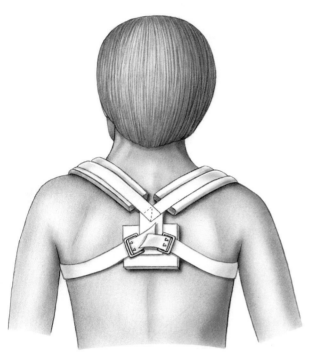

Figure 16-19.
Figure-eight dressing for clavicular fractures. Technique
with commercially available equipment.

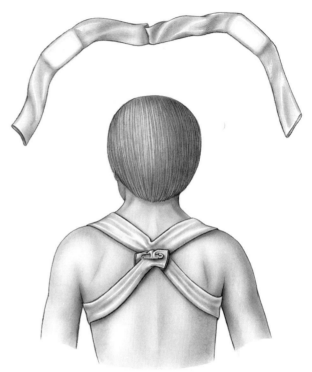

Figure 16-20.
Figure-eight dressing for clavicular fractures. Technique.

be relied on for immobilization of a joint unless used with a
splint. Although it may be therapeutic for first-degree ligament
sprains (tear of some but not all fibers of the ligament, manifested by joint tenderness without joint instability or effusion), it is *not* appropriate for second-degree ligament sprains
(tear of most of fibers of the ligament plus some joint capsule,
manifested by moderate joint instability and joint effusion or
hemarthrosis) or third-degree ligament sprains (complete
tear of the ligament and joint capsule, manifested by major
joint instability and hemarthrosis).

3. Equipment and Supplies (See Appendix for equipment
and supplies manufacturers and suppliers. Appendix is keyed
to italicized words in the equipment and supplies lists):

 • Commercially available elastic bandage *rolls* (2-, 3-, or
 4-inch).

4. Description of Procedure:

a. Ankle wrap:

 • Have the patient sit, holding the ankle at neutral position (with the help of an assistant's hand under the
 metatarsal heads if necessary) (Figure 16-21).
 • Use a 2- or 3-inch bandage for a small child and a 4-
 inch bandage for an adolescent. Holding the bandage at
 the left of the foot and so that the end comes from

underneath the roll, start the wrapping on the dorsum
of the foot.

 • Stretch the bandage no more than one half to two
 thirds of its total available stretch, and wrap it in a
 "figure-eight" manner, obliquely toward the ankle,
 around, and back to the foot.
 • Avoid transverse circumferential wraps. Overlap one
 half of the width of the previous wrap, and cover the
 foot and the ankle from just proximal to the base of the
 toes to 4 to 6 inches above the malleoli.
 • Secure the ends with the hooks attached to the wrap
 or with tape.
 • Removing and rewrapping: If the bandage has attached
 hooks, bend that end of the bandage backward to re-
 roll. This allows the hooks to be in the proper position
 when the bandage is reapplied.

b. Wraps for other joints:

 • For the wrist, use a 2- or 3-inch bandage; for the elbow,
 a 3- or 4-inch bandage; and for the knee, a 4- or 6-inch
 bandage.
 • The same wrapping principles are used: wrap
 obliquely, overlap one half of the previous wrap, and do

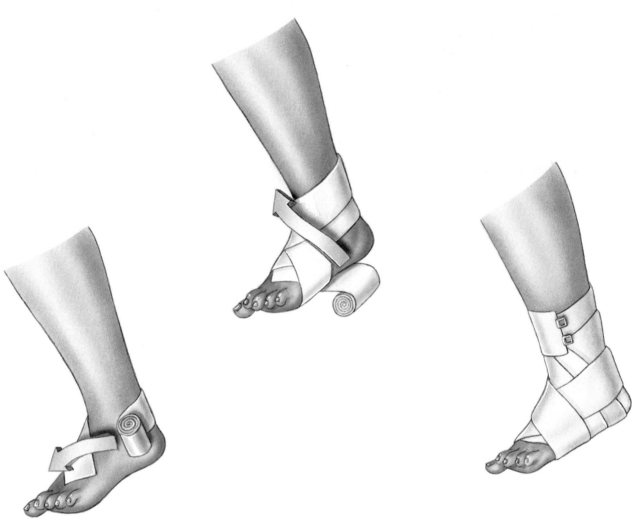

Figure 16-21.
Compression wrapping—Ankle wrap. Technique.

not stretch more than one half to two thirds of the available stretch.

5. Side Effects and Complications: Skin rashes, maceration, or ischemia can occur if the wrap is left in place for more than 24 hours without being rewrapped. Neurovascular compromise can result if the limb is wrapped too tightly, or further swelling occurs beneath the wrap. Removal of the wrap and rewrapping are indicated if any digits become swollen or numb, the capillary refill time exceeds 3 seconds, or the bandage slips or its edges become rolled.

D. Splinting

1. Purpose: The purpose of a splint is to immobilize an injured or inflamed joint.

2. Selection of Patients:

a. Indications: Patients with swollen, painful, or injured joints or limbs are candidates.

b. Contraindications and Precautions: Neurovascular compromise can occur with restrictive splints. Splinting of patients with second-degree or third-degree sprains (See Compression Wrapping, page 198) or possible fractures should be temporary, until consultation with an orthopedist is possible.

3. Equipment and Supplies (See Appendix for equipment and supplies manufacturers and suppliers. Appendix is keyed to italicized words in the equipment and supplies lists):

  • *Splints* made of canvas and felt are commercially available in various sizes for the knee and ankle. Available metal splints, except for aluminum *splints* for fingers, are useful *only* as temporary emergency splints. Padded aluminum *splints* are available for fingers. Plaster *splints* can be made easily and adapt to any joint. Inflatable *splints* for ankles and knees are very useful.

· Plaster *bandages* or *splints* (2-inch, 3-inch, 4-inch, or 6-inch)
· Universal *scissors*
· Cotton *padding*
· Water bucket
· Sterile gauze *bandage* (3- to 4-inch)
· Elastic *bandage*

4. Description of Procedure:

a. Elbow, Knee, Ankle (Posterior Splint):

· Use at least 10 to 15 thicknesses of plaster as wide as half the circumference of the joint, and long enough to reach from just below the axilla, groin, or knee to just above the wrist, ankle, or toes, respectively.

· Lay out two layers of cotton padding slightly longer than the splint length (Figure 16-22).

· Dip the plaster in a water bucket, pull the plaster over the edge of the bucket or rub it between your fingers to mesh the layers together, and lay the plaster on the padding.

· Cover the outside of the plaster with two additional layers of padding (Figure 16-22). Alternatively, the dry plaster may be pulled into a piece of tube stockinette of the same width as the plaster and slightly longer; the plaster-containing stockinette is then dipped in water. The padding prevents the subsequently applied bandage from adhering to the splint. A splint *not* stuck to the bandage allows you to inspect the skin and rewrap the

bandage if there is a painful fold or wrinkle or if the wrap is too tight.

· Before the plaster dries, apply the splint along the dorsal surface of the arm or leg (Figure 16-23). Leave the splinted elbow at 90-degree flexion and the forearm in neutral between pronation and supination. Have the splinted knee in slight (5–10-degree) flexion. Have the ankle splinted at a 90-degree angle.

· Wrap the splint into place with the gauze bandage, using the figure-eight technique described previously (See Compression Wrapping, page 198). Be careful not to pull the wrap too tightly, which would make the edges constricting.

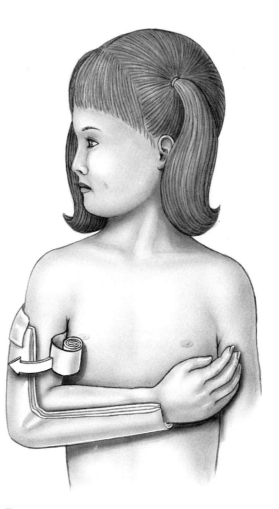

Figure 16-23.
Splinting—Posterior splint (elbow). Technique for applying the splint.

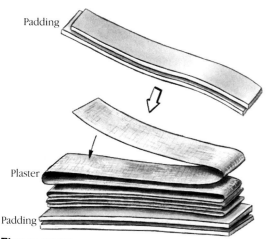

Figure 16-22.
Splinting—Posterior splint. Technique for preparing the splint.

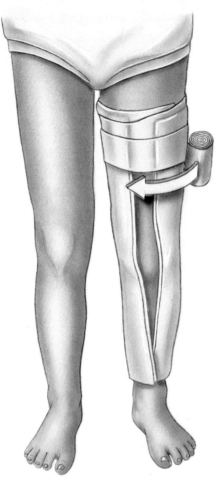

Figure 16-24.
Splinting—Medial and lateral splints (knee). Technique.

· Reinforce the wrap with elastic bandage if necessary (e.g., for swelling), wrapping figure-eight style and not too tightly (See Compression Wrapping, page 198).

b. Alternative splints for the knee (medial and lateral splint):

· The advantage of medial and lateral splinting is better resistance to flexion of the joint.

· The same process as above is used, but use a width that is less than half the circumference, and make two splints. Apply as shown in the illustration (Figure 16-24), overlapping the ends of the splints anteriorly and posteriorly on the distal leg. Have the splint extend proximally to 1 to 2 inches from the groin and distally to 1 to 2 inches above the malleoli.

· At the knee, the Jones compression dressing (See page 203) may allow you to provide better support, especially if the joint is swollen.

c. Forearm and Wrist (Volar splint):

· Apply the splint similarly to the posterior splint (See page 201). With the wrist in 20 degrees of dorsiflexion, apply the splint to the volar forearm and proximal palm (Figure 16-25). Keep the distal end of the splint proximal to the distal palmar crease to allow full flexion of the metacarpal–phalangeal joints. Mold over the thenar eminence to allow oppositon of the thumb to at least the index finger.

d. Fingers (Volar or dorsal splint):

· Use ½- or ¾-inch foam-padded aluminum splints. They are easily bent into the desired shape and you can trim them with scissors.

· Bend the splint to conform to the position of function of the splinted joint (20–30 degrees of flexion for the metacarpal–phalangeal joints and interphalangeal joints, and 20–30 degrees of dorsiflexion for the wrist).

· For a distal interphalangeal joint, cut the splint to the length from just distal to the proximal interphalangeal (PIP) joint to the tip (Figure 16-26).

· If a PIP joint is to be splinted, cut the splint to the length of the finger from the web space to the tip (Figure 16-27).

· For a metacarpal–phalangeal joint, include the wrist and stabilize it with a plaster volar splint over the aluminum one (Figure 16-28).

· Tape with ½-inch tape to the finger at each segment.

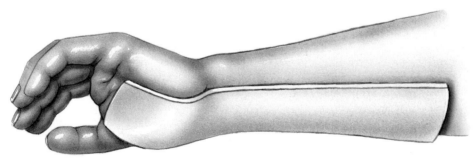

Figure 16-25.
Splinting—Volar splint (forearm and wrist). Technique.

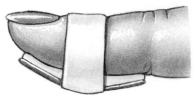

Figure 16-26.
Splinting—Volar splint (distal interphalangeal joint).
Technique.

e. Toes ("Buddy" taping):
   · Put a 2 × 2-inch dry gauze bandage between the toes. Tape the injured toe to the adjacent longer toe, if possible.
5. Side Effects and Complications: Skin rashes, maceration and irritation, or ischemia can infrequently occur.

E. Neck Collars
1. Purpose: The purpose of the procedure is to support a *mildly* injured neck.
2. Selection of Patients:
a. Indications: Patients with muscular spasm or neck pain *without* signs of neurologic deficit may benefit.
b. Contraindications and Precautions: Patients with signs or symptoms of neurologic deficit need a *firm* collar for immobilization *and* emergency evaluation.
3. Equipment and Supplies (See Appendix for equipment and supplies manufacturers and suppliers. Appendix is keyed to italicized words in the equipment and supplies lists):
   · Commercially available "firm" and soft *collars* come in various sizes. Alternatives:
      — Hand towel (home variety) of terry toweling, approximately 15 inches by 24 inches or
      — Orthopedic felt, ½ inch,
      — Tube stockinettes, 4- or 5-inch diameter.
      — Bandage *scissors*
   and
      — Large safety pins

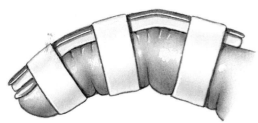

Figure 16-27.
Splinting—Dorsal splint (proximal interphalangeal joint).
Technique.

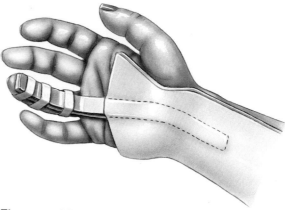

Figure 16-28.
Splinting—Volar splint (metacarpal–phalangeal joint).
Technique.

4. Description of Procedure:
a. Towel collar:
   · Fold the towel by thirds, longwise (Figure 16-29A).
   · Wrap the towel around the neck, overlapping it to fit snugly (Figure 16-29B).
   · Pin the towel in place (Figure 16-29C).
b. Felt collar:
   · Cut a piece of felt to size (4–5 inches shorter than the tube stockinettes to be used). The width should be equal to the distance between the medial end of the clavicles and the tip of the chin. The length should be equal to the circumference of the neck.
   · Place the felt inside a doubled tube stockinette created by pulling one tube stockinette inside another.
   · Overlap around the neck and pin.

F. Jones' Compression Dressing for a Knee
1. Purpose: The purpose of the procedure is to provide compressive immobilization of an injured knee, to help prevent swelling, and to hasten resolution of existing intra-articular effusion or extra-articular swelling of the limb.
2. Selection of Patients:
a. Indications: Patients with an injured thigh, knee joint, or proximal leg may benefit.
b. Contraindications and Precautions: Wrapping too tightly may lead to nerve or vascular compromise.
3. Equipment and Supplies (See Appendix for equipment and supplies manufacturers and suppliers. Appendix is keyed to italicized words in the equipment and supplies lists):
   · One roll (box) of Red Cross cotton *batting* (8–10 inches × 6–8 feet)
   · Elastic *bandages*—one 4-inch and two 6-inch (for ad-

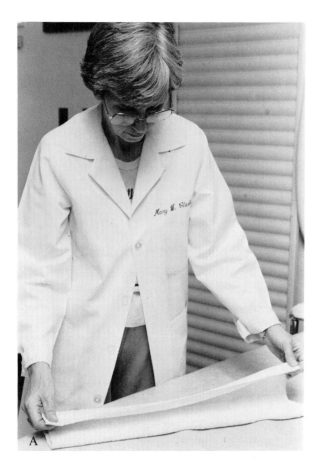

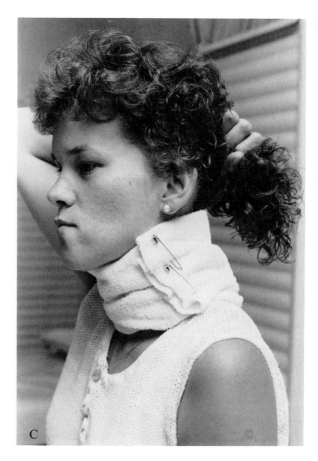

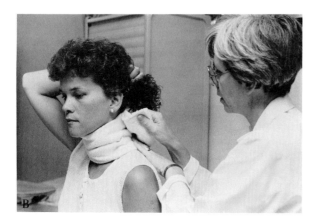

Figure 16-29.
Neck collars—Towel collar. Technique.

olescent or large child); one 3-inch and two 4-inch (for small child)
· Dressing supplies, for any open wound on the leg
4. Description of Procedure:
· Have the patient lie supine.

· Dress any open wound (See Minor Pediatric Surgical Procedures, page 217).
· Have an assistant hold the injured limb in the air by supporting the ankle. Have the patient's knee in maximum comfortable extension.

• Wrap the cotton batting around the limb, beginning at the ankle; wrap obliquely, overlapping about ½ the width of the cotton, all the way to the groin (Figure 16-30A).

• Using the larger elastic bandages (4–6-inch), begin *above* the ankle malleoli and wrap proximally over the cotton, pulling about two thirds to three quarters of the available stretch, and overlapping one third to one half the width of the wrap (Figure 16-30B). You will probably need two bandages. Stop 1 inch below the groin and roll the cotton back over the elastic edge (Figure 16-30C).

• Use the smaller elastic bandages (3- or 4-inch) and wrap the ankle in the usual ankle wrap (See page 200) (Figure 16-30C). You can rewrap as needed without re-doing the larger dressing.

5. Side Effects and Complications: Possible complications include neurovascular compression from tight wrapping or from progressive swelling. Skin rashes, maceration, or ischemia can occur.

G. Taping Techniques

"Taping" for support after injury or prophylactically for athletics is a specialized skill, best performed after much practice. Instructions are available in detail in many publications; one excellent source is *The Injured Athlete* by Daniel Kulund.[8]

H. Relief Padding for Pressure Areas

An irritated area of skin needs protection if the source of irritation (e.g., a shoe) is continuous. The best protection is "relief" in the sense that orthotists (brace makers) use the term: distributing pressure *around* the area relieves the pressure on the area itself.

Use adhesive-backed padding of some kind around the area, usually as a doughnut shape with a central hole cut to the size of the area to be protected. If over a bony prominence (e.g., a malleolus), the height (thickness) of the padding, when compressed, must be higher than the prominence.

1. Purpose: The purpose of relief padding is to relieve pressure from an irritated area of skin.

2. Selection of Patients:

a. Indications: Patients with red or blistered areas (frequently patients with insensitive skin, or dancers, gymnasts, or other athletes) benefit.

b. Contraindications and Precautions: None

3. Equipment and Supplies (See Appendix for equipment and supplies manufacturers and suppliers. Appendix is keyed to italicized words in the equipment and supplies lists):

• Bandage *scissors*
• Adhesive-backed *"moleskin"*
• *Benzoin*

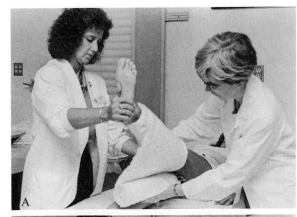

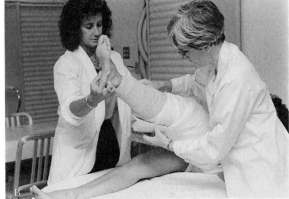

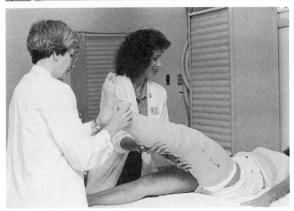

Figure 16-30.
Jones compression dressing for a knee. Technique.

4. Description of Procedure:

• Cut a circle of moleskin at least 2 to 3 cm greater in diameter than the area to be protected.

• Cut a central hole the *same size* as the area to be protected.

• Apply benzoin lightly to the skin *around* the area.

• Apply the moleskin; add layers of the same size until any prominence of skin or bone through the central hole is no longer prominent beyond the top of the padding when compressed (Figure 16-31). If desired, the top may be covered by a final layer without a central hole; leave the backing of the moleskin on the central area to prevent adherence to the lesion.

  • Instruct the parents to change the padding daily.

5. Side Effects and Complications: Blistering or an allergic response to the benzoin or the adhesive occurs unusually.

I. "Pyramid Dressing"

1. Purpose: The purposes of this dressing are to relieve *shear* stresses on skin, especially insensate skin and to prevent or heal pressure sores.

2. Selection of Patients:

a. Indications: Patients with grade 1 (reddened skin area, with or without superficial ulceration, of the epidermis only) or grade 2 (an open wound into subcutaneous fat, but not deeper) pressure areas may benefit.

b. Contraindications and Precautions: None

3. Equipment and Supplies (See Appendix for equipment and supplies manufacturers and suppliers. Appendix is keyed to italicized words in the equipment and supplies lists):

  • Bandage *scissors*
  • *Benzoin*
  • Adhesive-backed *foam,* ½-inch thick
  • Dressings if necessary

4. Description of Procedure:

  • Clean the wound if necessary; clean and dry the skin around the wound.

  • Apply benzoin for 2 to 3 cm around the wound.

• Cut three circles from the foam: one 4 to 6 cm larger in diameter than the wound; the others successively smaller by about 2 cm in diameter.

• Cut a central hole in all the foam pieces to match the size and shape of the wound as closely as possible (Figure 16-32).

• Apply the largest piece of foam around the wound; this is the bottom layer of the pyramid. Put the other two layers on top, matching the central holes carefully.

• If a dressing is necessary, place a gauze, dry or moistened with saline or other desired solution, in the central hole.

• Do *not* tape over the pyramid, unless you do so very loosely, without compressing the foam. Compressive taping decreases the dressing's ability to dissipate the shear forces that can damage the skin.

5. Side Effects and Complications: Rashes from the benzoin or adhesive may occur. The dressing frequently shifts or loosens; it must be reapplied one to three times per day, depending on the site.

J. Reductions

Radial Head Subluxation ("Pulled" or "Nursemaid's" Elbow)[9]

This injury usually involves a toddler and occurs when the child's arm is pulled suddenly overhead, often with the forearm in pronation (as in helping a child down a step) (Figure 16-33A). With the injury, the distal edge of the annular ligament slips partially over the radial head (Figure 16-33B). Pain and unwillingness to use the arm result. The displaced ligament often spontaneously reduces; but if not, a reduction without anesthesia can almost always be accomplished by manipulation in the office.

1. Purpose: The purpose of the procedure is reduction of radial head subluxation.

2. Selection of Patients:

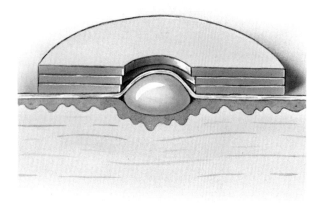

Figure 16-31.
Relief padding for pressure areas. Technique.

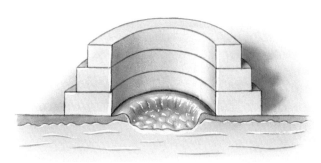

Figure 16-32.
Pyramid dressing. Technique.

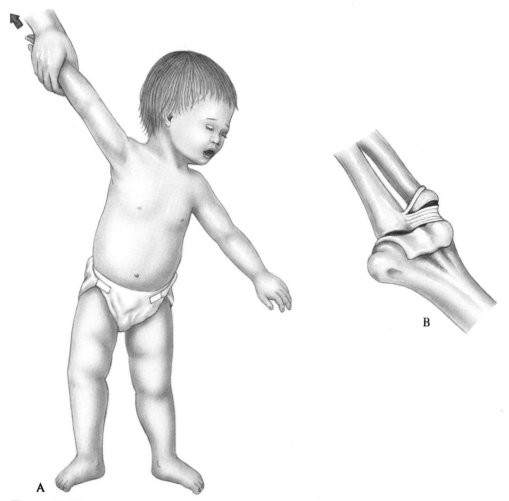

Figure 16-33.
Radial head subluxation (nursemaid's elbow). A, Typical pronation of forearm and direction of force creating injury. **B,** Anatomy.

a. Indications: Patients, usually 2 to 4 years of age (has been reported in patients 2 months to 7 years of age), with a typical history of a sudden longitudinal pull on the forearm (usually pronated) will benefit.

b. Contraindications and Precautions: A fracture or infection should be ruled out by careful palpation. With radial head subluxation, there should be localized tenderness lateral at the elbow over the radial head only. Palpation around the olecranon should reveal no palpable effusion in the elbow joint.

3. Equipment and Supplies: None
4. Description of Procedure:

• Tell the family the child will feel momentary pain followed, usually immediately, by the complete relief of discomfort.

• Have the patient sit on someone's lap, preferably a parent's.

• Sit in front facing the patient, and make eye contact, talk, and otherwise distract the patient.

• Hold the extended forearm distally with your hand (right hand for injured right elbow, left for left), placing the thumb of your other hand laterally over the radial head.

• Quickly supinate the forearm (turn the palm up) with

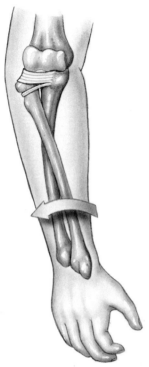

Figure 16-34.
Radial head subluxation (nursemaid's elbow). Standard technique.

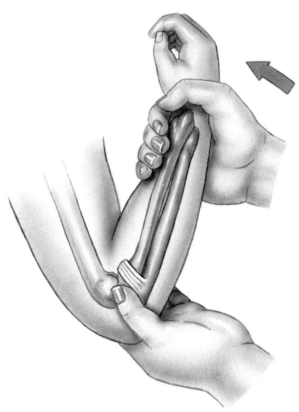

Figure 16-35.
Radial head subluxation (nursemaid's elbow). Alternative technique.

the hand that is on the patient's forearm. This may produce the "click" of reduction and provide relief of pain (Figure 16-34).

· If reduction was not achieved, flex the elbow, keeping the forearm supinated, and proceed to hyperflex beyond 100 degrees if necessary, pushing with your thumb over the radial head until a click is heard or felt (Figure 16-35). Some suggest you try a similar maneuver but rotate the forearm into full pronation rather than hyperflexion.

· With reduction the patient often immediately resumes full use of the arm, but the elbow sometimes remains painful. Support of the arm with a sling or sling and swathe (See pages 194 and 196) for 1 or 2 days may be appropriate.

5. Side Effects and Complications: A 5% to 30% recurrence rate is reported. There are no known long-term complications.

References

1. Weinstein SL. Adolescent Idiopathic Scoliosis, published by The University of Iowa, Iowa City. Sponsored by: American Academy of Orthopedic Surgeons and Scoliosis Research Society, 1988.

2. Bunnel WP. An objective criterion for scoliosis screening. J Bone Joint Surg 1984; 66A:1381–7.

3. Orr HW. On the Contributions of HO Thomas, Sir Robert Jones and John Ridlon, M.D. to Modern Orthopedic Surgery. Springfield, IL, Charles C. Thomas, 1949, pp 95–96.

4. Hoffer MM. Joint motion limitation in newborns. Clin Orthop 1980; 148:946.

5. Trendelenburg F, Deutsch, Med. Wschr. *21;* 21–4, 1895; *in* Rang M. Anthology of Orthopaedics. Edinburgh: Churchill Livingstone, Edinburgh, 1966, 139–43.

6. Hardcastle P, Nade S. The significance of the trendelenburg test. J Bone Joint Surg 1985; 67B:741–6.

7. Morscher E, Figner G. Measurement of leg length. In: Progress in Orthopaedic Surgery, Hungerford DS, ed. New York: Springer Verlag, 1977; pp 22–23.

8. Kulund D. The Injured Athlete. 2nd ed. Philadelphia: Lippincott, 1988.

9. Wilkins KE. Fractures in Children. Rockwood CA, Wilkins KE, King R, eds. Vol 3 of *Fractures*. Philadelphia: Lippincott, 1984, pp 556–62.

Chapter 17

Neurologic Procedures

Frank T. Saulsbury

I. Diagnostic Procedures

A. Transillumination

1. Purpose: Transillumination of the skull is a simple, non-invasive technique that is helpful in diagnosing a variety of conditions associated with increased fluid in the cranium. Such conditions include hydrocephalus, hydrencephaly, porencephaly, cerebral atrophy, and subdural effusion or hygroma.

2. Selection of Patients:

a. Indications: Successful transillumination is predicated on light passing through the skull. Calvaria greater than 2.5 mm thick do not transmit light. Under normal circumstances, the skull reaches 2.5 mm in thickness by 6 to 12 months of age; thus, transillumination is useful primarily in infants less than 1 year of age. Young infants with signs or symptoms suggestive of hydrocephalus, hydrencephaly, porencephaly, cerebral atrophy, subdural effusion, or hygroma are candidates.

b. Contraindications and Precautions: None

3. Equipment and Supplies (See Appendix for equipment and supplies manufacturers and suppliers. Appendix is keyed to italicized words in the equipment and supplies lists):

- A dark room
- A transilluminating light source. The Chun Gun, which has been shown to provide reproducible results,[1,2] can be used. This device delivers a constant bright light while dissipating heat. However, this instrument is no longer manufactured. Less cumbersome *transilluminators* (Figure 17-1) are easier to use, but normal values for transillumination with such devices are not available.

4. Description of Procedure:

- Infants should be studied in a completely darkened room.
- Allow 30 seconds for dark adaptation by the examiner.
- Apply the light source snugly to the area of the skull

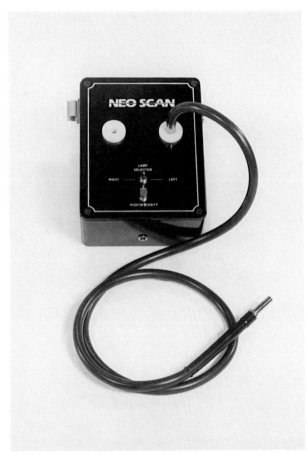

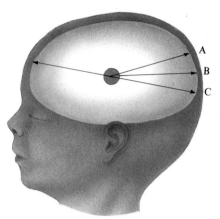

Figure 17-2.
Transillumination. Options for measuring the size of the rim of transillumination: **A,** Radius as measured from the center of the light beam to the outermost rim of transillumination **B,** Distance from the rim of the beam to the outermost rim of transillumination **C,** Diameter of the area of transillumination.

Figure 17-1.
Transillumination. Equipment and supplies: Examples of a transilluminating device (Neoscan).

to be examined, including the frontal, parietal, and occipital areas bilaterally as well as directly over the anterior and posterior fontanelles.

· The size of the rim of transillumination in each area should be measured. Some suggest measuring the radius of the area of transillumination (from the center of the light beam to the outermost rim of transillumination) or the distance from the rim of the beam to the outermost rim of the transillumination[1] (Figure 17-2). Others suggest measuring the diameter of the area of transillumination[2] (Figure 17-2).

5. Side Effects and Complications: None

6. Interpretation: Any asymmetry in the transillumination suggests an abnormality. Excessive, symmetric transillumination may also be abnormal. Cheldelin et al[1] reported normal values using the Chun Gun for transillumination of three areas

of the skull in children up to 18 months of age (Table 17-1). Likewise, Swick et al[2] reported normal values using the Chun Gun for skull transillumination for premature infants (Table 17-2). Increased transillumination is usually due to increased intracranial fluid. False-positive results may be seen in infants with subcutaneous fluid collections such as caput succedaneum, cephalohematoma, or intravenous fluid infiltration. False-negative results from transillumination may be seen in infants with skull thickness greater than 2.5 mm.

B. Lumbar Puncture

1. Purpose: Lumbar puncture is the safest and easiest procedure to obtain cerebrospinal fluid (CSF) for analysis.

2. Selection of Patients:

a. Indications: Lumbar puncture can be performed on children of any age. The procedure is indicated in children with signs or symptoms of central nervous system infections such as meningitis or encephalitis. It also may be a useful diagnostic adjunct in children with undiagnosed encephalopathy or with suspected subarachnoid bleeding. It is also used for administration of intrathecal chemotherapeutic agents.

b. Contraindications and Precautions: Lumbar puncture is contraindicated in children with increased intracranial pressure owing to space-occupying lesions. Under such circumstances, there is danger of herniation of cranial contents when spinal fluid is removed. Conversely, increased intracranial pressure owing to meningitis should not preclude the performance of a diagnostic lumbar puncture.

Lumbar puncture should not be performed through infected overlying skin.

Table 17-1. Normal Values for Transillumination of the Skull in Infants

Age	No. of Subjects	Frontal		Parietal		Occipital	
		cm	1 SD	cm	1 SD	cm	1 SD
Newborn	50	5.4*	0.4	4.8	0.4	4.5	0.5
Two months	50	5.6	0.6	5.1	0.5	5.4	0.7
Four months	50	5.7	0.7	5.0	0.3	5.1	0.5
Six months	50	5.5	0.6	5.0	0.5	5.1	0.5
Nine months	50	5.7	0.7	5.0	0.7	5.0	0.5
Twelve months	25	5.7	0.3	5.1	0.4	5.2	0.5
Eighteen months	25	5.4	0.4	4.9	0.5	4.7	0.5

* Distance as measured from center of light beam.

From Cheldelin LV, Davis PC Jr, Grant WW. Normal values for transillumination of skull using a new light source. J Pediatr 1975;87:937–8; with permission.

Lastly, lumbar puncture should not be performed in patients with severe, uncontrolled bleeding abnormalities.

3. Equipment and Supplies (See Appendix for equipment and supplies manufacturers and suppliers. Appendix is keyed to italicized words in the equipment and supplies lists):

- Disposable *lumbar* puncture set. Most hospitals and clinics stock sets that contain most of the necessary equipment:
  - Antiseptic solutions (povidone-iodine and isopropyl alcohol [70%])
  - Sterile drapes
  - A short-beveled needle with stylet (Figure 17-3). Twenty- or 22-gauge needles are used depending on the size of the patient. The selected length of the

needle (1½–2 inches) also depends on the size of the patient.
- A manometer (Figure 17-3)
- A three-way stopcock (Figure 17-3)
- Four sterile test tubes with stoppers (Figure 17-3)
- Sterile *gloves*
- *Lidocaine* (1%)

4. Description of Procedure:

Cooperation is seldom forthcoming from infants and children about to have a lumbar puncture. Therefore, adequate restraint is essential to maintain the proper position of the child and to insure the accurate identification of important landmarks. Sedation of the child, however, is rarely, if ever, necessary.

Table 17-2. Normal Values for Transillumination of the Skull in Premature Infants

Location	Gestational Age			
	30–32 wk (no = 8)	33–34 wk (no = 20)	35–36 wk (no = 36)	>36 wk (no = 31)
Anterior fontanelle				
Major axis (cm)	6.5 ± 1.6*	7.4 ± 0.9	7.7 ± 0.7	7.8 ± 0.9
Minor axis (cm)	5.9 ± 1.7	6.5 ± 0.7	6.8 ± 0.5	6.9 ± 0.7
Frontotemporal				
Major axis (cm)	5.8 ± 1.0	6.6 ± 0.6	6.6 ± 0.4	7.0 ± 0.7
Minor axis (cm)	5.2 ± 0.9	5.9 ± 0.5	6.1 ± 0.4	6.3 ± 0.6
Parieto-occipital				
Major axis (cm)	5.7 ± 1.2	6.5 ± 0.7	6.6 ± 0.5	6.8 ± 0.7
Minor axis (cm)	5.1 ± 1.1	5.8 ± 0.6	6.0 ± 0.6	6.3 ± 0.7

* Mean values ± 95% confidence limits.

From Swick HM, Cunningham MD, Sheild LK. Transillumination of the skull in premature infants. Pediatrics 1976; 58:658-64; with permission.

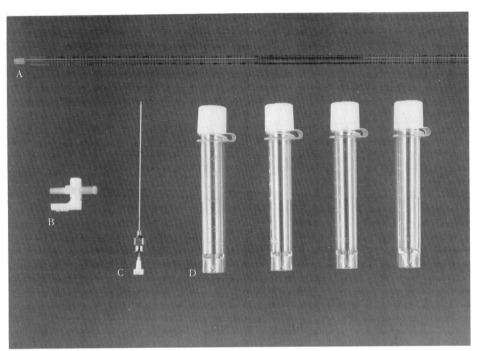

Figure 17-3.
Lumbar puncture. Equipment and supplies: **A,** Manometer; **B,** Three-way stopcock; **C,** Short-beveled needle with stylet; and **D,** Sterile test tubes with stoppers.

The position of the patient should be dictated by the mutual comfort of the patient, the assistant, and the operator. Under most circumstances, the lateral decubitus position is preferred (Figure 17-4). The patient is placed on his side with his back at the edge of and perpendicular to a firm supporting surface. The assistant restrains the patient by directing one arm under the flexed knees and the other arm around the neck and shoulders. In addition to restraint, the assistant will help maintain the lumbar spine in flexion, thereby widening the spaces between the lumbar spinous processes.

The sitting position is feasible for small infants who are unable to struggle and in older children who are cooperative and need no restraint. The small infant is restrained in the sitting position by grasping an elbow and knee in each hand and flexing the back (Figure 17-5). The older, cooperative child in the sitting position should be requested to lean his shoulders forward, thus arching his back toward the operator and widening the lumbar interspinous spaces.

  • Prepare the skin with appropriate antiseptic solutions, don sterile gloves, and drape the patient with sterile towels.
  • The preferred site for lumbar puncture is the L3–L4 interspace, located at the point at which an imaginary line drawn between the superior edges of the iliac crests crosses the spine (Figure 17-6). The interspace above and below may also be used.
  • Local anesthetic (lidocaine [1%]) infiltration of the skin and subcutaneous tissues is desirable in older children but is seldom necessary in small infants.
  • At this point, the operator should make certain that the assistant has the patient properly positioned. Less than ideal positioning increases the likelihood of an unsuccessful or complicated procedure.
  • The needle, with stylet in place (omission of the stylet may increase the chance of carrying a fragment of skin into the spinal canal, which could lead to the formation of a spinal epidermoid tumor), is inserted into the interspinous space in the midline and angled slightly cephalad. Proper alignment of the needle is aided by placing the tip of the inverted thumb of the non-inserting hand on the spinous process above the interspinous space being entered (Figure 17-7).
  • The needle is advanced slowly in the midline. A loss of resistance may be felt when the needle penetrates the ligamentum flavum (a longitudinal structure lying dorsal to the spinal cord). A second "give" or "pop" may be

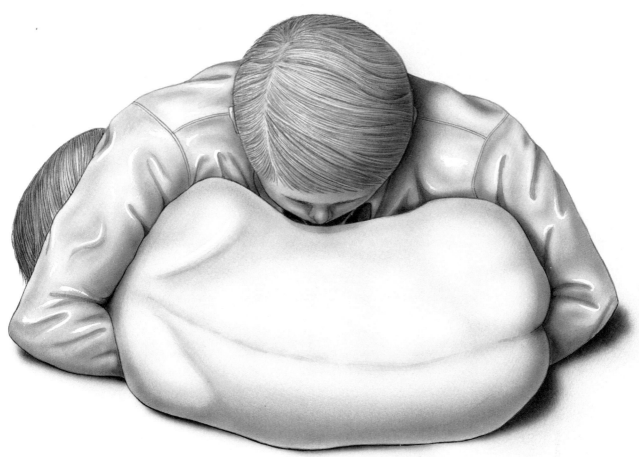

Figure 17-4.
Lumbar puncture. Lateral decubitus position.

noted when the needle penetrates the dura (Figure 17-8). These changes in resistance are not always felt, especially in infants.

· At this point, remove the stylet and observe for spinal fluid. If none is visible, rotate the needle 90 degrees in an attempt to free the opening of the needle tip from any occluding tissue. If no fluid is forthcoming, replace the stylet and advance the needle very slightly, rechecking for flow as before.

· When free flow of spinal fluid is established, the manometer is attached to the needle hub by means of a three-way stopcock. Fluid is allowed to fill the manometer and the height of the column is recorded. Normal pressure is 50 to 180 mm H_2O. The accurate measurement of pressure is possible only in the relaxed, cooperative patient. It is a worthless and virtually impossible measurement to perform in the crying, struggling infant.

· Aliquots of fluid are then collected in sterile tubes and sent for appropriate chemical, cytologic, and microbiologic tests. Ordinarily, the last tube, the least likely to be contaminated with red cells, is sent for cell count.

5. Side Effects and Complications: There are very few side effects of a properly performed lumbar puncture in patients without the previously outlined contraindications to the procedure. Although post–lumbar puncture headache may be encountered in adults and older children, this is rarely observed in younger children and infants. If headache occurs, maintenance of the patient in the recumbent position and administration of mild analgesics are all that are usually necessary.

Meningitis may result from a lumbar puncture performed through infected or inadequately prepared skin or from a lumbar puncture performed on a young infant with bacteremia.[3]

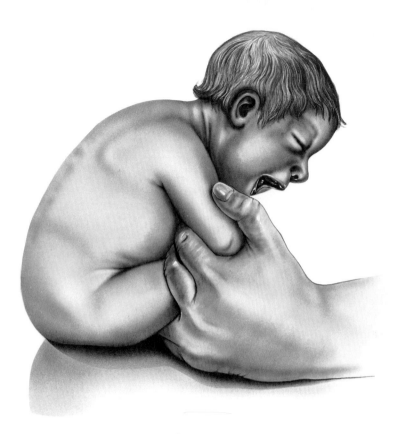

Figure 17-5.
Lumbar puncture. Sitting position
(feasible for small infants).

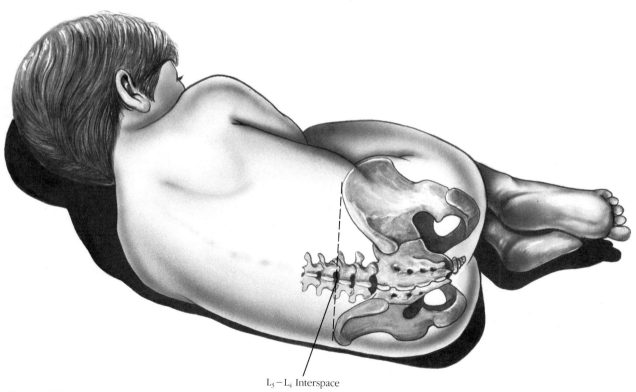

L₃ – L₄ Interspace

Figure 17-6.
Lumbar puncture. Technique for locating the preferred site (L3–L4 interspace).

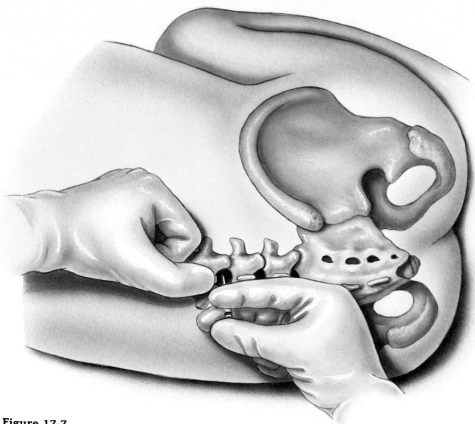

Figure 17-7.
Lumbar puncture. Technique for proper alignment of the spinal needle.

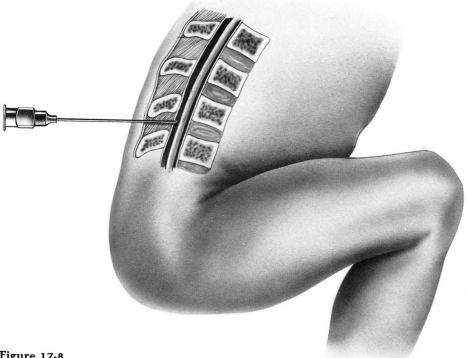

Figure 17-8.
Lumbar puncture. Proper position of the spinal needle in the spinal canal.

Table 17-3. Normal Values for Cerebrospinal Fluid Measurements

CSF Measurement	Newborn	Infant	Older Child
Pressure (mm H$_2$O)	50–90	40–150	70–200
Protein (mg/dL)	20–150	10–20	20–40
Glucose (mg/dL)	At least 50% of serum glucose at all ages		
Red blood cells (per μL)	0–500	0–5	0–5
White blood cells (per μL)			
Polymorphonuclear	0–5	0	0
Mononuclear	0–25	0–10	0–10
Total	0–30	0–10	0–10

6. Interpretation: Normal cerebrospinal fluid should be clear and colorless. Xanthochromia beyond the neonatal period is abnormal and is due to an elevation of spinal fluid protein (usually above 300 mg/dL) or bilirubin. Bloody spinal fluid may be the result of traumatic lumbar puncture or a recent subarachnoid hemorrhage. The two conditions can be distinguished by centrifuging the fluid and examining the supernatant. In traumatic taps, the supernatant is usually clear, and the amount of blood decreases in successive tubes. In subarachnoid hemorrhage, the supernatant is xanthochromic, and the amount of blood is constant in successive tubes. Normally, the spinal fluid contains no red blood cells and few, if any, white blood cells. A few hundred white or red cells will produce a slightly opalescent appearance to the fluid. Cloudy, white fluid indicates large numbers of white blood cells, as occurs in purulent meningitis.

The normal values for a number of cerebrospinal fluid measurements are shown in Table 17-3. Of note, the cerebrospinal fluid protein may normally exceed 50 mg/dL in infants up to 5 months of age.

References
1. Cheldelin LV, Davis PC, Grant WW. Normal values for transillumination of skull using a new light source. J Pediatr 1975; 87:937–8.
2. Swick HM, Cunningham MD, Sheild LK. Transillumination of the skull in premature infants. Pediatrics 1976; 58:658–64.
3. Teele D, Dashefsky B, Rakusen T, Klein JO. Meningitis after lumbar puncture in children with bacteremia. N Engl J Med 1981; 305:1079–81.

Chapter 18

Minor Pediatric Surgical Procedures

Eugene D. McGahren

Bradley M. Rodgers

I. Therapeutic Procedures

This chapter will describe the evaluation and treatment of minor pediatric surgical problems that are commonly encountered by the physician providing general medical care for children. These problems and their associated therapeutic interventions can be addressed with local anesthesia, perhaps with slight sedation in small children, and with follow-up care at home.

A. General Considerations

Proper Set-up. The patient must be comfortable, a sterile field must be easily maintained, and instruments must be easily accessible. An assistant and supportive medications should be available.

Patient Preparation. After a thorough history and physical examination have been completed, the patient and parents should have the risks and benefits of each procedure fully explained. Most older children prefer an explanation of what to expect for each step of the procedure. A written consent should be obtained before the procedure. The presence of parents during the procedure may have a calming influence on smaller children.

Patient Exam. Local anesthesia may be needed before the completion of the examination of a lesion or wound to allow better exploration. However, whenever the neurovascular status is in question, this examination must be completed before administration of anesthesia.

Procedure. The procedure should begin only after obtaining a proper history and completing an examination. Adequate anesthesia must be achieved. Sterile technique is always observed.

Dressings. Dressings are applied as appropriate to the wound. Initial dressings should remain in place 24 to 48 hours after the procedure and parents should receive specific instructions for care of the dressing and wound.

Follow-up. Return appointments are arranged before discharge.

B. Local Anesthesia

1. Purpose: Local anesthesia is administered for minor injuries for two reasons: a more complete examination is possible when there is less pain, and local anesthesia allows pain-free treatment.

2. Selection of Patients:

a. Indications: Virtually all minor procedures will require local anesthesia (Table 18-1). Additional sedation may be useful for smaller children (Table 18-2).

b. Contraindications and Precautions: If neurovascular injury is suspected, it must be assessed before the use of local anesthesia.

A careful history of allergies must be obtained before administration of any medication. Amide-linked anesthetics (lidocaine, mepivacaine, bupivacaine) are not necessarily cross-reactive with those containing para-aminobenzoic acid esters (procaine, chloroprocaine, tetracaine). For example, in a patient with a history of allergic reactions to lidocaine, one would not expect reactions from procaine anesthetic. Allergic signs and symptoms include rashes, urticaria, wheezing, and rarely, anaphylaxis. Allergic reactions may usually be treated with diphenhydramine (Benadryl) (2 mg/kg, intravenously) or epinephrine (1:1000, 0.01 mL/kg, with maximum dose of 0.3 mL). Toxic symptoms include drowsiness, coma, and seizures.

The physician should also inquire about a history of familial malignant hyperthermia. If a suggestive history is obtained, the ester-type local anesthetic agents are preferred (procaine, chloroprocaine, tetracaine). Dantrolene sodium should be available for intravenous administration in these patients (2–4 mg/kg).

Do not exceed maximum doses of local anesthetics.

Anesthetics containing epinephrine should be avoided for procedures involving digits, the nose, ear lobes, and genitals. These areas tend to have poor collateral blood flow and may suffer ischemic necrosis with the vasospasm induced by epinephrine.

Observe the patient for 1 to 1½ hours after infiltration for any adverse effects.

The use of TAC (tetracaine, adrenalin, and cocaine) topical anesthesia has potential significant adverse side effects that contraindicate its use in the pediatric patient.

3. Equipment and Supplies (See Appendix for equipment and supplies manufacturers and suppliers. Appendix is keyed to italicized words in the equipment and supplies lists):

· Local anesthetic (See Table 18-1, this page)
· 6-mL *syringe* (See Figure 20-7, page 262)
· 25- to 27-gauge *needle* (See Figure 20-7, page 262)

4. Description of Procedure: Methods include local infiltration and digital block.

a. Local infiltration:

· If a wound is to be anesthetized, place a few drops of anesthetic in the wound, and then infiltrate the edges with a 25- or 27-gauge needle attached to a 6-mL syringe. Advance the needle through the areas already anesthetized. Aspirate before injection to avoid intravascular administration.

· If the anesthesia is for removal of a lesion, try not to distort the anatomy.

b. Digital block:

· This technique may be less painful than local infiltration.

· Raise a dermal wheel of local anesthesia on the medial and lateral borders of the base of the proximal phalanx (Figure 18-1).

· Use a 27-gauge needle to infiltrate the deeper tissues in this region to the level of the periosteum, aspirating before injecting to avoid injection into the digital artery or vein.

· Avoid too much anesthetic, as this may cause a tourniquet effect with vascular occlusion and ischemic necrosis of the distal digit. For the same reason, never completely encircle a digit with local anesthesia.

· One to two milliliters of anesthetic agent should be

Table 18-1. Local Anesthetics

Name	Maximum Dose (mg/kg)	Onset of Action	Duration of Action (minutes)
Lidocaine (Xylocaine)	4	Fast	60–120
Bupivacaine (Marcaine)	3	Medium	180–600
Procaine (Novocaine)	11	Slow	30–45
Mepivacaine (Carbocaine)	4	Fast	90–180
Tetracaine (Pontocaine)	2	Slow	180–600
Chloroprocaine (Nesacaine)	11	Fast	30–45
Prilocaine (Citanest)	8	Fast	180–600

Table 18-2. Selected Agents for Sedation of Children for Outpatient Procedures

Drug	Route	Recommended Dose (mg/kg)	Maximum Total Dose	Dosage Schedule (minutes before procedure)
Chloral hydrate*	Oral	75.0	1.0 g	30–45
	Rectal	75.0	1.0 g	30–45
Midazolam†	Oral	0.3		10–15
	Rectal (in 5.0 mL saline)	0.3		10–15
	Intramuscular	0.05–0.15	5.0 mg	10–15
	Intravenous	0.02–0.04	0.2 mg/kg	Every 2–3 minutes until sedation achieved
Morphine‡	Intramuscular	0.1		20–30

* An occasional child will sleep up to 6 to 8 hours after drug administration.

† An occasional child will be resistant to the sedative effects. Respiratory depression and apnea can be associated with intravenous use.

‡ All narcotics cause dose-dependent respiratory depression. Naloxone hydrochloride should be immediately available; an initial dose of 0.01 mg/kg is given intravenously for morphine overdosage. If no response ensues, a subsequent dose of 0.1 mg/kg can be administered. Alternatively, the drug can be given intramuscularly or subcutaneously.

sufficient for a digital block. Test the effectiveness of the block by pricking the distal portion of the digit with the injection needle.

5. Side Effects and Complications: Complications include intravenous injection of the anesthetic agent, allergic reaction to the agent, and tourniquet effect of a circumferential injection of a digit.

C. Laceration Care

1. Purpose: Clean lacerations are repaired to expedite healing and minimize scarring. While any laceration could theoretically heal by secondary intention, that approach is only appropriate for contaminated wounds.

2. Selection of Patients:

a. Indications: Most simple lacerations can be treated in an outpatient setting.

b. Contraindications and Precautions: One must determine that deeper injuries are absent. Signs of a deeper injury might be detected in the initial neurovascular examination. Nonetheless, all lacerations should be carefully explored throughout their depth to evaluate deeper structures. Lacerations to

be sutured must be less than 6 hours old (less than 12 hours if on the face) and not the result of bites (except perhaps animal bites of the face). Antibiotics and tetanus prophylaxis will be needed in many cases. Animal bites may require rabies vaccination.

3. Equipment and Supplies (See Appendix for equipment and supplies manufacturers and suppliers. Appendix is keyed to italicized words in the equipment and supplies lists):

- Local anesthetic (See Table 18-1, page 218)
- 6-mL *syringe* (See Figure 20-7, page 262)
- 25- to 27-gauge *needle* (See Figure 20-7, page 262)
- Cleansing soap
- Sterile saline *solution*
- Povidone-iodine *solution*
- Sterile *gloves*
- Drapes
- 2 × 2- and 4 × 4-inch gauze *pads*
- Iris *scissors* (Figure 18-2)
- *Forceps* with teeth (Figure 18-2)
- Scalpel *handle* (Figure 18-2)
- Scalpel *blades* (no. 11, no. 15) (Figure 18-2)
- Needle *holder* (Figure 18-3)

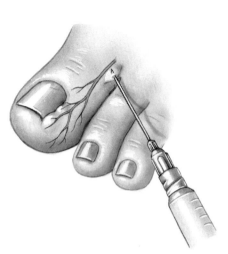

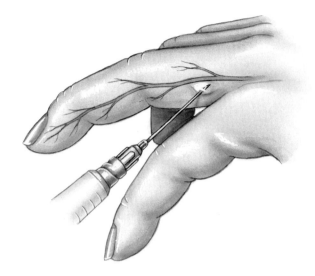

Figure 18-1.
Local anesthesia—Digital block. Technique.

- *Suture* material (Table 18-3)
- Suture *scissors* (Figure 18-3)
- Skin closure *strips* (Figure 18-3)
- *Benzoin*
- Surgical marking *pen*

- Antibacterial *ointment*
- Antibacterial impregnated *gauze*
- Adhesive *tape*
- Sterile conforming gauze *bandage*
- Hydrogen peroxide *solution*

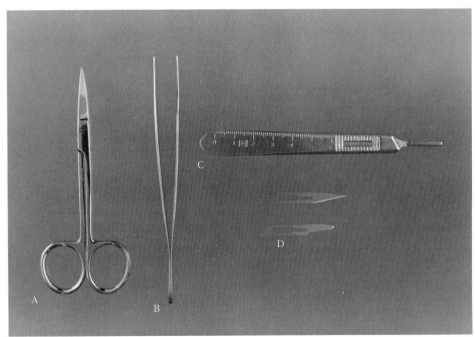

Figure 18-2.
Laceration care. Equipment and supplies: **A,** Iris scissors; **B,** Forceps with teeth; **C,** Scalpel handle; **D,** Scalpel blades (no. 11 and no. 15).

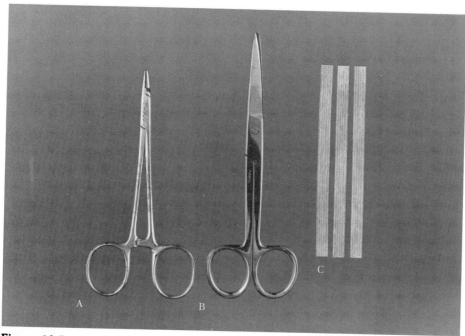

Figure 18-3.
Laceration care. Equipment and supplies: **A,** Needle holder; **B,** Suture scissors; **C,** Skin closure strips.

a. Types of sutures:

(1) Absorbable: These sutures are used for closure of subcutaneous tissues. They may occasionally be used for skin closure for a very small laceration in a noncosmetic area, (e.g., perianal region) when suture removal would present difficulties. They are also used for mucous membrane closure in the mouth.

(2) Nonabsorbable: Generally, this is a monofilament nylon with a cutting needle used for skin closure. It is minimally reactive. Silk should not be used for skin closure because of its reactivity. Silk holds knots well and is used to ligate blood vessels.

b. Types of suture needles:

(1) Tapered: This needle tapers to a sharp point, but does not have sharp cutting edges. It is used for closure of most deeper layers and the subcutaneous tissue, but not for

Table 18-3. Suture Material

Suture	Component	Manufacturer	Structure	Absorption	Uses
Silk	Silk	Ethicon	Braided	Nonabsorbable	Ligature
Ethilon	Nylon	Ethicon	Monofilament	Nonabsorbable	Skin
Plain Gut	Gut	Davis-Geck Ethicon	Monofilament	Absorbable (7 d)	Mucous membrane
Chromic Gut	Gut	Davis-Geck Ethicon	Monofilament	Absorbable (14 d)	Mucous membrane
Dexon	Polyglycolic acid	Davis-Geck	Braided	Absorbable (21 d)	Subcutaneous, mucous membrane
Vicryl	Polygalactin	Ethicon	Braided	Absorbable (21 d)	Subcutaneous
PDS	Polydioxamone	Ethicon	Monofilament	Absorbable (28 d)	Muscle, fascia

closure of the skin. The dermal tissue is too resistant for this needle to penetrate without excess pressure.

(2) Cutting: This needle tapers to a point, but also has sharp cutting edges. It is used for closure of the skin, as the cutting edges facilitate penetration of the tough dermal tissue.

4. Description of Procedure:
   · Achieve local anesthesia (See Local Anesthesia, page 218).
   · Scrub the wound with cleansing soap and saline, and then irrigate copiously with sterile saline.
   · Prepare the entire area with 2 × 2 gauze pads saturated with povidone-iodine and drape as a sterile field.
   · Don sterile gloves.
   · Examine the wound to be sure no significant underlying structures are damaged.
   · Remove all devitalized tissue. If contaminated or devitalized, sharply debride the edges of the wound with iris scissors or a scalpel to provide cleaner margins for closure.
   · Achieve hemostasis with digital pressure or suture ligature with silk. Secure the suture ligature by placing two bites of suture through the bleeding tissue in "figure-eight" fashion (Figure 18-4).
   · In placing stitches at any level, follow the curve of the needle during suture placement so as to avoid any excess trauma or tearing of the tissue. Accomplish this by gently rotating the needle holder in the direction of the needle with the wrist, as the needle is passed through the tissue.

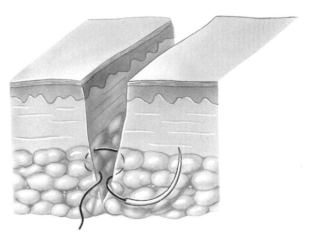

Figure 18-5.
Laceration care—Subcutaneous suture. Technique.

· If a layered closure is needed to obliterate the deeper dead spaces within the wound, first approximate the subcutaneous tissue with absorbable suture. Place these stitches perpendicular to the skin edges and with the knot buried (Figure 18-5).
· In cosmetic areas (e.g., the face) closely place simple interrupted sutures of 5–0 or 6–0 material.
· Wounds closed under tension require larger sutures (4–0). The type of closure depends on the location and strength needed.

a. Types of closures:
   (1) Simple interrupted: This method is used for cosmetic closures on the face and wounds with minimal tension and good natural skin apposition. Place simple interrupted sutures at right angles to the skin edges (Figure 18-6).
   · You should enter and exit the sutures 2 to 3 mm from the skin edges and place them approximately 4 to 5 mm apart. Extend the "bite" of the suture 2 to 3 mm into the subcutaneous tissue.
   (2) Vertical mattress: This method is used for added strength and enhanced eversion of the skin edges. It is particularly good in areas where there is a lot of skin movement and in areas of thick skin such as the back, the soles of the feet, the scalp, and the palms of the hands.
   · Place vertical mattress sutures perpendicular to the skin edges (Figure 18-7). These sutures must take deeper "bites" of the skin edges to achieve approximation.
   (3) Skin closure strips: These reinforced pieces of sterile tape can be used in place of sutures to approximate wound edges that are under minimal tension. Small shallow wounds with clean edges, particularly on the face and neck, are ideal wounds for this technique (Figure 18-8).

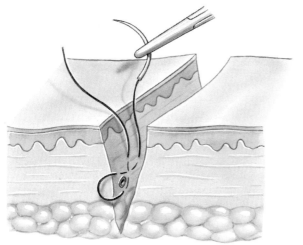

Figure 18-4.
Laceration care—Hemostasis. Technique.

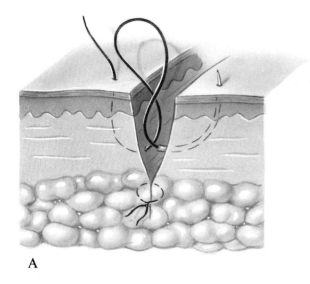

A

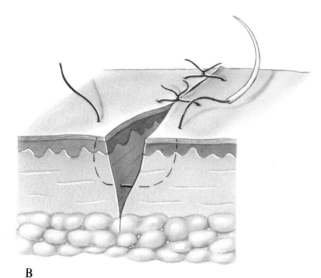

B

Figure 18-6.
Laceration care—Simple interrupted suture skin closure.
Technique.

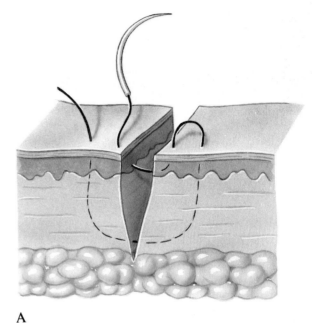

A

B

Figure 18-7.
Laceration care—Vertical mattress suture skin closure.
Technique.

Often you can use skin closure strips to reinforce wounds after skin sutures have been removed. Apply skin closure strips after benzoin has been placed on the skin surrounding the wound, and allow them to peel off on their own after 7 to 10 days.

- Remove sutures at a time to maximize healing and minimize scar:
  - Face: 3 to 5 days
  - Scalp: 7 to 10 days
  - Trunk: 7 to 10 days
  - Limbs: 10 to 14 days

b. Specific injury considerations:
  (1) Scalp:
  - Clip only enough hair to allow good visualization of the wound. Shaving of the area may cause local irritation to the skin and predispose to superficial infections.
  - If the galea is violated, close it with an absorbable suture after obtaining a skull film to be sure there is no underlying fracture.

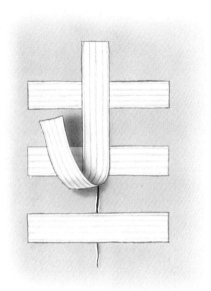

Figure 18-8.
Laceration care—Skin closure strips. Technique.

- Lidocaine with epinephrine is useful for hemostasis in scalp wounds. Hemostasis is important, as the area is vascular.

(2) Eyebrow:
- You should not shave or clip eyebrow hair, as quality of regrowth is uncertain. Also, eyebrows provide landmarks for your proper alignment of wound edges.

(3) Eyelid:
- You should refer all eyelid lacerations to a surgeon.

(4) Lip:
- You should refer to a surgeon all lip wounds that are not simple, straight lacerations.
- Close the vermilion border first, as this is the most important step in lining up the lip correctly. Assess the approximation of the vermilion border before infiltrating local anesthesia, because once infiltration is accomplished, the landmarks may be compromised.
- Before infiltrating anesthesia, draw a line with a surgical marking pen along the vermilion border on both sides of the laceration to indicate proper alignment of the border.
- Use nonabsorbable and monofilament suture for the vermilion border and outward.
- Use absorbable suture to loosely approximate mucosal tissue.
- Use a loose closure, or none at all, intra-orally to allow drainage.

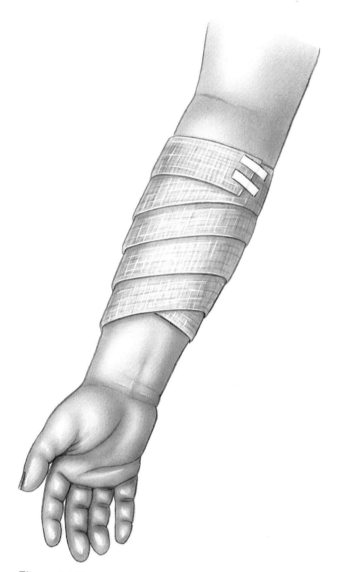

Figure 18-9.
Laceration care—Dressing care for an extremity. Technique.

(5) Face:
- Carefully assess damaged tissues, as the skin often rolls up.
- If skin edges are carefully identified, you can frequently appose them precisely.
- Place simple interrupted sutures 1 to 2 mm apart with approximately 1 mm of tissue edge taken in the "bite."
- Refer the patient if significant scarring is a possibility.

(6) Hand:

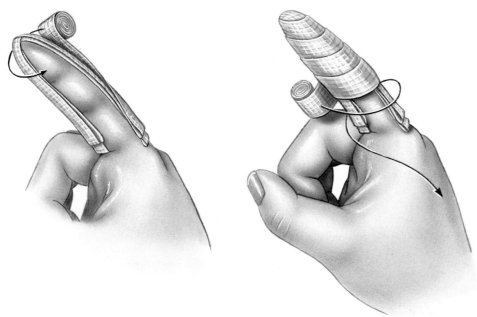

Figure 18-10.
Laceration care—Dressing care for a digit. Technique.

• Perform a thorough neuromuscular examination before anesthesia. There should be a low index for referral.
• Digital block (without epinephrine) for distal lesions is preferred.

c. Dressing care:
• Most dressings consist of several layers, each of which serves a specific purpose.
• Place an antibacterial ointment (e.g., povidone-iodine) immediately adjacent to the wound to provide some protection from contamination and to prevent the overdressing from sticking to the wound. For larger abrasions apply antibacterial impregnated gauze (e.g., Furacin or Xeroform) directly to the surface.
• Use the next layer of dressing to absorb wound drainage and apply even pressure to the wound. The layer consists of 2 × 2-inch or 4 × 4-inch gauze pads.
• Do not cut these gauze pads, to avoid fraying of the material into the wound.
• Secure these layers of dressing to the injured area with an outer layer. In many cases, this can be adhesive tape. To avoid trapping moisture in the wound and macerating it, do not apply the tape in occlusive fashion. Never encircle an extremity with tape, to avoid ischemia if swelling occurs.
• In more difficult areas (scalp, extremities, digits) secure the dressing using a circumferential wrap with a sterile conforming gauze bandage (e.g., Kling or Kerlix). Kling is a porous dressing with minimal stretch. Do not wrap it completely around an area in which swelling is expected because it may cause ischemia. Kerlix is a bulkier and more elastic dressing, which will absorb excess wound drainage. Use it in areas of movement and expected swelling.
• Secure dressings on extremities by wrapping the extremity with the bandage in an overlapping, oblique fashion to cover the wound and yet allow movement (Figure 18-9).
• Secure dressings of the digits by wrapping the bandage material several times in a longitudinal fashion and securing it with a circumferential, overlapping wrap that extends proximally onto the wrist (Figure 18-10).
• Likewise, secure head dressings by passing the bandage material over the crown of the scalp, overlapping in a radial fashion until the entire scalp is covered (Figure 18-11).
• Then secure the ends of the bandage by encircling the scalp between the forehead and occiput with a firm wrap of the bandage.
• Leave the initial dressing in place for 24 to 48 hours.
• Afterwards, clean the wound by gentle swabbing with hydrogen peroxide solution two to three times per day.
• Reapply the dressing if soiling or trauma to the wound

is feared. Instruct the patient to avoid showering or bathing of the wound until the sutures are removed or until 5 to 7 days after the injury.

5. Side Effects and Complications: One must observe the patient carefully for signs of excessive pressure from the dressing, such as local pain or paresthesias. One should watch for wound swelling, increased pain, redness, and purulent drainage as signs of infection. In addition, bluish swelling soon after closure suggests a hematoma, which may require reexploration and ligation of a vessel. Local cellulitis is initially treated with elevation, heat, immobilization, and antibiotics. If there is no improvement, or if fluctuance develops, the wound must be opened and allowed to heal by secondary intention. In this case, the wound is irrigated with saline and packed with saline moistened gauze and covered with dry gauze. This procedure is repeated two to three times per day until healing occurs. The probability of scarring is increased by closure with too much tension, suture bites being placed too wide apart, infection, and delayed suture removal.

D. Abrasion Care

1. Purpose: Proper abrasion care helps to avoid the development of infection and may help to minimize scarring in the affected area. Abrasions are essentially like burns, and depth must be evaluated. Furthermore, they often contain particulate matter that must be removed.

2. Selection of Patients:

a. Indications: Every abrasion should receive therapeutic care, and most can be treated in the office by the physician with follow-up care at home.

b. Contraindications and Precautions: Because abrasions are like burns, deep abrasions over areas such as the face, hands, and genitalia may require specialized care and, therefore, referral. The physician must rule out third-degree depth or an area of potential contracture with healing. In such cases, grafting may be required. The hands, face, and genital regions require special vigilance.

3. Equipment and Supplies (See Appendix for equipment and supplies manufacturers and suppliers. Appendix is keyed to italicized words in the equipment and supplies lists):

- Sedative (See Table 18-2, page 219)
- Local anesthetic (See Table 18-1, page 218)
- 6-mL *syringe* (See Figure 20-7, page 262)
- 25- or 27-gauge *needle* (See Figure 20-7, page 262)
- Soapy water
- Soft *brush*
- Sterile *gloves*
- Iris *scissors* (See Figure 18-2, page 220)

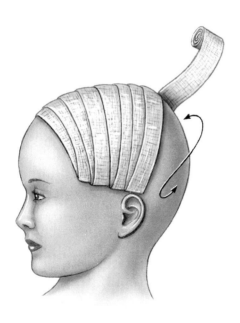
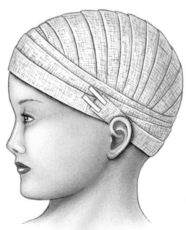

Figure 18-11.
Laceration care—Dressing care for the head. Technique.

- *Forceps* with teeth (See Figure 18-2, page 220)
- Povidone-iodine *solution*
- Antibacterial-impregnated *gauze*
- Antibacterial *ointment*
- 4 × 4-inch gauze *pads*
- Sterile conforming gauze *bandage*

4. Description of Procedure:

- Because abrasions are very painful to clean, you may need to use local anesthesia (See Local Anesthesia, page 218) for a small abrasion; you may need to use sedation for a large abrasion.
- First rinse the abrasion with soapy water and then scrub with a soft brush to remove all particulate matter.
- Then completely clean the abrasion with povidone-iodine solution.
- Don sterile gloves.
- Excise devitalized tissue with iris scissors and forceps.
- Apply antibacterial impregnated gauze or topical antibacterial ointment.
- Place dry gauze and a bulky wrap with sterile conforming gauze.
- Instruct the patient or parent to remove the dressing at home in 24 to 48 hours and to wash the abrasion twice a day with soapy water. They should then reapply a topical antibacterial ointment and a sterile gauze dressing.
- When the area has re-epithelialized, usually 3 to 4 weeks after injury, apply lanolin lotion or cocoa butter, which aid in replacing skin oils and preventing drying of the skin.

5. Side Effects and Complications: The persistence of pain or the development of erythema or fever may indicate infection and careful inspection of the abrasion is required. Particulate matter that is not adequately removed may cause subcutaneous abscesses and scarring.

E. Bites

1. Purpose: Proper treatment of bites, both animal and human, prevents infection and deforming scarring. In addition, diseases transmitted by bites, especially rabies, can be avoided.

2. Selection of Patients:

a. Indications: All bites require cleansing, and generally, healing by secondary intention, rather than by primary closure.

b. Contraindications and Precautions: Known or suspected human bites should never be closed primarily. Human bites introduce spirochetes, fusiform bacteria, and pepto-streptococci. These wounds often appear on the dorsum of the hand as a result of a punch to the mouth during a fight. Such wounds must be assumed to be human bites. Mistreatment can result in severe infection and loss of hand function; there-fore, many recommend referral of these injuries to a surgical specialist.

Animal bites to the face may require primary closure and should be referred to a plastic surgeon. For any animal bites, rabies prophylaxis must be administered if the offending animal is lost or shows signs of rabies. Otherwise, the animal can be observed for 10 days. If no signs of rabies are seen in the animal, no prophylaxis is needed.

3. Equipment and Supplies (See Appendix for equipment and supplies manufacturers and suppliers. Appendix is keyed to italicized words in the equipment and supplies lists):

- Sterile *gloves*
- Soapy water
- Sterile saline *solution*
- Antibacterial impregnated *gauze*
- 2 × 2- and 4 × 4-inch gauze *pads*
- Sterile conforming gauze *bandage*

4. Description of Procedure:

- Allow lacerations due to bites to heal by secondary intention, with the single exception of bites on the face noted above.
- Don sterile gloves.
- Clean the wound with soapy water and irrigate profusely with saline.
- Secure an antibacterial-impregnated dressing, covered with a dry sterile gauze, with a conforming gauze bandage.
- Administer appropriate antibiotic therapy and tetanus prophylaxis.
- Subsequent cleansing with ordinary soap may take place at home.

5. Side Effects and Complications: The wounds may become infected and close follow-up is necessary. Unsightly scarring may require subsequent revision.

F. Incision and Drainage

1. Purpose: Incision and drainage allows total cleansing of a contained infection and healing of the tissue by secondary intention.

2. Selection of Patients:

a. Indications: Drainage is required for any pocket of infection that is fluctuant and does not appear likely to drain spontaneously.

b. Contraindications and Precautions: Abscesses on the face, and neck, deep rectal abscesses, or abscesses with much extension (especially in the hand) need referral and drainage in the operating room.

3. Equipment and Supplies (See Appendix for equipment and supplies manufacturers and suppliers. Appendix is keyed to italicized words in the equipment and supplies lists):

- Local anesthetic (See Table 18-1, page 218)
- 6-mL *syringe* (See Figure 20-7, page 262)

- 25- to 27-gauge *needle* (See Figure 20-7, page 262)
- Povidone-iodine *solution*
- Sterile *gloves*
- Sterile drapes
- No. 15 scalpel *blades* (See Figure 18-2, page 220)
- Scalpel *handle* (See Figure 18-2, page 220)
- Cotton-tipped culture *swab* (See Figure 14-5, page 167)
- Fine curved *clamp* (Figure 18-12)
- Saline irrigation *solution*
- Bulb *syringe* (Figure 18-12)
- Povidone-iodine *solution*
- 2 × 2- and 4 × 4-inch gauze *pads*
- Sterile conforming gauze *bandage*

4. Description of Procedure
   - After administering local anesthesia (See Local Anesthesia, page 218), prepare the area with povidone-iodine.
   - Don sterile gloves.
   - Drape the area as a sterile field.
   - Make an incision with a no. 15 scalpel in a skin line (Figure 18-13) over the abscess (Figure 18-14).
   - Take a culture of the pus at the time of the incision.
   - Probe the cavity with a clamp and gently spread the clamp in all quadrants to open all pockets of infection (Figure 18-14).
   - Copiously irrigate the cavity with saline from a bulb syringe.
   - Pack the cavity tightly with gauze pads soaked with povidone-iodine solution, for initial hemostasis, and dress the wound with dry gauze covered with a conforming gauze bandage.
   - Remove the povidone-iodine–soaked gauze within 24 to 48 hours.
   - Irrigate the cavity and loosely repack it with povidone-iodine–soaked gauze. Repeat the process every 24 hours until the capacity is small, at which time you may place a simple dry dressing until there is complete skin healing.
   - Administer oral antibiotics.

   Two particular types of abscesses merit special consideration:
   a. Felon
      - This is a trabeculated abscess in the pulp of the distal finger. There is a danger of osteomyelitis in the distal phalanx if this infection is not treated properly. In the past, it was treated with a fishmouth, hockey stick, or "through and through" incision, but these approaches

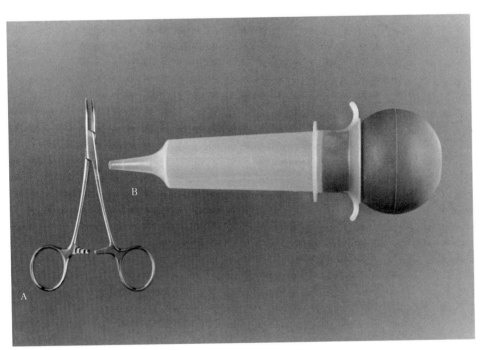

Figure 18-12.
Incision and drainage. Equipment and supplies: **A,** Fine curved clamp; **B,** Bulb syringe.

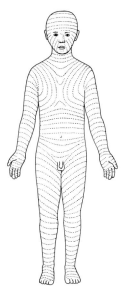
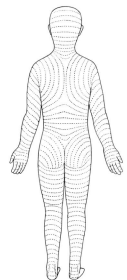

Figure 18-13.
Incision and drainage. Skin lines.

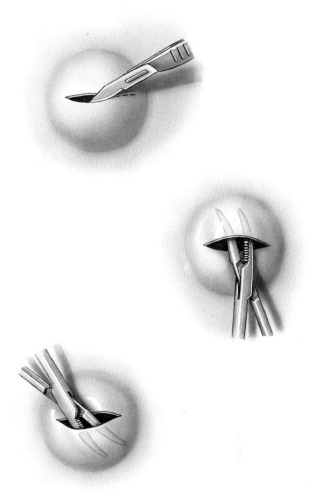

Figure 18-14.
Incision and drainage of an abscess. Technique.

were found to be inadequate and potentially dangerous. The "fishmouth" incision is one made completely around the distal aspect of the finger in the finger pulp and may result in finger tip necrosis. The "hockey stick" incision is an incision made along the lateral aspect of the digit and extending in hockey stick fashion onto the distal finger pulp. This incision may damage the digital vessels and nerves. The same is true for the "through and through" incision, which is made by placing separate incisions on the lateral and medial aspects of the distal digit and opening the space between them. Preferable to these incisions is a longitudinal incision made 1 cm long and 1 cm deep directly through the pulp of the distal digit in the midline of the palmar surface (Figure 18-15).

· Irrigate the wound with saline, and leave a small povidone-iodine–soaked gauze wick in place.

· Place a finger dressing with a conforming gauze bandage (See Figure 18-10, page 225).

· Remove the dressing and wick in 24 hours. Irrigate the wound twice a day until healing is complete.

· Leave a small wick in place until the cavity is obliterated.

· Use oral antibiotics.

b. Paronychia

This is an abscess of the tissue at the base of the nail.

· To treat, make an incision in the infected tissue and place a wick (Figure 18-16).

· Treatment is then similar to that of a felon.

· You may find it necessary to undermine the proximal nail or remove the nail for adequate drainage (See Removal of an Ingrown Toenail, page 230)

· In some minor cases, all you need to do is retract the infected tissue with a cotton swab for proper drainage.

· Use oral antibiotics.

5. Side Effects and Complications: Recurrent infection may occur, especially if drainage is not adequate.

G. Minor Burns

1. Purpose: Minor burns require proper treatment to minimize the potential for scarring and infection.

2. Selection of Patients:

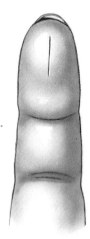

Figure 18-15.
Incision and drainage of a felon. Technique.

a. Indications: Most children with minor burns may be treated as outpatients. Minor burns consist of 15% or less partial-thickness burns (first- and second-degree) or 2% or less full-thickness burns (third-degree).

b. Contraindications and Precautions: Any child with larger burns, deep burns, or burns to the hand, face, perineum, or across joints should be referred to a specialist capable of managing such injuries. In addition, inpatient care is standard practice for managing burns in children less than 2 years of age; electrical, chemical, or inhalation burns; or burns inflicted as part of child abuse.

3. Equipment and Supplies (See Appendix for equipment and supplies manufacturers and suppliers. Appendix is keyed to italicized words in the equipment and supplies lists):
   · Sterile *gloves*
   · Soapy water (at body temperature)
   · Iris *scissors* (See Figure 18-2, page 220)
   · *Forceps* with teeth (See Figure 18-2, page 220)
   · Antibacterial impregnated *gauze*
   · 4 × 4-inch gauze *pads*
   · Sterile conforming gauze *bandage*

4. Description of Procedure:
   · Don sterile gloves.
   · In second- and third-degree burns, irrigate the burn area and gently clean with soapy water at approximately body temperature. The area will be very sensitive to cold or hot water.
   · Leave intact blisters unopened.
   · Debride dead skin from open blisters with forceps and iris scissors.
   · Dry the area and apply antibacterial impregnated gauze with a dry 4 × 4-inch gauze pad overdressing.
   · Then wrap the wound with a sterile conforming gauze bandage. An elastic bandage such as Kerlix is preferred to allow for swelling.
   · Systemic antibiotics are generally not needed for treatment of minor burns. Tetanus prophylaxis should be provided.
   · Wash the area with soapy water twice a day at home with reapplication of the gauze and a dry dressing until the skin has healed.
   · Frequent outpatient follow-up is prudent until healing occurs.
   · Lanolin or cocoa butter applied regularly for 1 to 2 months after healing helps preserve skin suppleness and reduce itching. Aloe-containing cream may be useful for alleviation of pain in the initial treatment of a first-degree burn.
   · You must be alert to the formation of scars, or contracting areas. If present, refer the patient, as grafts may then be necessary.

5. Side Effects and Complications: Local wound infections may occur and interfere with burn wound healing. Scarring is a possibility with deeper burns.

H. Removal of an Ingrown Toenail

1. Purpose: Ingrown toenails should be treated to avoid progressive infection or ulceration of the toe and to relieve pain.

2. Selection of Patients:

a. Indications: Development of swelling and redness along the edge of the toenail—almost exclusively involving the great toe.

b. Contraindications and Precautions: Special care should be exercised in the diabetic to adequately treat all infection.

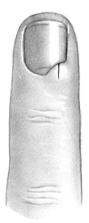

Figure 18-16.
Incision and drainage of a paronychia. Technique.

3. Equipment and Supplies (See Appendix for equipment and supplies manufacturers and suppliers. Appendix is keyed to italicized words in the equipment and supplies lists):

- Warm soapy water
- Local anesthetic (without epinephrine) (See Table 18-1, page 218)
- 6-mL *syringe* (See Figure 20-7, page 262)
- 25- to 27-gauge *needle* (See Figure 20-7, page 262)
- Povidone-iodine *solution*
- Sterile *gloves*
- Sterile drapes
- Fine curved *clamp* (See Figure 18-12, page 228) or straight *clamp*
- Straight *scissors* (Figure 18-17)
- No. 15 scalpel *blade* (See Figure 18-2, page 220)
- Scalpel *handle* (See Figure 18-2, page 220)

- Bone *curette* (Figure 18-17)
- Silver nitrate *applicators* (Figure 18-17)
- Cotton-tipped *applicator* (Figure 18-17)
- Cotton wisp
- Antibacterial *ointment*
- Antibacterial-impregnated *gauze*
- 2 × 2-inch gauze *pads*
- Sterile conforming gauze *bandage*

4. Description of Procedure:
- Administer a digital block (See Figure 18-1, page 220), after soaking the toe in warm soapy water for about 15 to 20 minutes.
- Prepare the toe with povidone-iodine.
- Don sterile gloves.
- Drape the area as a sterile field.
- Undermine the affected side of the nail with a fine clamp and cut the nail vertically with straight scissors such that one third of the nail is freed (Figure 18-18).
- Work loose the one third of the nail with a fine clamp and remove. Obliquely incise the skin at the base of the nail with a no. 15 scalpel to facilitate complete removal of this portion of the nail. It is important that the affected side of the nail bed is totally free of nail tissue, to prevent recurrence. It may be necessary for you to curettage the lateral nail bed and matrix with a small bone curette. The entire nail may need to be removed if the complete nail bed is infected or if the infection represents a recurrence.
- Control bleeding with finger pressure or a silver nitrate applicator.
- Place antibacterial ointment and antibacterial-impregnated gauze on the nail bed and wrap the toe with 2 × 2-inch gauze and a conforming gauze bandage.
- Instruct the patient to elevate the foot for 24 hours.
- Remove the dressing in 1 or 2 days and clean the toe with soapy water.
- Apply antibacterial ointment and a dry 2 × 2-inch gauze dressing twice a day.
- A loose fitting shoe is recommended.
- Alternatively, in mild cases, separate the swollen area from the nail with a swab and keep the nail elevated with a cotton wisp until the edge grows out.
- Instruct the patient to cut the nails straight across in the future and to wear appropriately fitting shoes.

5. Side Effects and Complications: Persistent infection may occur if the entire segment of nail is not removed.

I. Drainage of a Subungual Hematoma

A subungual hematoma is a hematoma underneath a nail, usually as a result of a forceful blow.

1. Purpose: Subungual hematomas require drainage for relief of pain and avoidance of infection.

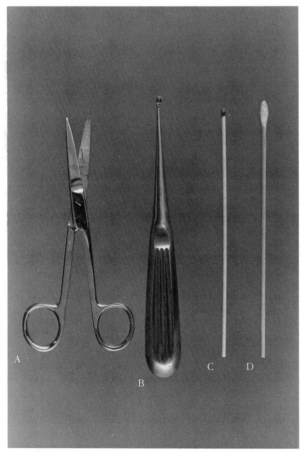

Figure 18-17.
Removal of an ingrown toenail. Equipment and supplies: **A,** Straight scissors; **B,** Bone curette; **C,** Silver nitrate applicator; **D,** Cotton-tipped applicator.

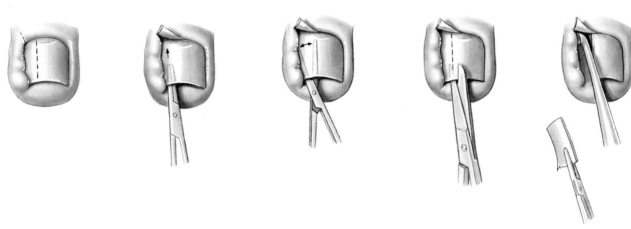

Figure 18-18.
Removal of an ingrown toenail. Technique.

2. Selection of Patients:

a. Indications: A subungual hematoma causing significant pain should be drained.

b. Contraindications and Precautions: Radiographs may be needed if the blow was of sufficient force to potentially fracture the underlying bone.

3. Equipment and Supplies (See Appendix for equipment and supplies manufacturers and suppliers. Appendix is keyed to italicized words in the equipment and supplies lists):
- Povidone-iodine *solution*
- Paper clip
- Heat source (such as alcohol lamp)
- No. 11 scalpel *blade* (See Figure 18-2, page 220)
- Antibacterial *ointment*
- Sterile bandage *strip*

4. Description of Procedure:

There are two widely used methods for draining a subungual hematoma. It is helpful to soak the finger or toe in warm water and cleanse with povidone-iodine before either procedure.

a. Method 1:
- Unfold a paper clip and heat it on one end.
- Press the heated end into the nail over the hematoma (Figure 18-19).
- The tip will rapidly melt through the nail and drain the hematoma.
- Apply antibacterial ointment and a sterile bandage strip.

b. Method 2:
- Make a small incision through the nail by rotating a no. 11 blade, leaving a hole for drainage (Figure 18-20).

5. Side Effects and Complications: Redrainage may sometimes be necessary if the hole closes off too quickly.

J. Toe Abrasion and Nail Avulsion

1. Purpose: Toe abrasions and nail avulsions require treatment to alleviate pain and avoid infection.

2. Selection of Patients:

a. Indications: Injuries to the toe that cause abrasion of the skin or disruption of the nail bed require treatment. These lesions usually result from stubbing injuries.

b. Contraindications and Precautions: If there is bone visible or any evidence of fracture, refer the patient to a specialist.

3. Equipment and Supplies (See Appendix for equipment and supplies manufacturers and suppliers. Appendix is keyed to italicized words in the equipment and supplies lists):

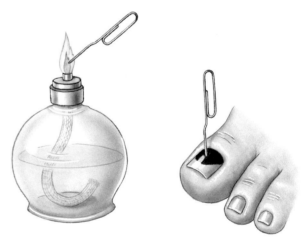

Figure 18-19.
Drainage of subungual hematoma—Paperclip method. Technique.

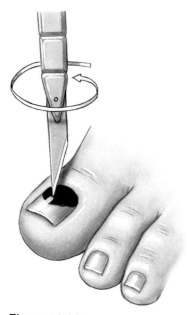

Figure 18-20.
Drainage of a subungual hematoma—Scalpel blade method. Technique.

- Local anesthetic (See Table 18-1, page 218)
- 6-mL *syringe* (See Figure 20-7, page 262)
- 25- to 27-gauge *needle* (See Figure 20-7, page 262)
- Warm soapy water
- Sterile saline *solution*
- Povidone-iodine *solution*
- Sterile *gloves*
- Sterile drapes
- Iris *scissors* (See Figure 18-2, page 220)
- *Forceps* with teeth (See Figure 18-2, page 220)
- Fine curved *clamps* (See Figure 18-12, page 228)
- No. 15 *blade* (See Figure 18-2, page 220)
- Scalpel *handle* (See Figure 18-2, page 220)
- *Suture* material (See Table 18-3, page 221)
- Needle *holder* (See Figure 18-3, page 221)
- Antibacterial impregnated *gauze*
- 2 × 2-inch and 4 × 4-inch gauze *pads*
- Sterile conforming gauze *bandage*
- Antibacterial *ointment*

4. Description of Procedure:
- Take radiographs of the toe first.
- After performing a thorough neurologic exam, administer a digital block (See Figure 18-1, page 220).
- Cleanse the toe thoroughly with soapy water (prior soaking helps) and irrigate with saline.

- Prepare the area with povidone-iodine.
- Don sterile gloves.
- Drape the area as a sterile field.
- Remove any foreign material with forceps and iris scissors.
- If the nail is damaged, undermine it with a fine clamp and remove (See Figure 18-16, page 230).
- If the nail bed is lacerated, close it with simple interrupted sutures of 5–0 absorbable material (e.g., Dexon) (See Figure 18-6, page 223).
- Place a dressing of antibacterial impregnated gauze, dry 2 × 2-inch gauze, and a conforming gauze bandage.
- Remove the dressing in 1 to 2 days and clean the wound with soapy water.
- Apply antibiotic ointment and apply a dry dressing.
- Instruct the patient to wear loose-fitting shoes.

5. Side Effects and Complications: Inadequate removal of foreign material or devitalized tissue may lead to secondary infection.

K. Foreign Body Removal

1. Purpose: The purpose of this procedure is to remove symptomatic foreign bodies in the skin and subcutaneous tissue.

2. Selection of Patients:

a. Indications: Symptoms and accessibility determine whether a foreign body should be removed in the office. Foreign bodies that are readily accessible and are causing symptoms, infection, or cosmetic deformity are best removed.

b. Contraindications and Precautions: In the office or emergency room, avoid exploration for a foreign body that cannot be seen or easily felt. Fluoroscopic guidance is helpful for radiopague foreign bodies.

3. Equipment and Supplies (See Appendix for equipment and supplies manufacturers and suppliers. Appendix is keyed to italicized words in the equipment and supplies lists):

- Sterile *gloves*
- Local anesthetic (See Table 18-1, page 218)
- 6-mL *syringe* (See Figure 20-7, page 262)
- 25- to 27-gauge *needle* (See Figure 20-7, page 262)
- Soapy water
- Povidone-iodine *solution*
- Sterile drapes
- No. 11 scalpel *blade* (See Figure 18-2, page 220)
- Scalpel *handle* (See Figure 18-2, page 220)
- Fine curved *clamp* (See Figure 18-12, page 228)
- Iris *scissors* (See Figure 18-2, page 220)
- *Suture* material (See Table 18-3, page 221)
- Needle *holder* (See Figure 18-3, page 221)
- Antibacterial *ointment*
- 2 × 2-inch gauze *pads*
- Sterile conforming gauze *bandage*

4. Description of Procedure:

- Anesthetize the area with local anesthesia (See Local Anesthesia, page 218).
- Wash the area with soapy water.
- Cleanse the area with povidone-iodine.
- Don sterile gloves.
- Drape the area as a sterile field.
- Make an elliptical incision with a no. 11 scalpel blade around the object or the wound of entry to allow best exposure.
- Remove the object by grasping it with a fine clamp.
- Debride the surrounding tissue with iris scissors if necessary.
- Allow the wound to heal by secondary intention.
- Cover the wound with antibacterial ointment and dress it with 2 × 2 gauze pads and a sterile conforming gauze bandage.
- In the case of a foreign body under a nail, elevate or remove the nail (See Figure 18-18, page 232) under digital block (See Figure 18-1, page 220) to allow removal of the foreign body.

5. Side Effects and Complications: Incomplete removal may result in continued symptoms or infection.

L. Removal of Fish Hooks

1. Purpose: Removal of embedded fish hooks in the office is done to avoid further pain and tissue damage.

2. Selection of Patients:

a. Indications: Office removal of fish hooks is necessary for those in which the barb is completely embedded or has penetrated the skin.

b. Contraindications and Precautions: Hooks embedded near the eye should be referred to a specialist.

3. Equipment and Supplies (See Appendix for equipment and supplies manufacturers and suppliers. Appendix is keyed to italicized words in the equipment and supplies lists):

- Sterile *gloves*
- Local anesthetic (See Table 18-1, page 218)
- 6-mL *syringe* (See Figure 20-7, page 262)
- 25- or 27-gauge *needle* (See Figure 20-7, page 262)
- Povidone-iodine *solution*
- Wire *cutters* (Figure 18-21)
- Fine curved *clamp* (See Figure 18-12, page 228)
- Heavy *suture* material (See Table 18-3, page 221)
- Antibacterial *ointment*
- 2 × 2-inch gauze *pads*
- Adhesive *tape*

4. Description of Procedure: There are two simple methods for removing embedded fish hooks. Either method generally requires local anesthesia (See Local Anesthesia, page xxxx). Tetanus prophylaxis should be provided.

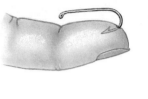
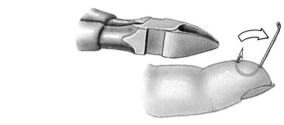
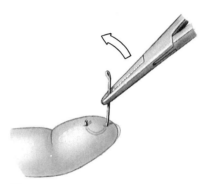

Figure 18-21.
Removal of a fish hook—Wire cutter method. Technique.

a. Method 1:

- Anesthetize the area with local anesthesia (See Local Anesthesia, page 218).
- Don sterile gloves.
- After preparing the area with povidone-iodine, grasp the shaft of the hook with a clamp and pass the barb completely through the skin (See Figure 18-21).
- Then cut the barb from the hook with wire cutters and rotate the shaft back to remove it from the skin.
- Apply a small 2 × 2-inch gauze dressing with antibacterial ointment and tape it over the remaining wound.

b. Method 2:

- Anesthetize the area with local anesthesia (See Local Anesthesia, page 218).
- Don sterile gloves.
- Prepare the area with povidone-iodine.
- In cases in which the barb is completely embedded within the subcutaneous tissues, encircle the shaft with a heavy ligature (Figure 18-22).

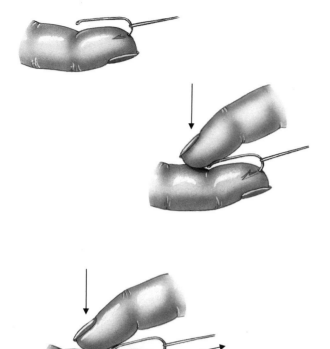

Figure 18-22.
Removal of a fish hook—Ligature method. Technique.

· Using the left hand, depress the shaft of the hook, disengaging the barb from the deep tissues.
· At the same time provide a jerk on the ligature away from the patient, which should remove the hook completely.
· Apply a small 2 × 2-inch gauze dressing with antibiotic ointment and tape it over the remaining wound.

M. Removal of Skin Lesions

1. Purpose: Removal of skin lesions in the office is generally done for cosmetic purposes.
2. Selection of Patients:
a. Indications: Lesions less than 1 cm in diameter may be removed in the office.
b. Contraindications and Precautions: Lesions larger than 1 cm or possible malignancies are best treated by wider excision and possible grafting in the operating room.
3. Equipment and Supplies (See Appendix for equipment and supplies manufacturers and suppliers. Appendix is keyed to italicized words in the equipment and supplies lists):

· Local anesthetic (See Table 18-1, page 218)
· 6-mL *syringe* (See Figure 20-7, page 262)
· 25- or 27-gauge *needle* (See Figure 20-7, page 262)
· Soapy water
· Povidone-iodine *solution*
· Sterile *gloves*
· Sterile drapes
· No. 15 scalpel *blade* (See Figure 18-2, page 220)
· Scalpel *handle* (See Figure 18-2, page 220)
· *Forceps* with teeth (See Figure 18-2, page 220)
· Iris *scissors* (See Figure 18-2, page 220)
· Formalin (10%) *solution*
· *Suture* material (See Table 18-3, page 221)
· Needle *holder* (See Figure 18-3, page 221)
· 2 × 2- and 4 × 4-inch gauze *pads*
· Adhesive *tape*

4. Description of Procedure:
· Infiltrate the area with a local anesthetic (See Local Anesthesia, page 218).
· Wash the area with soapy water and prepare with povidone-iodine.
· Don sterile gloves.
· Drape the area as a sterile field.
· Using a no. 15 scalpel blade, make an elliptical incision around the lesion, parallel to the skin lines (Figure 18-23).
· Take as small a margin of normal skin as possible.
· Elevate the lesion with forceps and divide the subcutaneous tissue beneath the lesion with iris scissors, thus removing the lesion.
· Place the specimen in 10% formalin and label carefully. All specimens removed in the office should be examined by a pathologist.
· Close the skin with a simple or mattress stitch with monofilament suture material (e.g., Ethilon) (See Figures 18-6 and 18-7, page 223).
· Dress the wound with sterile 2 × 2-inch gauze and tape.
· Observe routine postoperative wound care, as for a laceration.
· You do not need to use antibiotics for these procedures.
· Lesions that may recur or that may be malignant should be referred to a specialist.
5. Side Effects and Complications: Failure to provide adequate margins may lead to a recurrence of the lesion.

N. Venous Cut-down

1. Purpose: Peripheral venous cut-downs may be necessary for intravenous hydration in situations in which a percutaneous intravenous device cannot be secured.

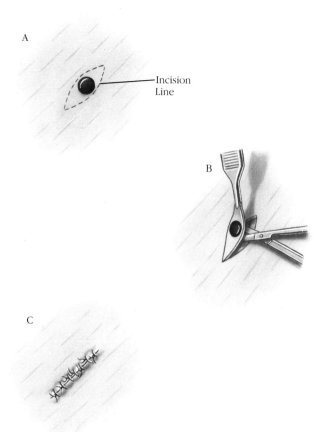

Figure 18-23.
Removal of a skin lesion. Technique.

2. Selection of Patients:

a. Indications: A venous cut-down involves cannulation of a vein under direct vision. It is employed when percutaneous cannulation is not possible. Cut-downs are performed in areas where movement of skin is minimal and in areas that can be kept clean. Preferred sites in children are the greater saphenous vein at the ankle and basilic and cephalic veins in the arm (Figure 18-24).

b. Contraindications and Precautions: There are no contraindications in the otherwise healthy child.

3. Equipment and Supplies (See Appendix for equipment and supplies manufacturers and suppliers. Appendix is keyed to italicized words in the equipment and supplies lists):
- Local anesthetic (See Table 18-1, page 218)
- 6-mL *syringe* (See Figure 20-7, page 262)
- 25- or 27-gauge *needle* (See Figure 20-7, page 262)
- Povidone-iodine *solution*
- Sterile *gloves*

- Sterile drapes
- No. 11 and no. 15 scalpel *blades* (See Figure 18-2, page 220)
- Scalpel *handle* (See Figure 18-2, page 220)
- *Forceps* with teeth (See Figure 18-2, page 220)
- Fine curved *clamp* (See Figure 18-12, page 228)
- Suture material (See Table 18-3, page 221)
- Needle *holder* (See Figure 18-3, page 221)
- Intravenous *cannula* (See Figure 21-1, page 276)
- 2 × 2-inch gauze *pads*

4. Description of Procedure:
- Infiltrate the skin over the vein with a local anesthetic (See Local Anesthesia, page 218).
- Wash the area with soapy water and prepare with povidone-iodine.
- Don sterile gloves.
- Drape the area as a sterile field.
- Make an incision with a no. 15 scalpel blade approximately 1 cm long perpendicular to the vein, in a skin line directly over the vein (Figure 18-25).
- Spread the tissues with a fine clamp until the vein is isolated and encircled with the clamp.
- Place a loop of absorbable suture (e.g., Dexon) around the proximal end of the vein and tie the distal end with similar suture.
- Pick up the vein with forceps and cut partially through the vein with a no. 11 scalpel blade with the cutting edge facing up.
- Insert the intravenous cannula into the vein under direct vision and tie the proximal ligature around the catheter.
- Introduce the catheter into the venotomy at a 45-degree angle with the vein. Use the beveled tip of the catheter to elevate the anterior wall of the vein so as to open the venotomy further. You can then more easily slip the catheter into the vein with gentle pressure.
- Secure the distal ligature around the catheter and close the incision with nylon sutures. Tie one of the skin sutures around the hub of the cannula to secure the cannula.
- Place a sterile dressing over the cut-down site and immobilize the limb with an armboard and dressing (See Infusion Procedures, page 275).

5. Side Effects and Complications: Swelling, redness, and increased pain indicate probable infiltration or phlebitis, and catheter removal may be necessary.

O. Central Venous Catheter Care

1. Purpose: Proper outpatient care of central venous catheters minimizes infection and facilitates their long-term use.

2. Selection of Patients:

a. Indications: Central venous access is selected for certain

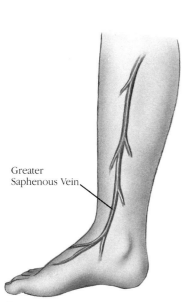
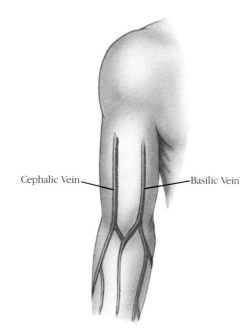

Greater
Saphenous Vein

Cephalic Vein

Basilic Vein

Figure 18-24.
Venous cut-down. Preferred sites.

patients for the administration of fluids, blood products, parenteral nutrition, or drugs. Central venous catheters are placed sterilely in the operating room and are designed for long-term use with minimal physical restriction to the patient. They may have one or more lumens and most are made of Silastic. These catheters are tunneled in the subcutaneous tissue and a Teflon cuff in the tunnel keeps them in place.

b. Contraindications and Precautions: The principal problems encountered with these catheters are 1) thrombosis, 2) leaking, and 3) infection. Care of the catheters is entrusted to parents and primary care physicians in most instances.

3. Equipment and Supplies (See Appendix for equipment and supplies manufacturers and suppliers. Appendix is keyed to italicized words in the equipment and supplies lists):

- Sterile towel
- 4 × 4-inch gauze *pads*
- Povidone-iodine *solution*
- Heparin *solution*
- Sterile *gloves*
- 6-mL *syringe* (See Figure 20-7, page 262)
- 21-gauge *needle* (See Figure 20-7, page 262)
- Fine curved *clamp* (See Figure 18-12, page 228)
- Povidone-iodine–impregnated *pads*
- Clean *gloves*
- Alcohol *pads*
- Povidone-iodine *ointment*

- 2 × 2-inch gauze *pads*
- Adhesive *tape*
- Transparent catheter *dressing*

4. Description of Procedure: The principal outpatient procedures are heparin flushing of the catheter, dressing changes, and injection cap change.

a. Heparin flush:

- Observe sterile technique at all times.
- Place a sterile towel on a table.
- Place 4 × 4 gauze pads on the towel and saturate with povidone-iodine.
- Place a sterile bowl on the towel, and pour "heparinized" saline flush (1 unit of heparin per 1 mL of saline) into the bowl.
- The parent or physician performing the flush should wear sterile gloves.
- Draw 3 mL of the heparin flush into a 6-mL syringe using a 21-gauge needle.
- With the catheter clamped, thoroughly prepare the protective injection cap and entire hub of the catheter with povidone-iodine–impregnated swabs.
- Unclamp the catheter and flush it with the heparin solution using a 21-gauge needle attached to a 6-mL syringe.
- Withdraw a small amount of blood into the syringe before injecting, to remove all of the air from the system.

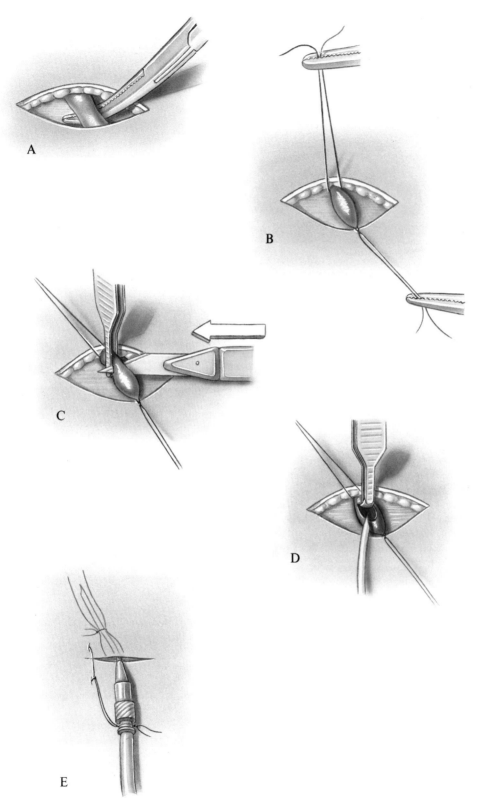

Figure 18-25.
Venous cut-down. Technique.

· Inject 2 to 3 mL of heparin solution.

· Withdraw the needle from the injection cap as the last of the solution is being injected.

· Reapply the catheter clamp.

b. Dressing change:

· Place materials for the dressing change (i.e., sterile gauze, povidone-iodine ointment, and alcohol swabs) on a sterile towel.

· Remove the old dressing with clean gloves.

· Change to sterile gloves.

· Clean the site with the alcohol swabs, and place povidone-iodine ointment at the catheter entrance site.

· Then place sterile gauze over the site.

· Secure the gauze with tape or transparent catheter dressing.

c. Injection cap change:

· Follow sterile procedure in a manner similar to that for the flush procedure.

· Prepare the cap with povidone-iodine solution.

Clamp the catheter, remove the old cap, and place a new sterile cap.

· Unclamp the line, and flush it as in (a).

5. Side Effects and Complications:

a. Thrombosis: If gentle attempts at flushing do not open the catheter, the patient should be referred to a surgeon for consideration of a urokinase flush or a change of the catheter.

b. Leakage: Flush the catheter with heparin, as in (a). Clamp the catheter between the leaking area and the patient's skin. The patient should be referred immediately to a surgeon, for repair of the catheter or replacement with a new system.

c. Infection: Purulent drainage, erythema, swelling, or tenderness indicate line infection. The catheter should be removed by a surgeon and the infection allowed to resolve before a new catheter is placed. Infected catheters often cause systemic signs of infection before local indications are apparent. Patients with infection of the catheter should be hospitalized and should receive systemic antibiotics.

Chapter 19

Allergy Evaluation and Treatment Procedures

Peter W. Heymann

Deborah D. Murphy

Approximately 10% to 20% of the general population experience symptoms caused by exposure to allergens in the environment. Because allergic diseases (i.e., those mediated by immunoglobulin E [IgE] antibodies) are common, an understanding of the procedures described in this chapter will help the practitioner identify allergic patients, determine in a given patient which allergens are most likely to precipitate symptoms, and decide which modes of therapy are most likely to be helpful. The emergency treatment of asthma and anaphylaxis also will be discussed.

Organ systems commonly associated with allergic symptoms include the respiratory tract, skin, and gastrointestinal tract, where mast cells coated with IgE antibodies predominate. Thus, a history for allergies should identify patients who have perennial or seasonal respiratory symptoms (chronic or recurrent cough, wheezing, nasal congestion, rhinitis, and conjunctivitis); skin symptoms (atopic dermatitis and urticaria); and gastrointestinal symptoms (chronic diarrhea, abdominal discomfort, and vomiting). Anaphylaxis may occasionally occur when allergens trigger mediator release from basophils (in the circulation) together with mast cells (in tissues). A history of atopy in the immediate family is important in identifying a potentially allergic child. In addition, a description of the home environment, including household pets, may suggest precipitating factors. Finally, because allergic individuals are prone to acquire infections when allergic symptoms are present, the practitioner should inquire about recurrent ear infections, upper respiratory and sinus infections, and pneumonias.

This chapter includes a description of the procedures that can be used in the evaluation and treatment of the allergic child in an office setting. Some of the procedures described require no technical skills, but are important to the evaluation.

I. Diagnostic Procedures

A. Evaluation of Nasal Eosinophilia

1. Purpose: The evaluation of nasal smears for the presence of eosinophils is of value in judging whether nasal symptoms may be allergy related. When present in children, nasal eosinophils not only suggest that the patient is likely to be allergic, but also suggest that the patient has had recent exposure to an environmental allergen.

2. Selection of Patients:

a. Indications: Nasal smears are indicated for patients with chronic or recurrent rhinitis, and particularly in patients who have rhinitis and asthma.

b. Contraindications and Precautions: None

3. Equipment and Supplies (See Appendix for equipment and supplies manufacturers and suppliers. Appendix is keyed to italicized words in the equipment and supplies lists):

- Cotton-tipped *applicator* (See Figure 14-5, page 167)
- Clear plastic *wrap*
- Clean glass microscope *slides*
- Hansel stain, for cytologic examination of nasal, bronchial, and conjunctival secretions. This stain contains methanol, eosin, methylene blue, and glycerin.

4. Description of Procedure:

a. Collection of nasal secretions:

- In some instances, you may need to have the patient restrained as you do to obtain a throat culture (See Figure 9-21, page 98).
- Typically, secretions in allergic rhinitis are clear and viscous rather than runny.
- In children too young to blow their nose, use a cotton swab, or nasopharyngeal swab, to collect secretions in sufficient quantity to visualize when smeared on a slide. Insert the swab along the floor of the nose, parallel to the turbinates (See Figure 9-22, page 99) rather than obtain secretions from the anterior nares. In patients with scant secretions, the swab may absorb most of the fluid, making it difficult to prepare a smear. In addition, swabbing the nares can be irritating.
- Have older patients blow their nose into plastic wrap just as one would into a tissue.
- Transfer the secretions directly to a slide and allow them to dry. Once dry, smears remain stable and do not have to be stained immediately.
- Some patients can be instructed to prepare smears at home. The slides can then be mailed to you or to a laboratory.

b. Hansel stain of secretions:

- Flood the slide with methanol for 20 to 30 seconds to dehydrate secretions.
- Pour off the methanol and flood with Hansel stain for 20 to 30 seconds.

- Rinse, flood with distilled water, and let stand for 20 to 30 seconds.
- Rinse with methanol before drying.
- Re-rinse with methanol if the slide is overstained.
- Allow the slide to dry.
- Examine the slide under oil immersion with $100 \times$ magnification.

5. Side Effects and Complications: None

6. Interpretation: The Hansel stain contains eosin. This dye is readily taken up by cytoplasmic granules in eosinophils. Under the microscope the granules appear bright red-orange in color (Figure 19-1A). The cytoplasm in neutrophils also may take up the stain, but granules are not distinct and the cytoplasm appears more homogeneous and light pink in color (Figure 19-1B). If Hansel stain reagents are not available, wet secretions can be covered with a coverslip and examined under high power using phase contrast microscopy. With practice, the granules of eosinophils can be distinguished.

There are no definitive guidelines as to how many eosinophils must be present to suggest allergy; however, some semiquantitative scales have been suggested (Table 19-1). The presence of eosinophils in nasal secretions indicates that eosinophilic chemotactic factors have been released (e.g., from mast cells) after allergen exposure in a sensitized individual. Although occasional eosinophils may be seen in normal secretions, the presence of moderate to many eosinophils is consistent with the diagnosis of allergic rhinitis. Nonallergic vasomotor rhinitis with eosinophils is uncommon in children.

The absence of eosinophils in nasal secretions can be misleading. For example, eosinophils in the nasal secretions are only increased during periods of, or for a short period after, allergen exposure. Thus, a grass-allergic individual may have few or no eosinophils present during an upper respiratory tract infection in midwinter. During the grass pollen seasons, however, eosinophils may be abundant.

When patients with chronic allergic rhinitis develop superimposed infections, nasal secretions become purulent, and neutrophils rather than eosinophils predominate. After the infection has cleared, or has been treated, eosinophils are again apparent if allergen exposure persists.

To judge nasal secretions properly, negative nasal smears should be repeated 1) at a time when allergen exposure is most likely in patients with seasonal rhinitis, 2) after purulent secretions have cleared spontaneously or after antibiotic therapy in patients with purulent rhinorrhea, and 3) after patients treated with steroids, which inhibit nasal eosinophilia, have stopped taking the steroids.

B. Evaluation of Blood Eosinophilia

1. Purpose: When elevated, eosinophils in the blood can support the diagnosis of allergic disease. However, other causes (e.g., parasitic disease) must be considered.

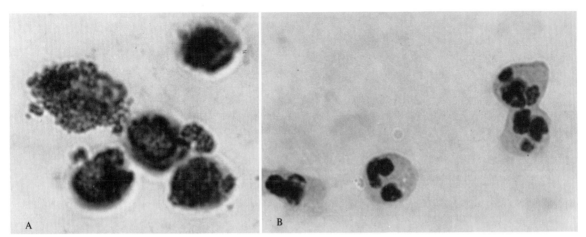

Figure 19-1.
Evaluation of nasal eosinophilia. A, Eosinophils; **B,** Neutrophils.

2. Selection of Patients:
a. Indications: The procedure is indicated for patients with respiratory, skin, or gastrointestinal symptoms suggestive of allergy. The procedure is often done in conjunction with evaluation of nasal eosinophilia.
b. Contraindications and Precautions: None
3. Equipment and Supplies (See Appendix for equipment and supplies manufacturers and suppliers. Appendix is keyed to italicized words in the equipment and supplies lists):
  • Standard equipment and supplies for obtaining venous blood sample (See Venous Bloods, Blood Collection Procedures, page 261)
4. Description of Procedure:
  • Obtain a 2- to 3-mL venous blood sample (See Venous Bloods, Blood Collection Procedures, page 261) in a tube containing ethylenediaminetetra-acetic acid (EDTA) to prevent coagulation.

Table 19-1. Scale for Interpreting Nasal Smears

	Grade
No eosinophilia (<5% eosinophils)	−
Slight eosinophilia (5–9% eosinophils)	+/−
Moderate eosinophilia (10–49% eosinophils)	+
Marked eosinophilia (≥ 50% eosinophils)	+ +

From Mygind N. Nasal Allergy. Blackwell Scientific Publications, Oxford, UK, 1978, with permission.
Values (+) and (+ +) are consistent with nasal allergy, particularly in children. A (±) grade has little diagnostic significance (a repeat sample may be helpful). A (−) grade is found in most normal subjects.

  • Obtain a complete blood count (including differential count) or a total eosinophil count.
5. Side Effects and Complications: There are no complications other than possible bleeding or bruising at the blood drawing site.
6. Interpretation: Like eosinophils in the nose, eosinophils in the peripheral circulation can vary. In addition, parasitic infections with tissue involvement also can elicit an eosinophilic response. When eosinophils are elevated in allergic children, they commonly represent 5% to 20% of the total white cell count. With parasitic infections, eosinophils may be markedly increased (up to 20% to 40% of the total white cell count). There are also other less common causes for blood eosinophilia (e.g., hypereosinophilic syndrome, neoplasms, drug reactions). It is important to remember that nonallergic children with asthma also can have increased eosinophil numbers in their blood.

One must be careful in judging eosinophils in the blood of patients (e.g., asthmatics) who have received an injection of epinephrine. Epinephrine releases marginated white cells, including eosinophils, into the peripheral circulation, thus elevating their numbers for several hours. Also, steroids decrease the peripheral eosinophil count. It is best to reserve judgment regarding peripheral eosinophils for at least 24 hours after epinephrine has been given and 48 to 72 hours after steroids have been discontinued. Normal values for peripheral blood eosinophils are 0% to 5% of the white blood cell count and, for total eosinophil count, 0.05 to 0.4 × 10^9 per liter of blood.

C. Allergy Skin Testing
1. Purpose: Skin testing is still the most frequently used method to diagnose IgE-mediated allergies. These tests are a

reliable and reproducible measure of allergen-specific IgE antibody. They are also extremely sensitive. In some cases, picogram (10^{-12} g) quantities of allergen are capable of eliciting a positive skin test response. Results of skin tests are used 1) to define which allergens can be avoided, 2) to plan the best approach for treating patients with medications, and 3) to select appropriate allergens for immunotherapy when allergen avoidance and medications are not successful in controlling symptoms.

2. Selection of Patients:

a. Indications: Any child who is suspected of being allergic (as judged by history, physical exam, nasal smear, peripheral eosinophil count, or total IgE level) and who requires medication frequently to control perennial or seasonal symptoms should be evaluated. In particular, children who miss school, who cannot sleep well at night, or whose exercise tolerance is limited because of their symptoms deserve a thorough evaluation. A careful history is important to determine which skin test reagents should be included in the evaluation. Allergic individuals with respiratory symptoms commonly show sensitivity to inhalent allergens (e.g., indoor dust and outdoor pollen allergens). After 2 to 4 years of age, children with respiratory symptoms suggestive of allergy are tested with extracts containing allergens indigenous to a geographic area (Table 19-2). Other allergens are added as indicated by the patient's history. Food sensitivity, however, is more common in infants and toddlers than in older children or adults. Most often, food allergens produce symptoms in the skin (atopic dermatitis) and gastrointestinal tract (diarrhea, vomiting, and abdominal discomfort). Occasionally, they cause anaphylactoid reactions and, less commonly, respiratory symptoms alone in the absence of skin or gastrointestinal symptoms. Thus, infants with allergic signs and symptoms are often tested with common food allergens (Table 19-2) known to stimulate IgE-specific antibody at an early age. Other allergens are then added as judged by the patient's history. Skin tests for insect venom (honey bee, wasp, hornet, and yellow jacket) allergies and drug (e.g., penicillin and cephalosporin) allergies are indicated only when a history of symptoms after exposure is obtained.

b. Contraindications and Precautions: Although adverse reactions resulting from skin testing are now rare, tests should be carried out in a medical setting where epinephrine and other appropriate drugs and supportive care are available. It is unwise to test patients who are actively wheezing, as symptoms may become worse in patients who are sensitized to allergen(s) used for testing. Some allergists wait approximately 4 to 6 weeks before testing a patient who has had an adverse reaction to a drug or insect sting. Antihistamines interfere with skin test reactions and should *not* be given within 48 to 72 hours before testing. Other medications, including steroids, are not known to alter skin test responsiveness.

Table 19-2. Common Inhalant and Food Extracts Used For Skin Testing*

A. Inhalant Extracts

1. *Indoor allergens*
   - Crude house dust
   - Dust mite *(Dermatophagoides sp)*†
   - Domestic animals (cat and dog)
   - Cockroach (mixed species)†
   - Molds (e.g., *Aspergillus* and *Penicillium*)

2. *Outdoor allergens*
   - Grasses (mixed and Bermuda)†
   - Tree mix†
   - Ragweed
   - Plantain
   - Molds (e.g., *Alternaria* and *Cladosporium*)

B. Food Extracts‡

Egg	Peanut
Milk	Wheat
Soy	Fish

* In North America, individuals who are skin-test negative to the above extracts and who have a normal total IgE level are unlikely to be allergic.

† To limit the number of skin tests, mixed species extracts are often used to initially evaluate children. Testing using individual species can be planned subsequently if indicated.

‡ The six extracts listed are foods that most commonly stimulate IgE-mediated allergy. Other foods are added as judged by the patient's history.

Occasionally patients with extensive eczema or urticaria have no areas of uninvolved skin available for reliable testing. In food-allergic infants with atropic dermatitis, an elemental formula can be tried for 2 to 3 weeks before testing to improve the condition of the skin, provided no other foods are present in the diet. A short course of steroids can also be tried to improve skin lesions before testing. Skin tests are understandably contraindicated during pregnancy. During pregnancy and in patients with severe eczema or urticaria, *in vitro* allergy tests (e.g., the radioallergosorbent test [RAST]) can be considered as a diagnostic alternative.

3. Equipment and Supplies (See Appendix for equipment and supplies manufacturers and suppliers. Appendix is keyed to italicized words in the equipment and supplies lists):

- Alcohol *pads*
- Marking pen
- Commercial *extracts* (inhalant, food, venom, or drug allergens)
- Buffered saline with phenol *solution*
- 26-gauge *needles,* sterile metal *scarifier,* or disposable plastic *scarifier* (Figure 19-2)
- Histamine acid phosphate *solution*

4. Description of Procedure:

a. Prick skin tests:

- Proper selection of an area of skin for testing is an

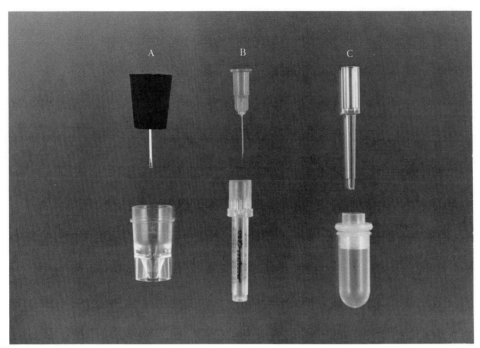

Figure 19-2.
Allergy skin testing. Equipment and supplies: **A,** Metal scarifier with two prongs; **B,** 26-gauge needle; **C,** Plastic scarifier with tines.

important factor in determining patient comfort as well as ease in interpreting positive and negative results. It is important, for example, to choose an area not affected by eczema, urticaria, or any other irritation of the skin. Children less than 1 year of age are often tested on their backs while lying face down across their parents' legs. The hands and feet can be held by the parent if restraining becomes necessary. Evaluations are usually limited to skin prick tests in infants, and intradermal testing is not done commonly until after age 2. Prick testing is not very painful and is often limited to 5 to 10 food and inhalent allergens when testing infants. After 2 years of age, children are often tested on an arm (biceps area) or thigh, and the extremity being tested is restrained as described for blood drawing (Blood Collection Procedures, page 258).

· Cleanse the skin with alcohol and allow it to dry.

· Separate test sites by at least 1 inch. Use a marking pen to label each test site.

· To perform a test, apply a drop of allergen extract to a hair-free area of the skin.

· As controls to judge a positive and negative response, apply histamine acid phosphate (0.1 mg/mL) and buffered saline adjacent to the test sites, respectively.

· Insert a 26-gauge needle through a drop and gently prick and lift the skin, being careful not to induce bleeding (Figure 19-3). Metal scarifiers, which must be autoclaved after use, or disposable plastic scarifiers, can be used instead of 26-gauge needles and do not often cause bleeding. When inserting a scarifier through a drop of extract, press it firmly onto the skin and then rotate it 45 degrees, allowing allergen to penetrate the epidermis and come into contact with skin mast cells. Use separate needles or scarifiers for each test so that each drop of allergen extract on the skin is never contaminated with allergen from a previous test. Importantly, use disposable needles, disposable scarifier with tines, or autoclaved metal scarifiers for each patient, to eliminate the possibility of blood contamination and the risk of transferring the human immunodeficiency virus or hepatitis B virus.

· Read the tests 10 to 15 minutes after applying the extracts. Before reading the results, remove all allergens and control solutions by gently wiping the skin with alcohol·pads. Positive skin reactions are characterized by a raised wheal surrounded by erythema (Figure 19-4). The diameter of the raised wheal is measured in millimeters and graded from 0 to 4+ (Table 19-3). Results are then recorded in the patient's medical re-

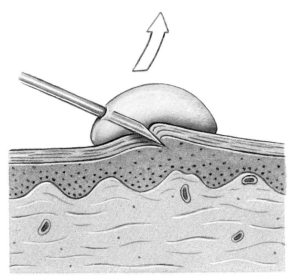

Figure 19-3.
Allergy skin testing—Prick skin test. Technique.

**Table 19-3. Grading System for Skin Test Reactions
(Mean Wheal Diameter)**

Prick	Grade	Intradermal
< 2 mm	0	< 5 mm
2–3 mm	±	5–6 mm
3–4 mm	1+	6–8 mm
5–7 mm	2+	8–10 mm
7–10 mm	3+	> 10 mm
7–10 mm/with pseudopod(s)	4+	> 10 mm/with pseudopod(s)

cord. The erythema (i.e., flare response), together with itching, is indicative of histamine release from skin mast cells and is also observed with the positive histamine control test. Occasionally induration caused by trauma to the skin and blood vessels is noted with a negative test; however, erythema and itching will not be noted. Measuring and recording the diameter of erythema is not recommended and is not thought to correlate well with the degree of sensitization. In general a wheel less than 3 mm in diameter is *not* considered to be significant.

· One should remember that antihistamines taken by the patient 48 to 72 hours before testing can suppress the skin test response. When prick skin tests are negative, carry out intradermal tests (see below). Note: *Scratch* skin tests are very similar to *prick* tests. A scratch test is carried out by scratching the skin with a needle or scarifier and then applying a drop of allergen extract to the scratch. Occasionally, the scratch may cause bleeding and thus contaminate the dropper used to apply the extract. Although no cases of acquired immunodeficiency syndrome or hepatitis have been transferred from one patient to another using this method, scratch tests currently are not recommended.

b. Intradermal skin tests:

· Intradermal tests are carried out in older children (2 years of age or older) after skin prick tests have been evaluated. Only negative prick tests are repeated intradermally. Most allergists reserve intradermal testing for evaluating hypersensitivity to inhalant, drug, and insect venom allergens. Intradermal tests for food allergy usually are not performed.

· Dilute 1:100 in buffered saline each allergen extract (concentrations are noted as weight per volume [w/v], protein nitrogen units [PNU], or, in some cases, allergen units [AU]).

· Using a tuberculin syringe with a 26-gauge needle attached, inject intradermally an exact volume (0.02–0.04 mL), which introduces approximately 100- to 1000-fold more allergen into the skin than by the prick test (Figure 19-5). Use the same method as described for the tuberculin Mantoux test (PPD) (See Administration of Tuberculin Skin Tests, page 28).

· Inject intradermally as a positive and negative control the same volumes of histamine acid phosphate (0.275 mg/mL) and buffered saline, respectively.

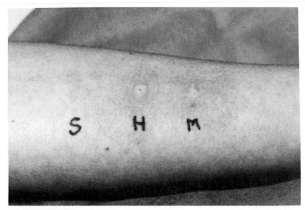

Figure 19-4.
Allergy skin testing. Positive reaction to mite allergen (M). Positive control [histamine (H)]. Negative control [saline (S)].

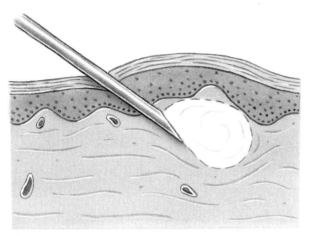

Figure 19-5.
Allergy skin testing—Intradermal skin test. Techique.

• Read the tests 10 to 15 minutes after the intradermal tests are completed (see Figure 19-4; Table 19-3) and record the results in the patient's medical record. As with prick tests, a positive intradermal reaction is characterized by a raised pruritic wheal surrounded by erythema. A wheal diameter < 5 mm is not usually considered to be significant.

5. Side Effects and Complications: After testing, patients should be observed for at least 30 to 40 minutes so that any symptoms of anaphylaxis can be recognized early and properly treated. Anaphylactic reactions after skin testing, however, are not common.

6. Interpretation: When allergic individuals become sensitized to an allergen (e.g., ragweed pollen), they produce IgE (reagenic) antibodies specific for that allergen. Although these antibodies can be measured in the serum, only IgE antibodies attached to mast cells or basophils are clinically important. After exposure (e.g., to an inhaled allergen, or to an allergen injected into the skin for testing), allergen molecules bind to IgE antibodies fixed to mast cells, resulting in the release of histamine and other mediators (Figure 19-6). The response to mediators in the skin results in vasodilation, edema, and erythema (wheal and flare) within 2 to 15 minutes (type I Gel and Coombs reaction, or immediate hypersensitivity). This reaction, which looks like a hive and itches, may be followed by a late-phase reaction 3 to 12 hours later. This latter reaction is distinct from a type IV Gel and Coombs reaction, or delayed hypersensitivity, which develops 24 to 72 hours after an exposure.

Most allergic patients have more than one positive skin reaction. Although positive tests are accurate markers of sensitization, not all positive results are clinically significant. A patient's history must be carefully evaluated together with skin test results to judge which tests are important. Follow-up visits to monitor a patient's progress also may help delineate which tests are meaningful. A ragweed-allergic patient, for example, will have a positive skin test and an increase in symptoms during the ragweed season. The same patient may have a positive skin reaction for grass allergen (indicating sensitization), but may have subclinical or minimal symptoms during the grass pollen season. Thus, the grass skin reaction is not judged to be clinically important as far as further treatment is concerned. In summary, when skin test responses are evaluated together with the patient's history, the practitioner can:

1. Make sensible recommendations regarding allergen avoidance when patients are allergic to indoor dust or animal allergens.
2. Prescribe medications to prevent or control symptoms during periods of increased allergen exposure and avoid the unnecessary use of daily medications throughout the year.
3. Prescribe allergen immunotherapy when indicated.

The same commercially produced extracts that are used for skin testing are also used for immunotherapy. All extracts are standardized in either protein nitrogen units (PNU) or allergen units (AU) per milliliter, and companies must submit their extracts to the Food and Drug Administration for approval together with skin test data demonstrating reactivity and safety in a selected group of patients. Variability in allergen content, however, has been shown to exist among extracts (particularly house dust extracts) produced by different companies. Batch-to-batch variability among extracts produced by the same company also has been shown. New approaches to standardization using allergen-specific immunoassays have now been proposed. These assays should make it possible to measure the allergen concentration of extracts quantitatively, thus improving the quality control of extracts used for diagnosis and treatment.

D. *In Vitro* Measures of IgE Antibody

1. Purpose: Measurements of IgE antibody in the serum can be used:

1. as a screening tool for identifying patients likely to be allergic individuals.
2. to measure IgE antibodies produced against specific allergens (e.g., grass, ragweed, mite allergen) via the radioallergosorbent test (RAST).

2. Selection of Patients:

a. Indications: As with skin testing, children who require medication frequently to control perennial or seasonal symptoms suggestive of allergy should be evaluated.

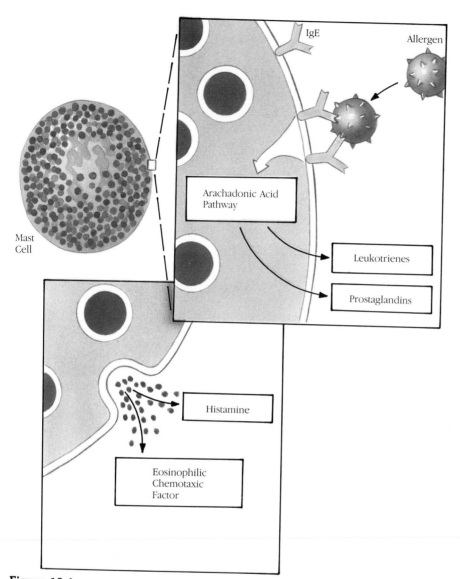

Figure 19-6.
Allergy skin testing—Mast cell activation. Histamine and other inflammatory
mediators are released after the bridging of IgE antibodies on mast cell membranes by
allergen molecules. Chemotactic factors also are released and attract eosinophils to
tissue sites where allergic reactions occur.

Total Serum IgE Measurements. Unlike nasal or peripheral eosinophil counts, IgE levels tend to vary less significantly
in a given individual and remain elevated for prolonged
periods after sensitization and allergen exposure. Total IgE
measurements are higher in allergic individuals with asthma
and rhinitis and markedly elevated in children with allergic
eczema (See Interpretation, below). Measurements of total

IgE, therefore, can be used to judge whether further allergy
testing might be indicated.

Although skin testing remains the preferred method of
evaluating patients for specific allergen sensitivities, not all
individuals can be conveniently tested. As an alternative, *in
vitro RAST analyses* may be preferred 1) in patients with
extensive eczema, or any skin condition, which involves po-

tential skin test sites; 2) in patients recently treated with antihistamines; 3) when allergy evaluations are required during pregnancy. As with skin testing, children whose symptoms cause morbidity or who require medication frequently to control perennial or seasonal symptoms suggestive of allergy should be evaluated.

Two advantages to RAST testing are that a large number of analyses can be carried out using blood obtained from a single needle stick, and adverse anaphylactic reactions are not a problem. These tests, however, are not available in all hospitals or clinical centers and when ordered commercially are generally more expensive than skin tests. The use of radiolabeled reagents prohibits RAST analyses from being carried out in a clinical practice. Thus, serum usually is sent to commercial or research laboratories and results may not be available for several days. Similar assays using fluorometric techniques and enzyme-labeled reagents have been developed to obviate the need for radiolabeled reagents and may make it possible to measure allergen-specific IgE antibody in sera from allergic patients in a clinical setting.

b. Contraindications and Precautions: None

3. Equipment and Supplies (See Appendix for equipment and supplies manufacturers and suppliers. Appendix is keyed to italicized words in the equipment and supplies lists):

  · Standard equipment and supplies for obtaining a venous blood sample (See *Venous Bloods, Blood Collection Procedures*, page 261).

4. Description of Procedure:

  · Obtain a venous blood sample (See *Venous Bloods, Blood Collection Procedures*, page 261). Approximately 3 to 5 mL of blood should be sufficient for total IgE measurement and RAST analyses. Allergen-specific IgE antibodies in the serum are measured by RAST, as shown in Figure 19-7.

5. Side Effects and Complications: There are no complications other than possible bleeding or bruising at the blood drawing site.

6. Interpretation: Total IgE levels > 100 international units (IU) per milliliter are usually considered elevated (1 IU = 2.4 nanograms of IgE) in adults. However, IgE levels between 20 and 100 IU/mL may occur in patients who have elevated IgE antibodies for specific allergens. Thus, patients who have an impressive personal or family history of allergy-related symptoms should be tested (skin testing or RAST) for allergies even if their total IgE level is not markedly elevated. Be aware that total IgE levels in infants and young children (less than 2–3 years of age) who have allergy-related symptoms are often low by adult standards. After 3 years of age, however, IgE levels are generally higher in allergic children, and the range of total IgE levels can be remarkable. IgE levels in excess of 1000 IU/mL are often seen in sera from patients with extensive atopic dermatitis or allergic bronchopulmonary aspergillosis.

One should also note that total IgE levels can be markedly elevated in patients with helminth infections and immunodeficiencies.

Although skin tests are more sensitive than RAST analyses for measuring IgE antibodies to specific allergens, RAST testing for IgE antibodies to inhalant and insect venom allergens are comparable to skin tests in judging clinically important sensitivities. At present, RAST evaluations for measuring IgE antibodies to foods, molds, and most drug allergens (other than those performed in some research laboratories) are not helpful or reliable for routine diagnostic purposes. Extracts used for RAST have the same limitations as extracts used in skin testing with respect to standardization. It must be emphasized that, like skin tests, positive RAST results must be interpreted in the context of the patient's history to judge which results are clinically meaningful.

II. Therapeutic Procedures

A. Allergen Avoidance

1. Purpose: After the patient's history and allergy tests have been assessed to judge which allergic sensitivities are clinically important, the first line of management is to recommend decreased allergen exposure whenever possible. The goal is to decrease symptoms and reliance on medications.

2. Selection of Patients:

a. Indications: Patients whose symptoms are caused or aggravated by indoor dust, dust mite, animal, food, or drug allergens benefit most from allergen avoidance. Avoidance of outdoor allergens (e.g., pollens and weeds) often is not practical.

b. Contraindications and Precautions: Practitioners should vary their recommendations in keeping with the severity of a patient's symptoms, the costs involved, and changes in lifestyles required with some allergen avoidance regimens. For example, not all patients are willing to get rid of their cat or dog and not all dust-allergic patients can afford to remove wall-to-wall carpeting.

3. Equipment and Supplies: None

4. Description of Procedure: Printed educational materials for patients regarding allergen avoidance can be obtained from the American Academy of Allergy and Immunology, 611 East Wells Street, Milwaukee, WI 53202 (telephone number 1-800-822-2762). Recommendations specific for house dust and mold control can also be obtained from Allergy Control Products, Inc., 96 Danbury Road, Ridgefield, CT 06877 (telephone number 1-800-422-3878).

5. Side Effects and Complications: None

6. Interpretation: Allergic symptoms often take time to improve after allergen avoidance, particularly when allergen exposure over time has caused chronic inflammation. For

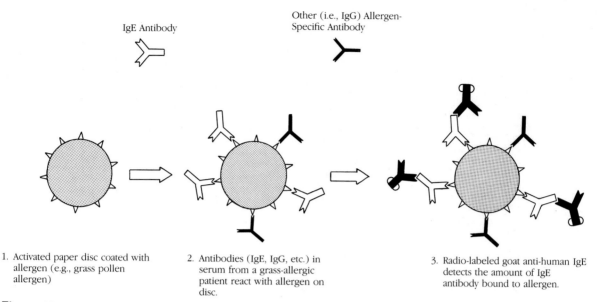

IgE Antibody

Other (i.e., IgG) Allergen-Specific Antibody

1. Activated paper disc coated with allergen (e.g., grass pollen allergen)

2. Antibodies (IgE, IgG, etc.) in serum from a grass-allergic patient react with allergen on disc.

3. Radio-labeled goat anti-human IgE detects the amount of IgE antibody bound to allergen.

Figure 19-7.
***In vitro* measurements of IgE antibody.** *In vitro* (RAST) test for allergen-specific IgE antibody.

example, when allergic asthmatics are monitored in allergen-free environments, bronchial hyperreactivity may not return toward normal for three to six weeks.

B. Emergency Management of Asthma and Anaphylaxis

1. Purpose: The purpose of this procedure is to treat patients seen in a clinic, office, or emergency department who have signs and symptoms of severe anaphylaxis or asthma.

2. Selection of Patients:

a. *Anaphylaxis:* Although less common in children than adults, anaphylaxis must be recognized and treated early to prevent mortality. The clinical manifestations of anaphylaxis leading to respiratory tract obstruction and cardiovascular collapse evolve rapidly because of the sudden release of large amounts of diverse mediators from mast cells and basophils. Symptoms usually begin within minutes after exposure to an exciting agent and reach peak intensity within 30 to 60 minutes.

Often, pruritic cutaneous eruptions (acute urticaria), generalized swelling (angioedema), and skin erythema are the earliest signs of anaphylaxis and begin either at the site of allergen exposure (e.g., insect sting) or on the face and upper body. Other allergy-related signs and symptoms (hoarseness, stridor, wheezing, nasal congestion, rhinorrhea, conjunctival hyperemia, nausea, vomiting, diarrhea, and crampy, abdomi-

nal pain) also may develop rapidly. However, at least one of the following must be present to establish the diagnosis of anaphylaxis: 1) respiratory tract obstruction involving the upper (angio- or laryngeal edema) or lower (bronchospasm and interstitial edema) airways; 2) acute hypotension (drop in blood pressure and tachycardia predisposing to cardiac arrest) resulting from sudden peripheral vasodilatation, increased postcapillary permeability, and loss of intravascular volume.

The most common causes of allergic (IgE-mediated) anaphylaxis include exposures to *Hymenoptera* stings (bees, wasps, hornets, yellow jackets, and fire ants); drugs (particularly penicillin and cephalosporin antibiotics given intravenously or intramuscularly); hormone preparations (insulin, chymopapain); transfusions of blood products; injections of foreign proteins in vaccines (e.g., horse serum); food allergens (especially peanuts, other nuts, eggs, and shellfish); and injections of extracts used to treat allergies (e.g., immunotherapy). Anaphylaxis can also be caused by substances that stimulate direct release of mediators from mast cells and basophils without involving IgE antibodies. Examples include opiate medications (codeine, morphine) and iodinated radio-contrast media used in radiologic studies.

b. *Acute asthma attack:* Patients who present with wheezing or who show signs of retractions, anxiety, or irritability characteristic of air hunger require immediate attention and eval-

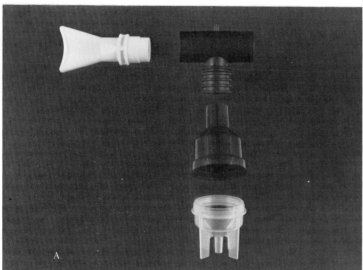

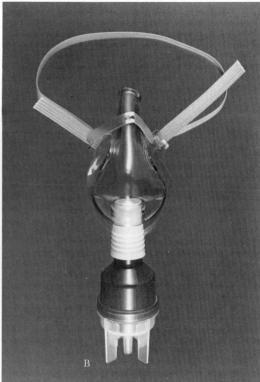

Figure 19-8.
Emergency management of asthma and anaphylaxis. Equipment and supplies: **A,**
Nebulizer, T-tube, and mouthpiece; **B,** Nebulizer attached to face mask.

uation for asthma. A brief history focused on duration of symptoms, previous attacks, possibility of foreign body aspiration, other respiratory illness, medications taken, and precipitating causes should indicate whether the patient is an asthmatic. In addition to lung auscultation, the physical examination should focus on signs of severe obstruction, including retractions, pulsus paradoxus greater than 20 mm Hg, significant agitation or lethargy, a quiet chest in an otherwise distressed patient, and obvious cyanosis. Cyanosis is a late sign of hypoxemia in asthma and is indicative of marked respiratory failure.

Most children with an asthma attack develop mild to moderate airway obstruction that responds to beta-adrenergic agonist medications. A peak expiratory flow rate (PEFR), which can be used to assess obstruction and monitor the course of treatment, can be performed by most school-aged children. When patients do not respond to beta-adrenergic agonist drugs, their attack is often defined as status asthmaticus and more intensive monitoring and treatment is indicated.

3. Equipment and Supplies (See Appendix for equipment and supplies manufacturers and suppliers. Appendix is keyed to italicized words in the equipment and supplies lists):

- Standard equipment for administering intravenous medications should be immediately available (See Infusion Procedures, page 275).
- Emergency treatment rooms are usually equipped with wall compressed air units for administering nebulized medications as well as outlets for compressed oxygen. If compressed air units are not available, portable air compressor *units* can be purchased and used very effectively in a clinic, office, or home to nebulize medications for treatment of children who have bronchospasm as well as chronic symptoms of asthma.
- *Nebulizer* for mixing medications with saline (Figure 19-8A and 19-8B).
- *T-tube* with *mouthpiece* attachment (Figure 19-8A) or *face mask* (Figure 19-8B)
- Saline *solution* for nebulization

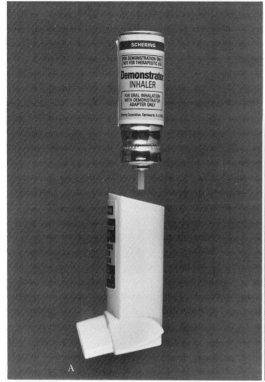
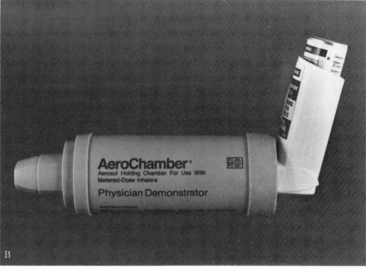

Figure 19-9.
Emergency management of asthma and anaphylaxis. Equipment and supplies: **A,**
Metered dose inhaler; **B,** Spacer attached to metered dose inhaler.

- Tweezers
- *Tourniquet* (See Figure 20-6, page 261)
- Emergency *kits* for administering epinephrine at home
- Metered dose *inhaler* (Figure 19-9A and B)
- *Spacer* (Figure 19-9B)

4. Description of Procedure:

a. *Anaphylaxis:* General treatment measures to prevent cardiorespiratory arrest in patients with suspected anaphylaxis should include:

- If a sting has occurred, examine the sting bite and remove the stinger, if present, with tweezers. Only honey bees have a barbed stinger, which often remains in the sting site with venom sacs attached. Remove the stinger, being careful not to compress the venom sac. Other venomous insects rarely leave their nonbarbed stingers behind.
- Place a tourniquet above the sting site, but release and then reapply the tourniquet approximately every 15 minutes.

- Put the patient in a supine position with his legs elevated (Trendelenburg position) and his neck slightly extended. Monitor the pulse and the blood pressure frequently.
- Until hypoxia is ruled out, oxygen should be administered routinely either by nasal cannula (5 L/minute) or face mask (40%–60% O_2) to sustain the $PO_2 \geq 60$ mm Hg.
- A beta-adrenergic agonist is the drug of choice for the initial management of anaphylaxis. Typically, epinephrine is given as soon as possible and the dose is repeated after 10 minutes if the first has not resulted in improvement. Prompt benefit often occurs within minutes. The risk of serious side effects (arrhythmias, hypertension) from properly administered epinephrine is low in children.
- If epinephrine is not effective, begin intravenous fluid administration with either Ringer's lactate or normal saline to rapidly expand the intravascular volume and to

Table 19-4. Drugs Used for the Emergency Treatment of Anaphylaxis and Asthma

	Route of Administration†	Dosage	Comments
A. Anaphylaxis			
1. Epinephrine 1:1000 (Aqueous)	SQ	0.01 mL/kg/dose (max. single dose = 0.3 mL)	Duration of action is 10–15 minutes. Dose may be repeated q 15 minutes × 3.
2. Diphenhydramine	PO	1–2 mg/kg	H_1 antihistamine. Duration of action is 6 to 8 hours. Can be given orally early in the course of mild to moderate anaphylaxis. Contraindicated in neonates and infants.
	IV or IM	2 mg/kg slowly (max. single dose = 75 mg)	
3. Cimetidine	IV	4 mg/kg (max. single dose = 300 mg) infused over at least 5 minutes	H_2 antihistamine; dilute each dose in 20 mL 0.9% NaCl.
4. Aminophylline	IV	6 mg/kg (loading dose) in 100 mL saline over 20 minutes	If continuous drip necessary, see recommendations for treating asthma.
5. Steroids			
a. Hydrocortisone (Na succinate)	IV	4–8 mg/kg/dose; then 10 mg/kg/day q 6h	Onset of action is 4 to 6 hours. Helpful for treating persistent symptoms (See text).
b. Methylprednisolone	IV	2 mg/kg/dose q 6h for max. of 48 to 72 hours	
6. Isoproterenol by constant infusion	IV	Begin with 0.1 μg/kg/min. Increase q 10 minutes by 0.1 μg/kg/min if blood pressure is stabilized. Max. dose = 1.5 μg/kg/min.	Continuous infusion recommended for intensive care setting only. Monitor for arrhythmias and hypotension. Lower infusion rate when heart rate > 200 bpm or arrhythmia occurs. Use with care in congestive heart failure.
B. Acute asthma attack			
1. Inhaled beta-adrenergic agonists			
a. Albuterol (0.5%)	N	0.03 mL/kg (max. single dose = 10 mL) 4 hr*	These nebulized medications should be added to 2.5 mL saline in the nebulizer chamber and inhaled continuously over 10 to 20 minutes.
b. Terbutaline (1 mg/mL)	N	0.01–0.02 mL/kg (max. single dose = 1.0 mL) 4 hr*	
c. Metaproterenol (5%)	N	0.01–0.02 mL/kg (max. single dose = 0.3 mL) 4 hr*	
d. Isoproterenol (1:200)	N	0.01–0.02 mL/kg (max. single dose = 0.5 mL) 1 hr*	
2. Injected beta-adrenergic agonists			
a. Epinephrine 1:1000 (aqueous)	SQ	0.01 mL/kg/dose (max. single dose = 0.3 mL)	Dose may be repeated q 15 min × 3.
b. Terbutaline (1 mg/mL)	SQ	0.01 mL/kg (max. single dose = 0.3 mL)	Dose may be repeated q 15–20 min × 2.
c. Epinephrine 1:200	SQ	0.005 mL/kg/dose (max. single dose = 0.15 mL)	Duration of action is approximately 8 hours.
3. Isoproterenol by constant infusion	IV	0.1 μg/kg/min, increasing by 0.1 μg/kg/min q 15 min until respiratory effort improves or HR is ≥ 200 bpm	Indicated for patients in respiratory failure. Patients should be in an intensive care setting on a cardiac monitor.

Table 19-4. Drugs Used for the Emergency Treatment of Anaphylaxis and Asthma (continued)

	Route of Administration†	Dosage	Comments
4. Aminophylline	IV	6 mg/kg (loading dose) in 100 mL saline over 30 minutes followed by 1 mg/kg/hr constant infusion	If patient has recently taken theophylline, bolus dose should be reduced by one half.
5. Inhaled atropine sulfate (0.1 mg/mL)	N	0.05–0.1 mg/kg (max. single dose = 1.0 mg) q 4h	Added to 2.5 mL saline in nebulizer. Not studied extensively in children. May not add to further bronchodilation if other drugs are used appropriately.
6. Steroids			
a. Hydrocortisone (Na succinate)	IV	4–8 mg/kg/dose; then 10 mg/kg/day q 6h	Important for properly treating the effects of chronic inflammation. Onset of action may be 4–6 hours.
b. Methylprednisolone	IV	2 mg/kg/dose × 1. Maintenance: 1 mg/kg/dose q 6h	
7. Sodium bicarbonate	IV	1 mEq/kg/dose	Given to correct for metabolic acidosis. May be repeated × 1 after checking a blood gas.

† SQ = subcutaneous; PO = by mouth; IV = intravenous; N = nebulized
* Duration of action

facilitate intravenous drug administration. Other medications used to treat anaphylaxis including dosages, route of administration, and duration of action, are listed in Table 19-4.

• If marked improvement is not apparent after giving epinephrine, a vasopressor may be needed (e.g., norepinephrine) as well as combined H_1 and H_2 antihistamine therapy. Theophylline should be administered to treat the pulmonary manifestations of anaphylaxis. Corticosteroids (e.g., hydrocortisone or methylprednisolone) are also indicated, but the onset of action is 4 to 6 hours after the initial dose. Although not effective in treating the immediate effects of anaphylaxis, steroids are helpful in treating the late-phase inflammatory effects of the mediators released and are also helpful in cases where the allergic or chemical cause of anaphylaxis cannot be removed rapidly or eliminated from the body (e.g., food allergen in the gastrointestinal tract).

• If the patient is unresponsive, maintain a patent oropharyngeal airway with a plastic mouthpiece and prepare to intubate and treat cardiac arrest (See Chapter 24) if necessary.

• If a food or drug ingestion leading to anaphylaxis is suggested, a nasogastric tube should be placed and the gastric contents removed by lavage (See Chapter 23). A cathartic should be given and, for some drug ingestions causing anaphylaxis, activated charcoal considered. These measures, however, should not be initiated until the patient has been stabilized.

• If the patient is unstable, cardiac monitoring, blood pressures, oxygen saturation via oximetry, and blood gases to judge the onset or presence of respiratory failure and metabolic acidosis should be followed closely. Steps should be taken to prepare for intubation or cricothyrotomy and assisted ventilation. When stable enough to be moved, the patient should be transferred to an intensive care setting and, once stable, monitored for an additional 12 hours.

• After successfully treating the patient, proper management must include the prevention of future anaphylactic episodes. For example, avoidance of the drug or food allergen causing the acute event is most important, and a Medical Alert bracelet should be prescribed if the patient is at high risk for future exposures. Patients (if old enough) and parents also should be taught how to use one of the available emergency kits for the administration of epinephrine at home. Patients and parents should be taught both the indications for giving epinephrine as well as the methods of self-administration, and they should review the procedure on a regular basis as long as the patient is at risk. Practice is particularly important for patients who have insect sting hypersensitivity, keeping in mind that sensitized children are at a lower risk of severe anaphylaxis after a sting than adults.

b. *Acute asthma attack*—Most children who are treated for an asthma attack have symptoms of wheezing, coughing, and an increased respiratory rate without evidence of respiratory distress. For these patients, the use of aerosolized beta-adrenergic agonists specific for beta$_2$-receptors in the lungs (e.g., albuterol, terbutaline, metaproterenol) represents the first-line treatment, which often leads to marked improvement. As compared with injected beta-agonists (epinephrine or terbutaline), the advantages to using aerosolized drugs include the use of smaller doses of medication, reduced cardiovascular side effects, onset of action similar to epinephrine but with a longer duration of action, and no pain. These medications are given by nebulizers powered by wall oxygen delivery or inexpensive portable compressor–nebulizer units available for office and home use. Children older than 3 or 4 years of age can usually inhale their medication through a T tube (Figure 19-10A), whereas younger children (preferably sitting in their mother's lap) do better with a face mask attached to the nebulizer (Figure 19-10B). In general, metered dose inhalers (MDI) do not represent a reliable delivery system for administering adrenergic agents in an office or hospital setting. Although ideal for treating exercise-induced asthma and mild episodes of wheezing at home, most children who present with acute wheezing to a medical facility have already tried their MDIs at home, or will have never used one and will therefore not be familiar with their proper use. Clearly, if no other treatment is available, an MDI should be used, preferably using a holding chamber or spacer attachment, which obviates the need to activate the inhaler at the beginning of a deep inspiration.

After a patient's wheezing clears by auscultation, a measurement of the PEFR often demonstrates residual abnormalities in air flow. These abnormalities reflect inflammation commonly caused by infection, allergen exposure, tobacco smoke exposure, or other environmental triggers of asthma. Thus, in addition to sending the patient home on a long-acting bronchodilator (e.g., epinephrine 1:200), almost all patients should be sent home on a short course of steroids (prednisone tablets or liquid, 2 mg/kg, orally, every morning) for 5 days. Unless a more prolonged course of steroids is used (≥ 7 days) a tapered dosage schedule is not usually necessary.

If wheezing does not improve significantly after two doses of an inhaled adrenergic agonist, it is unlikely that a third dose will dramatically improve symptoms. The following approach to treatment is then recommended for patients suspected to have status asthmaticus:

• If there is any doubt that the nebulized, adrenergic medications were properly inhaled, give epinephrine or terbutaline subcutaneously to confirm that the patient is "beta-agonist–resistant." Injected adrenergic agents should actually be used instead of the inhaled medications (at least for the first dose), if the patient has evidence of poor air exchange (e.g., retractions, absence of wheezing or poor breath sounds by auscultation).

• Supplemental oxygen should be administered routinely if the above signs of poor air exchange are evident or if the arterial PO$_2$ is less than 70 mm Hg while breathing room air. Humidified oxygen, 5 to 7 L/min, administered by nasal cannula or mask is usually sufficient. Indications for obtaining a blood gas include the presence of retractions, diminished breath sounds by auscultation, or beta-adrenergic unresponsiveness.

• Most children who have status asthmaticus require hospitalization or observation and management in an emergency room setting. In particular, wheezing infants (less than 2 years of age) who present with respiratory distress and who have a less than complete response to adrenergic drugs and children whose asthma has recurred within 48 hours should be hospitalized.

• To insure adequate observation, vital signs should be checked every 15 to 30 minutes until the patient's respiratory efforts are stabilized. Although children with status asthmaticus are at significant risk for respiratory failure, it occurs in less than 1% of hospitalizations.

• Intravenous fluids (e.g., D$_5$ ¼ normal saline) should generally be started at 1 to 1½ times maintenance. In patients unresponsive to beta-agonists, aminophylline is given intravenously as a 6 mg/kg bolus. If theophylline has been taken within 24 hours by the patient, the bolus dose should be reduced by one half. A constant infusion of aminophylline (1 mg/kg per hour) should then be continued. It is helpful to know that a change of 1 mg/kg in the infusion rate will change the peak serum level 2 μg/mL and that a 50% change will usually change the steady-state theophylline concentration by a factor of 2. To judge whether the serum theophylline concentration is in the therapeutic range (10–20 μg/mL), theophylline levels are recommended one half hour after the initial loading dose and then 6 to 12 hours later. Further determinations every 12 to 24 hours will guide therapy until the patient is taking theophylline by mouth. Concurrent with the administration of aminophylline, hydrocortisone or methylprednisolone should be given (See Table 19-4, page 252).

• During an asthma attack, the PCO$_2$ initially decreases in a tachypneic patient. With early signs of respiratory failure, the return of the PCO$_2$ toward normal is worrisome and a PCO$_2$ above normal is an ominous sign. Frequent administration of inhaled aerosolized beta ag-

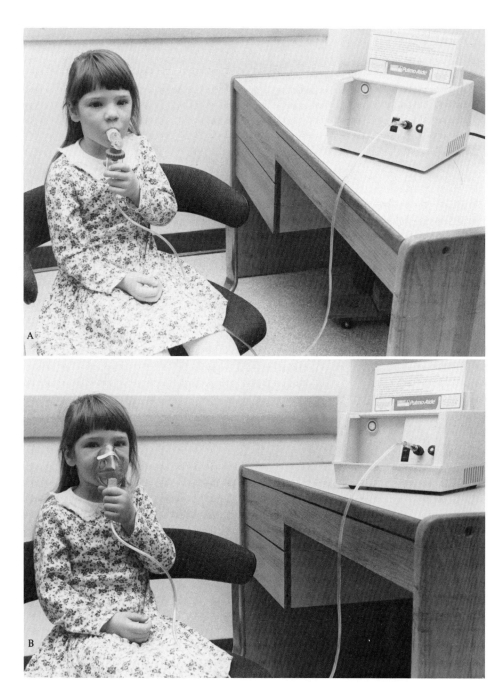

Figure 19-10.
Emergency management of asthma. A, Technique for inhalation using air compressor unit with nebulizer, T-tube, and mouthpiece. **B,** Technique for inhalation using air compressor unit with nebulizer and face mask.

onists every 30 to 60 minutes, or continuously if necessary, has been recommended for treating impending respiratory failure. Conventional treatment of patients with respiratory failure involves more aggressive treatent with intravenous isoproterenol or terbutaline (See Table 19-4, page 252), which is often used to obviate the need for mechanical ventilation. All patients thought to have impending respiratory failure should be managed in an intensive care setting and monitored by electrocardiogram. Progression to respiratory failure despite the measures described above indicates a need for intubation and mechanical ventilation.

· When hospitalized patients improve, oral theophylline is begun at a dose extrapolated from the intravenous requirement (24-hour aminophylline dose times 0.85 divided by the dosing interval of the oral preparation). If a slowly absorbed theophylline is given, wait 4 hours to discontinue aminophylline. Oral prednisone, in a single morning dose of 2 mg/kg/day for 5 days should be prescribed. Inhaled adrenergic agonists, using a metered dose inhaler or nebulizer, also should be continued, or oral adrenergic agonists if inhaled medications are not feasible. A return outpatient visit is recommended in 2 weeks.

5. Side Effects and Complications:

a. *Anaphylaxis:* If patients do not respond rapidly to epinephrine, consider the following regarding the patient's status:

(1) Marked hypotension (poor capillary filling, weak and rapid pulse, and subnormal blood pressure) leading to metabolic acidosis is the most serious cause of beta-adrenergic hyporesponsiveness. Intravenous fluids to expand the intravascular volume should be started as soon as possible and sodium bicarbonate (1 mEq/kg per dose intravenously) is given to correct the acidosis. Sodium bicarbonate may be repeated if necessary after checking a blood gas. After correcting the hypovolemia and acidosis, patients may become more responsive to epinephrine, but are at risk for developing cardiac arrhythmias from subsequent doses of epinephrine and aminophylline. Therefore, cardic monitoring is required. Once an intravenous line is established, other medications (e.g., H_1 and H_2 antihistamines, theophylline, and steroids) can be given. Consider moving the patient to an intensive care setting as soon as feasible, then start an isoproterenol drip if the blood pressure has not been normalized.

(2) Patients taking beta-adrenergic blocking medications (e.g., propanalol) and patients with cardiac disease or asthma can also respond poorly to beta-agonist drugs.

b. *Acute asthma attack:* Asthmatic patients with lower respiratory tract infections (most commonly viral and occasionally mycoplasma) are at increased risk for status asthmaticus and respiratory failure. Bacterial sinus infections reportedly also make asthma more difficult to treat. Chest radiographs are indicated for asthma patients who are "beta-agonist unresponsive" or who are febrile or who have rales on lung auscultation. Patients with evidence of infiltrate or atelectasis on chest radiograph are unlikely to improve with routine management and should be hospitalized. Afebrile patients who respond readily to beta-agonist therapy do not require a chest radiograph. Pneumomediastinum and pneumothorax are uncommon, but should be considered in patients unresponsive to therapy. Foreign body aspiration, particularly in young children, may also present as an initial episode of acute wheezing unresponsive to asthma medications.

A complete blood count may help assess the role of infection, provided that adrenergic drugs, which induce a granulocytosis, have not been given. Ketonuria and an elevated specific gravity are commonly found on urinalysis. Electrolytes are often normal; however, in patients with respiratory failure, metabolic acidosis may be evident, in keeping with findings on blood gas analysis. Patients with metabolic acidosis often require intensive care management, cardiac monitoring, and treatment with sodium bicarbonate.

C. Immunotherapy

1. Purpose: The purpose of immunotherapy is to decrease the severity of symptoms caused by allergen exposure in patients who cannot be successfully managed by allergen avoidance and medications. Included are patients who request immunotherapy to avoid using daily medications, particularly if those medications have led to undesirable side effects.

2. Selection of Patients:

a. Indications: Injection therapy has been efficacious when used selectively in patients with sensitivities to inhalent and venom allergies. Rapid desensitization is occasionally used to desensitize patients with a drug (e.g., penicillin, insulin) allergy when immediate treatment is required and no other drug can be used as an alternative.

b. Contraindications and Precautions: Immunotherapy is not effective or recommended for the treatment of food allergies. During pregnancy, immunotherapy should not be started, nor should dosages be increased. Maintenance immunotherapy, however, may be continued during pregnancy.

3. Equipment and Supplies (See Appendix for equipment and supplies manufacturers and suppliers. Appendix is keyed to italicized words in the equipment and supplies lists):

· 25-gauge *needles* (See Figure 3-2, page 24)

· Tuberculin *syringes* (See Figure 3-2, page 24)

· Alcohol *pads*

· Allergen *extracts* used for immunotherapy are the same as those used for skin testing (See Allergy Skin Testing, page 242). Storage of extracts at 4°C in a standard refrigerator is usually recommended; however, many extracts are also stable at room temperature.

· Diluent (buffered saline *solution*)

4. Description of Procedure:

· Inhalant allergen immunotherapy (e.g., ragweed) involves weekly subcutaneous injections (See Administration of Subcutaneous [SQ] Immunizations and Medications, page 23) of increasing amounts of extract, often covering a period of 4 to 6 months before a maintenance dose is reached. Although different extracts can be mixed in a single injection, large volumes (≥ 0.5 mL) are not advised. Instead, split injections are recommended for large doses.

· After an injection, observe patients for at least 30 to 45 minutes, in the event that an adverse reaction to the injection occurs.

· Protocols for immunotherapy may vary somewhat in different allergy practices. Once patients are on maintenance immunotherapy, decrease the frequency of the injections to every 2 weeks.

5. Side Effects and Complications: Anaphylactic reactions to allergy injections are now rare because of improvements in the quality of extracts used. Nevertheless, patients do vary in their sensitivities, and physicians should be prepared to treat anaphylaxis. It is not advisable for patients to administer their own injections at home.

Small local reactions do occur and indicate that a patient is reacting to allergen in the extract. It is not necessary to decrease the dose of allergen for such reactions. When large localized reactions occur ($>$ 1 inch in diameter), increasing the allergen dose is not advisable and antihistamines (e.g., diphenhydramine or terfenadine) are often given to patients shortly before their next injection.

In the event of a systemic reaction to an injection (e.g., generalized hives, nasal symptoms, wheezing), reduce the subsequent dose by one half and then increase it slowly with subsequent injections. Discuss such changes in protocol with the patient's allergist.

Late systemic reactions (e.g., urticaria, wheezing, but not anaphylaxis) can also occur after a patient leaves the clinic or office (e.g., 3–11 hours after the injection). Inform the patients of this possibility and advise them to notify you if such reactions occur. The next injection of allergen should again be reduced by one half. A few patients continue to have reactions with reduced doses of extract, leading to discontinuation of immunotherapy or acceptance of a treatment regimen using decreased amounts of allergen.

6. Interpretation: The efficacy of allergen immunotherapy is difficult to predict for any one patient. Patients treated for insect venom allergy or allergic rhinitis caused by pollen allergens commonly experience significant improvement. Decreases in medications required and improvements in pulmonary function should be expected in asthmatics if immunotherapy is working properly. Such improvements do not occur rapidly and changes should not be judged until patients have received maintenance immunotherapy for several months. Injections are discontinued after 1 year if no improvement occurs, and after 2 to 4 years if significant improvement is noted. One should keep in mind that the severity of allergic reactions in children tends to improve with advancing age; therefore, observed clinical improvement may not be due to immunotherapy alone. Should a patient's clinical status decline after the cessation of injections, immunotherapy should be started again.

Chapter 20

Blood Collection Procedures

Marie Lynd

Richard W. Kesler

Restraint

Adequate immobilization of the child should be insured before invasive procedures are begun. One or more assistants may be needed. It is better to have extra assistants than for the child to become free, risking injury to the child during the procedure or requiring repeated procedures.

A board with self-adhering straps may be used on small children if an attendant is not available. The supine child is strapped onto the board, leaving the selected blood collection site visible.

Occasionally it may be necessary to tape an arm board to an arm or leg to help decrease movement across a joint (See Figures 21-4 and 21-5, pages 279 and 280).

It is unusual for a parent to function as an assistant during an invasive procedure on their children. During and after the procedure, however, a parent may be able to provide comfort to the child.

The use of sedation for blood collection procedures is discouraged.

A. Capillary Bloods
1. Purpose: Capillary blood samples are commonly used to determine hematocrit, glucose, and bilirubin. Blood chemical analyses, drug levels, and complete blood counts can be obtained if the laboratory is equipped to process such specimens.
2. Selection of Patients:
a. Indications: Capillary blood can be obtained from any infant or child by the fingerstick method. Heel punctures are preferable in newborns and can be used in children up to several months of age.
b. Contraindications and Precautions: Capillary samples should not be obtained if there is an infection or a hematoma at the site. Sites of increased blood flow (e.g., hemangioma)

or decreased blood flow (e.g., scar tissue) should not be used. Capillary blood samples should not be performed in immunocompromised patients, because of the risk of soft tissue and blood stream bacterial infection.

3. Equipment and Supplies (See Appendix for equipment and supplies manufacturers and suppliers. Appendix is keyed to italicized words in the equipment and supplies lists):

- Warm, wet towel
- Alcohol *pads*
- *Microlancet* (Figure 20-1)
- 2 × 2-inch gauze *pads*
- Blood collection *tubes* (hematocrit tubes or capillary tubes) (Figure 20-1)
- Clay *sealer* (Figure 20-1)
- Sterile adhesive bandage *strips*

4. Description of Procedure:

a. Fingerstick method:

- Assemble all materials before starting.
- Put the child's fingers in a dependent position and wrap the fingers for 3 to 5 minutes in a warm, wet towel to increase blood flow.
- Immobilize the child's arm and hand by placing your left arm over the child's forearm and grasping the child's wrist and hand with your hand (Figure 20-2).

- In the larger infant and uncooperative child, restraint of the torso and free arm may be necessary (See Venous Bloods, Antecubital fossa, page 262).
- Isolate one finger away from the others, and choose a site for puncture on the ventral aspect of the finger, near the fingertip (Figure 20-3).
- Prepare the site by wiping it with an alcohol pad.
- Allow the site to dry.
- Using a swift motion and firm pressure, introduce a lancet at an angle perpendicular to the lateral aspect of the finger. Stick several times before removing the lancet from the skin surface.
- Wipe away the first drop of blood with a gauze pad.
- Gently "milk" the blood from the hand toward the fingertip, collecting the blood in a capillary tube (Figure 20-4). Avoid excessive force with the "milking" because of the possibility of contaminating the specimen with tissue fluid and increasing cell hemolysis.
- Release the finger for several seconds.
- Repeat the "milking" action and release.
- When the collection is complete (two thirds to three quarters of the tube is filled), seal the capillary tube with clay. This is done by placing a fingertip over the non–blood-containing end of the tube and pressing the

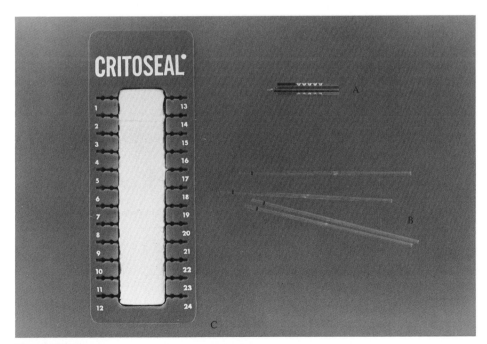

Figure 20-1.
Capillary bloods. Equipment and supplies: **A,** Microlancet; **B,** Blood collection (hematocrit or capillary) tubes; **C,** Clay sealer.

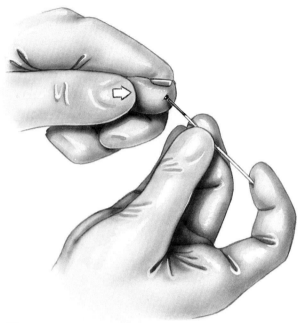

Figure 20-4.
Capillary bloods—Fingerstick method. Technique.

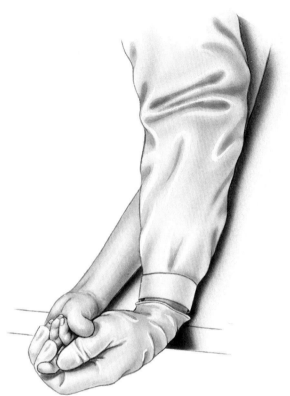

Figure 20-2.
Capillary bloods—Fingerstick method. Restraint of patient.

blood-containing end of the tube into the clay sealer. This method should avoid trapping air bubbles between the clay and the blood.
· Apply pressure to the puncture site with a gauze pad.
· Cover the wound with a sterile adhesive bandage.

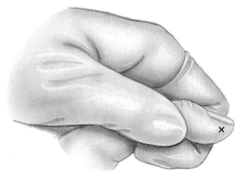

Figure 20-3.
Capillary bloods—Fingerstick method. Technique.

b. Heelstick method:
· Assemble all materials before starting.
· Wrap the baby's foot in a warm, damp towel for 5 minutes to increase capillary flow.
· Immobilize the foot with the left hand, keeping it in a dependent position (below the leg) (Figure 20-5).
· Select a site for puncture on the lateral aspect of the foot, one third of the distance between the plantar surface of the heel and the malleolus (Figure 20-5).
· Prepare the site with an alcohol pad.
· Allow the site to dry.
· Introduce a lancet at an angle perpendicular to the lateral aspect of the sole. Use a swift motion with firm pressure.
· Repeat the stick before removing the lancet from the skin surface.
· Wipe away the first drop of blood with a sponge.
· For 5 seconds, gently squeeze the blood from the toes and leg towards the heel with a "milking" motion.
· Collect the blood in a container or tube.
· Release the pressure on the foot for 5 seconds.
· Repeat the "milking" action. Alternate the "milking" with a release of pressure.
· When the sample is complete, seal the hematocrit tube with clay (See Capillary Bloods, Fingerstick method, page 259).

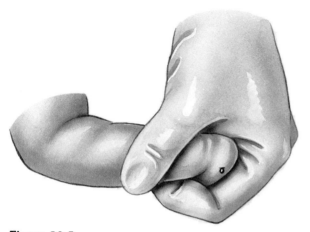

Figure 20-5.
Capillary bloods—Heelstick method. Restraint of patient and technique.

- Apply local pressure to the puncture site with a sponge until the bleeding stops.
- Cover with a bandage.

5. Side Effects and Complications: A minor hematoma may appear at the puncture site and may be minimized by firm pressure on the site until the bleeding stops.

B. Venous Bloods

1. Purpose: Venous blood samples are used to determine hematologic values, blood chemical composition, and serum drug concentrations.

2. Selection of Patients:

a. Indications: It is possible to obtain a venous blood sample from any age child. At one time or another virtually every child requires having a venous sample drawn.

b. Contraindications and Precautions: Venous bloods should not be obtained from the femoral vein in children less than 1 year of age because of the risk of introducing infection into the hip joint. In all patients, it is best to reserve this site for emergencies, because adequate samples are available from other sites. Femoral veins and neck veins should be avoided in children with known clotting abnormalities or thrombocytopenia; until evaluation for hemophilia is complete, these veins should be avoided in young males with a family history of bleeding disorders.

3. Equipment and Supplies (See Appendix for equipment and supplies manufacturers and suppliers. Appendix is keyed to italicized words in the equipment and supplies lists):

- *Tourniquets* (Figure 20-6):

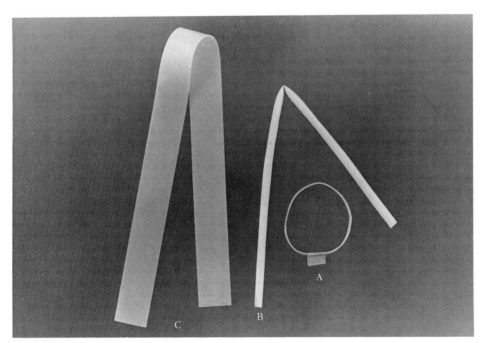

Figure 20-6.
Venous bloods. Equipment and supplies: Tourniquets (**A,** Rubberband with tape tab; **B,** Small drainage tubing; **C,** Flat rubber strip).

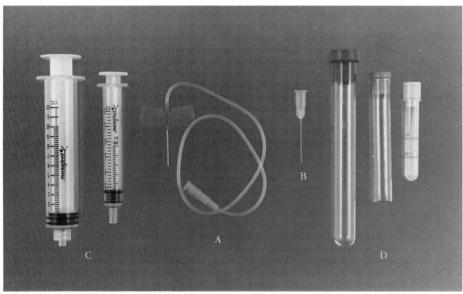

Figure 20-7.
Venous bloods. Equipment and supplies: **A,** Butterfly needle; **B,** Straight needle; **C,** Syringe; **D,** Blood collection tubes.

— Rubberband, for newborns
— Small drainage tubing, for infants and toddlers
— 1-inch flat rubber strips, for school-age children
· Non-sterile *gloves*
· Alcohol *pads*
· 2 × 2-inch gauze *pads*
· Needles—23-gauge butterfly *needle* (Figure 20-7); 23-gauge straight *needle* (Figure 20-7)
· 3- to 12-mL *syringe* (Figure 20-7)
· Blood collection *tubes* (Figure 20-7)
· Sterile adhesive bandage *strips*
· Razor
· Towel roll or sheet roll

4. Description of Procedure: The ideal site varies with age (Table 20-1). The procedure varies slightly with the site chosen. In all cases, the child should be restrained and needed materials should be readily available before starting.

a. Antecubital fossa:
· The superficial veins form an "M" pattern across the antecubital fossa (Figure 20-8). In some patients these veins are visible. If subcutaneous tissue prevents visualization of the veins, you can locate them by palpating the crease of the antecubital fossa. The three large veins have a "bouncing" reaction to palpation.
· You can use the following method of body restraint for obtaining blood from the antecubital fossa or from

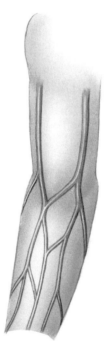

Figure 20-8.
Venous bloods—Antecubital fossa. Superficial venous system.

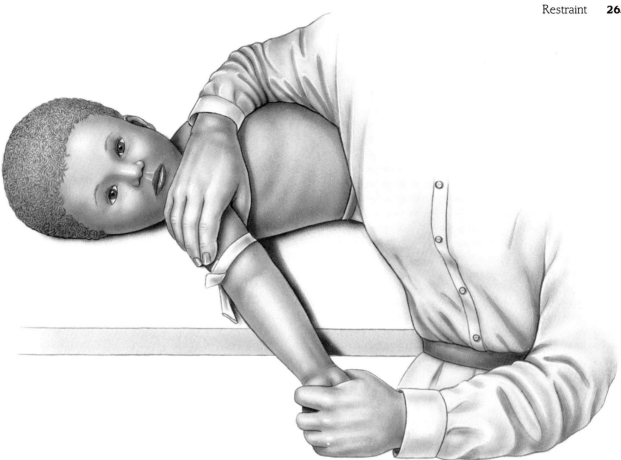

Figure 20-9.
Venous bloods—Antecubital fossa. Restraint of patient.

the wrist, hand, or finger: With the child lying supine, have an assistant stand next to the child's side and face the child's head, lean somewhat over the child's torso, and place his or her elbow adjacent to the far side of the child's chest or upper abdomen (Figure 20-9). The child's left arm and torso are thus restrained. The assistant's right arm can be used to help restrain the child's upper body, and the hand of that arm can be placed on the child's arm from which blood will be withdrawn.

· When blood is being withdrawn from the antecubital fossa, have the child's hand and forearm fully supinated. Have the assistant use his or her left hand to grasp the child's supinated wrist or hand, further preventing rotation of the forearm and assisting in maintaining the elbow in an extended position.

· You may need a second assistant to restrain the lower extremities.

· Place a tourniquet on the upper arm.

· After locating the vein, place a small ink mark on the vein outside of the field to be prepared, to serve as a useful landmark.

· Don gloves.

· Prepare the area with an alcohol pad.

· Allow the area to dry.

· Remove the cap from the tubing end of the 23-gauge butterfly needle.

· Grasp the child's extended arm with the left hand, providing additional restraint (Figure 20-10).

Table 20-1. Ideal Sites for Obtaining Venous Blood Specimen, According to Age of Patient

Age of patient:	Newborn to 1 year	1 to 3 years	More than 3 years
Site of choice:	Antecubital fossa	Antecubital fossa	Antecubital fossa
Other sites:	Hand Foot Scalp External jugular vein	Hand Foot	Hand

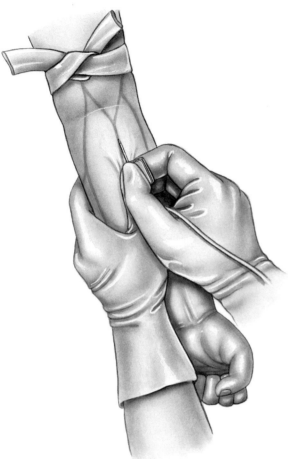

Figure 20-10.
Venous bloods—Antecubital fossa. Restraint of patient and technique.

• Hold the needle by the butterfly grip with the needle bevel up.

• Introduce the needle directly over the vein at a 30-degree angle to the skin surface (Figure 20-10).

• Puncture the skin surface quickly. Reidentify the vein, stabilize it by pulling the skin taut, and enter it with a separate motion. Some prefer using a single motion to enter the skin and vein.

• If blood return is not immediate, pull back slightly (without withdrawing the needle through the skin). Palpate the vein above the insertion of the needle. Reposition the needle as needed.

• When blood return is obtained, attach the syringe to the butterfly tubing and withdraw blood.

• When the sample is complete, remove the tourniquet,

cover the puncture site with a sponge, and remove the needle from the skin.

• Apply pressure to the site.

• Cover the wound with a bandage strip.

• Remove the butterfly needle from the syringe.

• Immediately transfer the blood from the syringe to collection tubes.

b. Hand:

• The dorsal aspect of the hand contains a network of veins that appear to fan out distally from a point in the center of the wrist to the web spaces between the fingers (Figures 20-11 and 20-12). Proximally, these unite to form two larger veins on the distal surface of the wrist. The basilic vein is located in the center of the wrist, near the skin creases. The cephalic vein ("intern's vein") crosses the anatomic snuff box and is easily palpable between the bony prominences of the lateral wrist. The basilic and cephalic veins may be easier to locate than antecubital veins in a chubby 1-year-old, but are not as well anchored and tend to roll. The ventral surface of the wrist contains several small caliber, easily visualized veins.

• The method for restraining the child is very similar to that used for antecubital sticks (See Figure 20-9, page

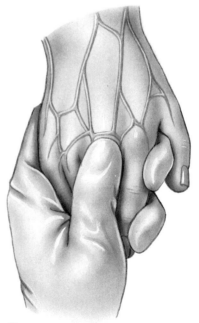

Figure 20-11.
Venous bloods—Hand. Venous network and restraint of patient.

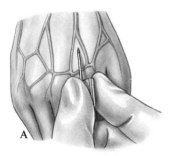

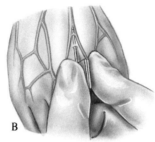

Figure 20-12.
Venous bloods—Hand. A and **B,** Technique.

263). When blood is being drawn from the hand, pronate the child's hand and flex the wrist. Have the assistant restraining the upper body place the hand of his or her inner arm over the child's upper arm, as is done for antecubital sticks (See Figure 20-9, page 263). Have the

assistant use his or her free hand to press the forearm to the table, preventing supination or other movement.

· You may need a second assistant to restrain the lower extremities.

· Don gloves.

· Restrain the child's hand by grasping her four fingers with your left hand (Figure 20-11). You can leave her thumb free. You may use your thumb to pull the skin taut over the vein selected for venipuncture.

· After immobilization and preparation of the site with alcohol, introduce a 23-gauge butterfly needle, bevel up, at an angle nearly parallel to the skin surface and at a point distal to the selected vein (Figure 20-12A). Then tunnel the needle up to the selected vein and enter it (Figure 20-12B).

c. Foot:

The great saphenous vein lies proximal and anterior to the medial malleolus (Figure 20-13). A venous network on the dorsal and lateral surfaces of the foot forms an arch between the great saphenous vein medially and small saphenous vein laterally.

· With the child lying supine, instruct an assistant, standing next to the child's side and facing the child's feet, to lean over the femurs to immobilize the upper legs (Figure 20-14). Have the assistant isolate and immobilize the idle lower leg so the operator and venipuncture site are not kicked.

· You may need a second assistant to hold the calf of the lower leg being used for blood collection.

· Don gloves.

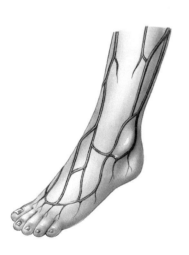

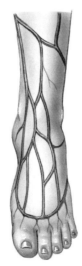

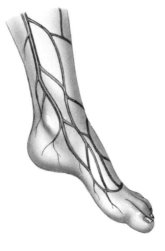

Figure 20-13.
Venous bloods—Foot. Venous network of saphenous veins.

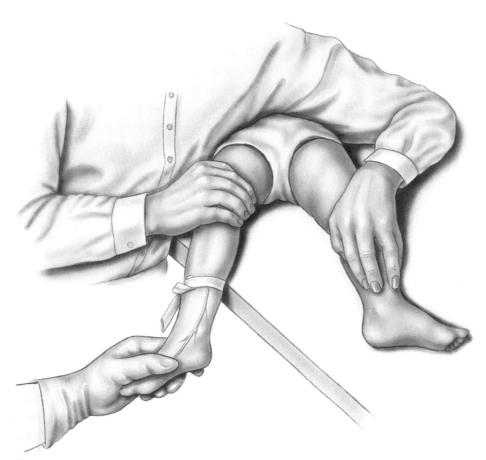

Figure 20-14.
Venous bloods—Foot. Restraint of patient and technique.

· Place the leg medial side up against a table. With your left hand, hold the foot in plantar flexion to better visualize and stabilize the veins. Extend the foot over the table to allow the right hand to move parallel to the skin when approaching the vein.

· Obtain blood samples from the foot in a manner similar to the method for antecubital sites (See page 262). Because the veins of the foot are more superficial, hold the needle at an angle nearly parallel to the skin in a manner similar to the method used for the hand veins.

d. Scalp:

Scalp veins are visible on the parietal surface above the ear and in the frontal area (Figure 20-15). To identify scalp veins, apply a rubber band around the forehead and occiput to act as a tourniquet. Apply a small tab of tape to the rubber band to help reposition or remove the rubberband later. Palpate the anterior fontanel and avoid this area.

· Place the infant supine with the infant's head turned to one side (Figure 20-16). Have an assistant immobilize the torso with the weight of his or her body and have the assistant use both hands to hold the infant's head firmly against the table. Have the assistant take care not to place his or her fingers near the infant's eyes or nose. Have him or her gently cover the infant's eyes when the rubber band is removed later.

· If necessary, shave a small area of scalp hair to better visualize the vein.

· Confirm by palpation that a vessel is a vein. If pulsations are present, it is an artery.

· Don gloves.

· Prepare the area with an alcohol swab and allow the alcohol to dry.

· Use the left hand to stretch the skin taut at the selected site, thus anchoring the selected vein (Figure 20-17).

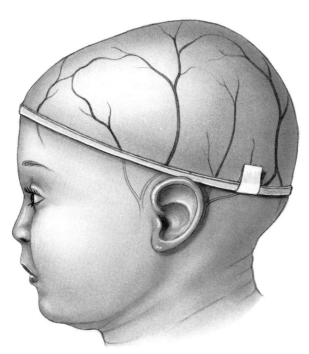

Figure 20-15.
Venous bloods—Scalp. Network of scalp veins.

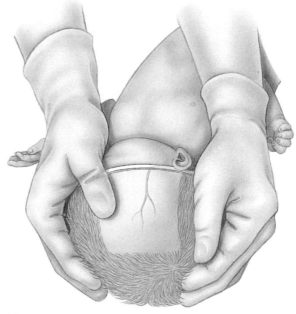

Figure 20-16.
Venous bloods—Scalp. Restraint of patient.

· Use a 23-gauge butterfly needle held bevel up, close to parallel to the skin (Figure 20-18).
· Enter the skin directly above the vein and enter the vein with the same motion.
· Withdraw a sample with a syringe.
· When the sample is complete, protect the baby's eyes and cut or otherwise remove the rubberband.
· Apply a gauze pad to the puncture site and remove the needle.
· Apply pressure to the puncture site until the bleeding stops.

e. External jugular:
This site should be reserved for experienced phlebotomists.
   The external jugular vein crosses perpendicular to the sternocleidomastoid muscle in a line between the angle of the mandible and the middle of the clavicle (Figure 20-19). The vein runs superficial and lateral to the carotid artery, which should be located by palpation and avoided.
   · Have the child lie supine with a towel or sheet roll beneath the shoulders to help extend the neck (Figure 20-19). Alternatively, place an infant supine with the head slightly over the end of the examination table (Figure 20-20).

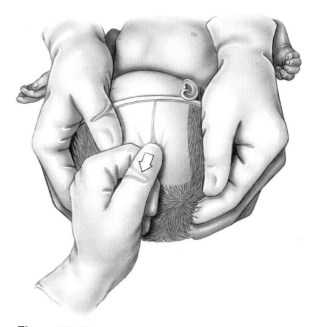

Figure 20-17.
Venous bloods—Scalp. Technique.

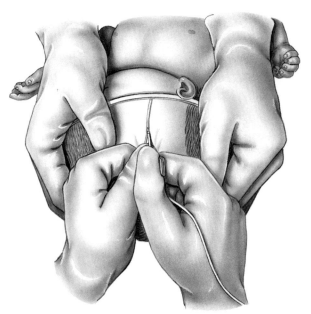

Figure 20-18.
Venous bloods—Scalp. Technique.

· Have an assistant immobilize the patient's torso with the weight of his or her body and use his or her hands to turn the patient's head to one side and hold it to the table.

· Identify the vein, don gloves, and prepare the area with povidone-iodine followed by alcohol.

· With the left hand stretch the surrounding skin taut to anchor the vein.

· Introduce the needle in a direction from the jaw towards the clavicle immediately above the vein at an angle nearly parallel to the skin (Figure 20-19).

· When blood return is obtained, place the syringe on the butterfly tubing.

· When the sample is complete, cover the site with a gauze pad and remove the needle.

· Set the child upright.

· Exert pressure at the site until the bleeding stops.

5. Side Effects and Complications: Bleeding occasionally and infection rarely may result from phlebotomy.

C. Blood Cultures

1. Purpose: Blood cultures are obtained to detect the presence of microorganisms in the circulation.

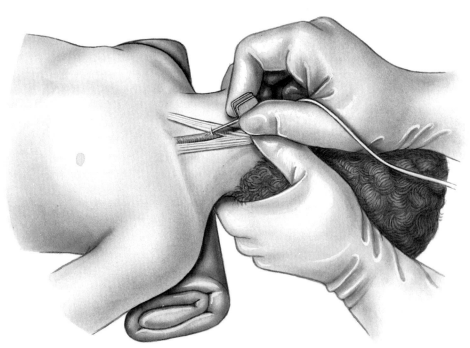

Figure 20-19.
Venous bloods—External jugular. Anatomy, positioning of patient, and technique.

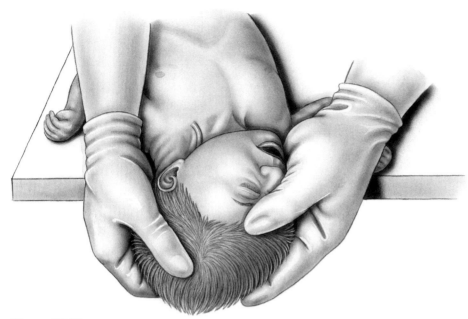

Figure 20-20.
Venous bloods—External jugular. Restraint of infant.

2. Selection of Patients:
a. Indications: Blood cultures may be indicated in the evaluation of febrile infants and children.
b. Contraindications and Precautions: Contraindications include overlying skin infection. Femoral and neck sites should not be used if the child has a known clotting disorder or if the child is a young male with a family history of hemophilia.
3. Equipment and Supplies (See Appendix for equipment and supplies manufacturers and suppliers. Appendix is keyed to italicized words in the equipment and supplies lists):
In addition to supplies for venous blood collection (See Venous Bloods, Equipment and Supplies, page 261), the following are required:
  · Alcohol *pads*
  · Two blood culture bottles
  · Non-sterile *gloves*
  · Povidone-iodine *solution*
  · 21- to 23-gauge butterfly *needle* (See Figure 20-7, page 262)
  · 2 × 2-inch gauze *pads*
  · 19-gauge *needles* (See Figure 20-7, page 262)
  · *Tourniquets* (See Figure 20-6, page 261):
    — Rubberband, for newborns
    — Small drainage tubing, for infants and toddlers
    — 1-inch flat rubber strips, for school-age children
4. Description of Procedure:
  · The best site varies with the age of the patient (See Venous Bloods, page 261). Because the site cannot be

palpated after preparation, you may find it easier to use visible veins such as those on the ventral surface of the wrist for obtaining cultures. Arterial blood may be used (See Arterial Bloods, page 271).
  · Choose the site by visual inspection. Palpate the vein to identify its course. A small ink mark on the vein outside of the field to be prepared can serve as a useful landmark.
  · Wipe the tops of two blood culture bottles with a sterile alcohol pad.
  · Restrain the child (See Venous Bloods, pages 263 and 266).
  · Don gloves.
  · Prepare the site by applying povidone-iodine solution, using a circular motion from the center to the periphery of the site.
  · Repeat for a total of three applications.
  · Wipe the central area of the prepared site with an alcohol pad. Allow it to dry. Do not touch the prepared area.
  · Apply a tourniquet.
  · Have the assistant hold the open end of the butterfly needle tubing without contaminating the hub.
  · Introduce the butterfly needle through the skin without contaminating the site.
  · If blood return is not immediate, pull back slightly, not pulling the needle out of the skin.
  · Reposition the angle of the needle and attempt again.

• When blood return occurs, attach the tubing to the syringe and withdraw the sample.
• Remove the tourniquet.
• Cover the site with a gauze pad and remove the needle.
• Remove the syringe from the butterfly needle tubing.
• Cap the syringe with a straight needle and inoculate the first culture bottle.
• Inoculate the second culture bottle.

5. Side Effects and Complications: Bleeding occasionally and infection rarely may result from a phlebotomy for blood cultures. Cutaneous reactions to the povidone-iodine or alcohol can occur.

D. Heparin Locks

1. Purpose: Blood may be drawn repeatedly from an existing heparin lock system dwelling in a vein.

2. Selection of Patients:

a. Indications: This method can be used in any patient requiring multiple venous blood samples.

b. Contraindications and Precautions: Placing and maintaining an intravenous line in a small child with limited or difficult access is often more difficult than simple phlebotomy. The risk of dislodging a functional intravenous line by using it to withdraw a blood sample may make the "heparin-lock" route undesirable. Blood cultures should not be obtained from heparin locks, because there is an increased risk of contaminating the samples.

3. Equipment and Supplies (See Appendix for equipment and supplies manufacturers and suppliers. Appendix is keyed to italicized words in the equipment and supplies lists):
• Heparin lock butterfly *needle* with a plastic cap already attached to the tubing *or* any butterfly *needle* or *angiocatheter,* plus a small plastic *cap* (Figure 20-21)
• *Tourniquets* (See Figure 20-6, page 261):
  — Rubberband, for newborns
  — Small drainage tubing, for infants and toddlers
  — 1-inch flat rubber strips, for school-age children
• Non-sterile *gloves*
• Alcohol *pads*
• Povidone-iodine solution
• 2 × 2-inch gauze *pads*
• 23-gauge straight *needles* (See Figure 20-7, page 262)
• Several 3- to 10-mL *syringes* (See Figure 20-7, page 262)
  — One filled with 3 mL normal saline
  — One filled with 1 to 3 mL of a heparin solution (heparin diluted with bacteriostatic saline to produce a 10 to 50 U/mL solution)

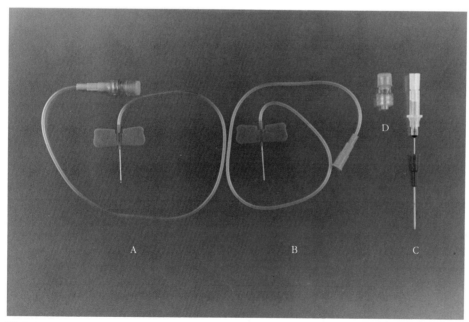

Figure 20-21.
Heparin lock. Equipment and supplies: **A,** Butterfly needle with cap; **B,** Butterfly needle; **C,** Angiocatheter; **D,** Cap.

- Adhesive *tape*
- *Armboard*

4. Description of Procedure:

Limited recent data suggest that saline may be substituted for heparin in peripheral intermittent infusion devices without significant effect on patency or duration of the system or on complications in the patient.[1]

- A vein in the antecubital fossa or hand is usually selected.
- Don gloves.
- Prepare the site with povidone-iodine followed by alcohol.
- Insert a heparin lock system in the same manner as a butterfly needle or flexible angiocatheter (See pages 262, 264, 277, and 278) and secure it with tape and an armboard (See Infusion Procedures, page 275).
- Once the line is in place, flush it with saline (1–3 mL) to clear it.
- If the cap does *not* have a "well" to fill with solution, flush the intravenous line with 1 mL of heparin solution, then attach the cap to close the system.
- Tape the short tubing onto the arm.
- If the cap *has* a hollow "well," fill it through a needle with normal saline from the prepared syringe. Then connect the cap to the tubing to close the system without introducing air. Insert the needle of the heparin syringe through the plastic cap and use 1 to 3 mL to fill the cap and clear the line. Remove the needle and syringe.
- A repeat infusion of 1 mL of heparin should be given every 3 to 8 hours to keep the line patent.
- Once the system is in place, samples may be obtained as follows:

(1) Apply a tourniquet proximal to the heparin lock.
(2) Swab the cap of the heparin lock with alcohol.
(3) Put a 23-gauge straight needle on a 3-mL syringe.
(4) Push the needle through the cap.
(5) Withdraw 2 to 3 mL of fluid and discard the fluid.
(6) Attach another syringe to the hub of the needle and withdraw the desired sample.
(7) Remove the tourniquet.
(8) Remove the syringe and needle.
(9) Flush the line with 1 to 3 mL of normal saline followed by a heparin flush.
(10) Cap or clamp the line.
(11) Ideally, the system should be removed and replaced, if necessary, before 72 hours.

E. Arterial Bloods

1. Purpose: Arterial blood samples are needed to determine the partial pressure of gases. They also may be used for cultures in lieu of venous blood samples.

Table 20-2. Ideal Sites for Obtaining Arterial Blood Specimen, According to Age of Patient

Age of patient:	Newborn to 1 year	More than 1 year
Site of choices:	Radial artery	Radial artery
Other sites:	Dorsalis pedis artery Posterior tibial artery	

---

2. Selection of Patients:

a. Indications: The procedure can be used in all but a few specific patients. The best arterial site varies with a patient's age (Table 20-2).

b. Contraindications and Precautions: Clotting disorders, local skin infection, and hematomas are relative contraindications to arterial sticks. Femoral sites should not be routinely used in children less than 1 year of age, because of the risk of introducing infection into the hip joint.

3. Equipment and Supplies (See Appendix for equipment and supplies manufacturers and suppliers. Appendix is keyed to italicized words in the equipment and supplies lists):

- Heparin *solution*
- 3-mL *syringe* (See Figure 20-7, page 262)
- Non-sterile *gloves*
- Povidone-iodine *solution*
- Alcohol *pads*
- 23-gauge butterfly *needle* (See Figure 20-7, page 262)
- 2 × 2-inch gauze *pads*
- Ice-filled container

4. Description of Procedure:

- Prepare a heparinized syringe by withdrawing 2 mL of heparin into a 3-mL syringe. Coat the inside of the

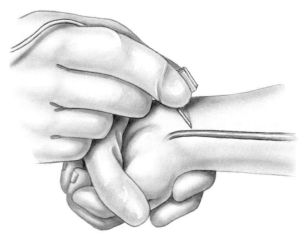

Figure 20-22.
Arterial bloods—Radial artery. Anatomy, restraint of patient, and technique.

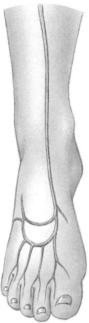

Figure 20-23.
Arterial bloods—Dorsalis pedis artery. Anatomy.

syringe cylinder with heparin. Attach a sterile butterfly needle and expel heparin through the butterly needle until the syringe is empty.

· Gather supplies and restrain the child.
· Palpate the pulsations of the artery. A small ink mark on the artery outside the prepared field can serve as a useful landmark.
· Don gloves.
· Using one hand, immobilize the child's limb.
· Prepare the site with povidone-iodine applied in a circular motion. Follow with alcohol and allow it to dry.
· Use a 23-gauge butterfly needle. Have the assistant ready to collect the sample in the heparinized syringe.

a. For the radial artery:

The radial artery is located on the ventral surface of the wrist, proximal to the thumb, at about the level of the skin creases (Figure 20-22). It lies deep below the skin but superficial to the radius. Dorsiflex the wrist to help identify the artery.

· Have an assistant immobilize the child in a manner similar to that for collecting venous bloods from the hand (See Figure 20-11, page 264). The method differs in that the child's hand is fully supinated and the wrist is dorsiflexed.
· You may need a second assistant to immobilize the lower extremities.
· Grasp the child's supinated wrist and hand with your left hand, containing the child's fingers and thumb (Figure 20-22).
· Insert a butterfly needle at a 60- to 90-degree angle to the skin (Figure 20-22). Quickly insert the needle deeply in one motion. Some prefer to insert the needle through the skin in one motion and insert it into the artery with a separate motion.

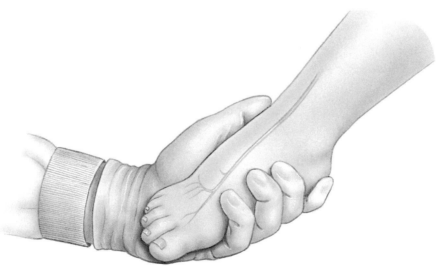

Figure 20-24.
Arterial bloods—Dorsalis pedis artery. Restraint of patient.

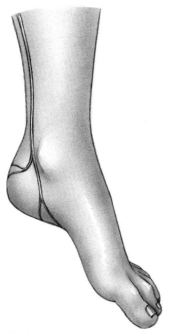

Figure 20-25.
Arterial bloods—Posterior tibial artery. Anatomy.

· If blood return is immediate, have an assistant collect a sample. The assistant should not be the one providing essential restraint.

· If the blood return is not immediate, slowly withdraw the needle, observing for the sudden appearance of blood, indicating that the needle is in the artery.

· When the sample is complete, cover the site with a gauze pad.

· Withdraw the needle.

· Hold the site with firm pressure for at least 5 minutes.

· Hold the blood-filled syringe with the plunger at the bottom.

· Tap air bubbles to the top of the syringe, cover the tip of the syringe with a gauze pad (to prevent your spraying blood), and expel the bubbles.

· Tightly cap the syringe.

· Place the syringe in ice for transport.

b. For the dorsalis pedis artery:

The dorsalis pedis pulse can be palpated on the dorsal surface of the foot, midway between the ankle and toes and between the great toe and the second toe (Figure 20-23). It lies deep to the intrinsic muscles of the foot. Identification of the dorsalis pedis artery is aided by holding the foot in plantar flexion.

· Have an assistant immobilize the child in a manner similar to that for collecting venous blood from the foot (See page 265).

· Don gloves.

· Grasp the foot with the palm of the left hand pressed to the plantar surface of the foot, the fingers on the medial surface, and the thumb on the lateral surface of the foot (Figure 20-24).

· Introduce the needle at an angle nearly perpendicular to the skin.

· Proceed as for the radial artery (See page 272).

c. For posterior tibial artery:

The posterior tibial artery is palpated posterior to the medial malleolus (Figure 20-25). Identification of the artery may be easier if you flex the foot dorsally.

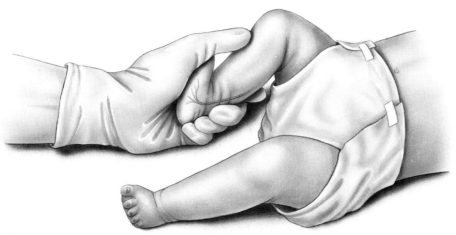

Figure 20-26.
Arterial bloods—Posterior tibial artery. Restraint of patient and technique.

• Have an assistant immobilize the child in a manner identical to that for the dorsalis pedis artery (See page 273).
• Don gloves.
• Grasp the foot with the left hand and hold the foot in a dorsiflexed position (Figure 20-26).
• Introduce the needle at a 60-degree angle to the skin.
• Proceed as for the radial artery (See page 272).

5. Side Effects and Complications: Hematomas and infection may result from an arterial puncture. Loss of perfusion to the limb distal to the puncture site could occur if thrombosis or spasm occurs. The risk of ischemic damage is minimized by checking for collateral circulation before performing an arterial puncture.

Reference

1. Lombardi TP, Gundersen B, Zammett LO. Efficacy of 0.9% sodium chloride injection with or without heparin sodium for maintaining patency of intravenous catheters in children. Clin Pharmacol 1988; 7:832–6.

Chapter 21

Infusion Procedures

Marie Lynd

Richard W. Kesler

Karen A. Bringelsen

Restraint

Adequate immobilization of the child should be insured before invasive procedures are begun. One or more assistants may be needed. It is better to have extra assistants than for the child to become free, risking injury to the child during the procedure or requiring repeated procedures.

A board with self-adhering straps may be used on small children if an attendant is not available. The supine child is strapped onto the board, leaving the proposed blood collection site visible.

Occasionally it may be necessary to tape an arm board to an arm or leg to help decrease movement across a joint.

It is unusual for a parent to function as an assistant during an invasive procedure on their children; however, a parent may be able to provide comfort to the child during the procedure.

The use of sedation for a minor procedure such as insertion of an intravenous line should be discouraged; however, the use of a local anesthetic at the site can decrease discomfort.

I. Infusions

A. Intravenous Infusions

1. Purpose: The intravenous route is used to administer fluid and electrolyte solutions, blood products, and medications.

2. Selection of Patients:

a. Indications: A percutaneous intravenous line may be inserted in any infant or child with adequate circulation who requires intravenous fluids or medications.

b. Contraindications and Precautions: Intravenous lines should not be inserted routinely in the femoral vein in infants less than 1 year of age, because of the risk of introducing infection into the hip joint. Femoral veins and neck veins should be avoided in children with known clotting abnormalities or thrombocytopenia, and in young males with a family history of bleeding disorders, until evaluation for hemophilia is complete.

3. Equipment and Supplies (See Appendix for equipment and supplies manufacturers and suppliers. Appendix is keyed to italicized words in the equipment and supplies lists):

· *Tourniquets* (See Figure 20-6, page 261):
  — Rubberband, for newborns
  — Small drainage tubing, for infants and toddlers
  — 1-inch flat rubber strips for school-age children
· Non-sterile *gloves*
· Alcohol *pads*
· 2 × 2-inch gauze *pads*
· *Needles*
  — 24-gauge intravenous catheter ("intercath") (Figure 21-1)
  — 22-gauge intravenous catheter ("intercath") (Figure 21-1)
  — 23-gauge butterfly scalp *needle* (Figure 21-1)
· 3-mL *syringe* (See Figure 20-7, page 262) filled with normal saline *solution*
· "T" *connector* (Figure 21-1) attached to 3-mL *syringe* (See Figure 20-7, page 262)

· Razor
· *Armboard* (Figure 21-1)
· *Lidocaine* (1%), 1 mL, in a tuberculin *syringe*
· Adhesive *tape* cut before the procedure
· Transparent catheter *dressing*
· Paper cup or plastic medication cup
· Povidone-iodine *pads*
· Towel roll or sheet roll
· Sterile conforming gauze *bandage*

4. Description of Procedure:

The procedure varies slightly with the site chosen. The ideal site varies with the age of the child (Table 21-1).

· You can use a 24-gauge needle in any age child. It is the preferred size for the small-caliber veins of the infant. Blood products may be administered via a 24-gauge needle. You can use a 22-gauge needle for antecubital and great saphenous veins in infants and for larger caliber hand veins in children. You can use a 23-gauge butterfly scalp needle for scalp veins in infants.

· In all cases, assemble all materials and properly restrain the child before starting.

· Draw a normal saline flush solution into a 3-mL syringe. Then attach a T-connector and fill it with saline. Use the saline to check for proper placement of the line

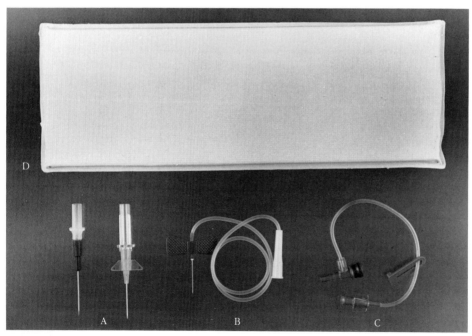

Figure 21-1.
Intravenous infusions. Equipment and supplies: **A,** Intravenous catheters (one without and one with wings); **B,** Butterfly scalp needle; **C,** "T" connector; **D,** Armboard.

Table 21-1. Ideal Sites for Intravenous Infusions, According to Age of Patient

Age of patient:	Newborn to 1 year	1 to 3 years	More than 3 years
Site of choice:	Hand	Hand	Hand
Other sites:	Foot	Foot	Antecubital fossa
	Antecubital fossa	Antecubital fossa	
	Scalp		
	External jugular vein		

before beginning the infusion. Flushing the hub of the intravenous catheter with saline before attempting to place it will help you quickly recognize when the vein has been entered.

· Don gloves, prepare the site with an alcohol swab, and, if you choose, raise a small subcutaneous wheal with 0.1 to 0.3 mL of lidocaine (1%) to provide local anesthesia.

a. Hand:

The dorsal aspect of the hand contains a network of veins that appear to "fan" out distally from a point in the center of the wrist to the web spaces (See Figures 20-11 and 20-12, page 265). These unite to form two larger veins on the distal surface. The basilic vein is located in the center of the wrist, near the skin creases. The cephalic vein ("intern's vein") crosses the anatomic snuff box. It is easily palpable at the bony prominence of the wrist, proximal to the thumb. Though palpable, the basilic and cephalic veins are difficult to visualize. The ventral surface of the wrist contains several small caliber, easily visualized veins.

· Properly restrain the child (See Venous Bloods, page 261).

· If desired, place an armboard beneath the wrist (to immobilize the joint). If the child is uncooperative, you can tape across the fingers and forearm to attach the armboard in a splint-like fashion (See Figure 21-4, page 279).

· Apply a tourniquet of proper size to the forearm.

· Choose a visible vein, preferably one that branches in an inverted "Y" pattern. If no veins are visible, identify the course by palpation. A small ink mark parallel to the vein and outside the field to be prepared can be a useful landmark.

· Prepare the site with an alcohol pad. Neutropenic patients should have the skin prepared with povidone-iodine and alcohol.

· Stretch the skin taut to keep the veins from rolling.

· Consider using lidocaine (1%) at the skin site.

· Insert the intravenous needle, bevel up, into the skin at an angle nearly parallel to the skin surface (Figure

21-2A). Begin at a point 1 cm distal to the vein to anchor the needle in the skin.

· If possible, enter the skin distal to a branch point and advance the needle into the vein at the site of intersection.

· Enter the skin surface quickly, then slowly advance the catheter and needle as a unit toward the vein. When the vein is entered, the first drop of blood will stain the saline in the hub pink.

· Keeping the needle stationary, carefully advance the plastic catheter forward (Figure 21-2B). Slightly twisting the catheter may help you advance it. The catheter should slide easily until the hub hits the skin if you have the catheter in the vein.

· If resistance is met, pull the plastic catheter back and reposition it while keeping the needle stationary.

· If a hematoma forms, or the vein cannot be entered, release the tourniquet, cover the site with a gauze pad, and remove the catheter.

· When the plastic catheter is properly positioned, remove the needle (while holding the catheter in place).

· Have the assistant remove the tourniquet.

· Use a small strip of tape to secure the hub at the skin, while still holding the catheter carefully.

· Attach the flushed T-connector to the hub and have the assistant flush 1 mL of normal saline through the line.

· Inspect and palpate the site for signs of infiltration such as hematoma or local swelling. The line should flush easily. It may or may not have a brisk blood return.

· If resistance is met, check that the tourniquet has been removed and that restraints are not acting as tourniquets. Change the position of the limb if needed. Check for a kink in the catheter and correct its position. Do not begin an infusion unless the line flushes easily.

· When the line is flushing easily, tape the hub securely to the skin with a 2-cm length of tape placed perpendicular to the catheter (Figure 21-3A).

· After taping the hub directly to the skin, slip a longer strip of tape, adhesive side up, below the hub (Figure 21-3B).

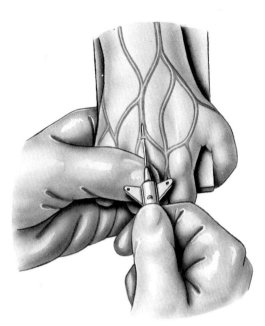 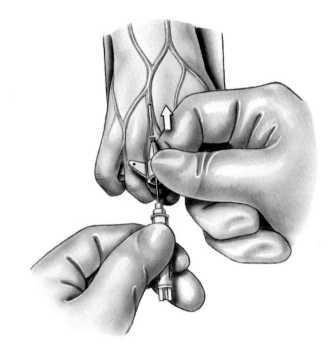

Figure 21-2.
Intravenous infusions—Hand. Technique.

· Crisscross the tape over the hub onto the skin to anchor the hub.

· Place another 2-cm length of tape perpendicular to the catheter, over the hub.

· Remove the syringe and attach the infusion set up.

· Tape all connections.

· Tape the tubing to the arm.

· Rolled 2 × 2-inch gauze pads laid parallel to the hub and taped in place will prevent the hub from "catching" on other objects and being dislodged (Figure 21-3C). Alternatively, place transparent catheter dressing over the needle and hub.

· For additional protection, cover the hub with a paper cup or medicine cup, but keep the site of the catheter tip exposed so signs of infiltration can be seen.

· If not previously done, tape the armboard to the wrist to immobilize the joint. A gauze pad in the palm helps to keep the hand in proper position. Tape the fingers securely. Tape the thumb separately (Figure 21-4).

b. Foot:

The great saphenous vein runs about the width of one's finger proximal and anterior to the medial malleolus (See Figure 20-13, page 265). There is a venous network on the dorsal and lateral surfaces of the foot forming an arch between the great saphenous vein medially and small saphenous vein lat-

erally. The small caliber veins of the foot are easily visualized and are relatively stationary. The large caliber great saphenous vein is often not visible, but is readily palpable.

· The method for inserting and securing an intravenous line in the foot is the same as in the hand.

· When the line is flushing easily, tape the hub to the skin with a 2-cm length of tape, placed perpendicular to the catheter (See Intravenous Infusions, Hand, page 277).

· After taping the hub directly to the skin, slip a longer strip of tape, adhesive side up, below the hub.

· Crisscross the tape over the hub onto the skin to anchor the hub.

· Place another 2-cm length of tape perpendicular to the catheter, over the hub.

c. Antecubital fossa:

The superficial veins form an "M" pattern across the antecubital fossa (See Figure 20-8, page 262). While not always visible, they are easily palpable. They are not as stationary as the veins of the hand and foot. It is difficult to restrict movement at the elbow of an active child, so this site is less desirable than the hand for continuous intravenous infusions. The method for inserting a catheter varies slightly at this site. Because the vein is deeper, the needle is inserted at about a 45-degree angle to the skin. It is more difficult to visualize

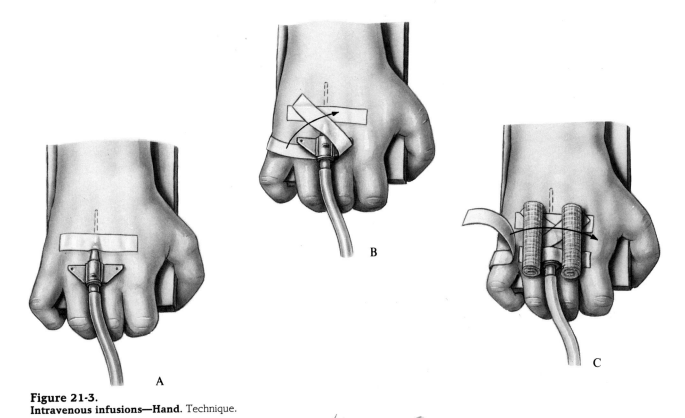

Figure 21-3.
Intravenous infusions—Hand. Technique.

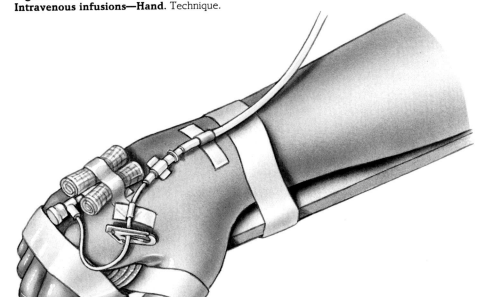

Figure 21-4.
Intravenous infusions—Hand. Technique.

signs of infiltration in these deep veins. Palpation of the site after infusion of 1 to 3 mL of normal saline is needed to verify placement.

- When the line is flushing easily, tape the hub to the skin with a 2-cm length of tape, placed perpendicular to the catheter (Figure 21-5).
- Slip a longer strip of tape, adhesive side up, below the hub.
- Crisscross the tape over the hub on to the skin to anchor the hub.
- Place another 2-cm length of tape perpendicular to the catheter, over the hub.
- Immobilize the elbow joint by taping the arm to an armboard (Figure 21-5). Some prefer to immobilize the joint before insertion of the needle.

d. Scalp:

Scalp veins are visible in an infant on the parietal surface above the ear and in the frontal area (See Figure 20-15, page 267).

- To identify a scalp vein, apply a rubberband around the forehead and occiput to act as a tourniquet. Apply a small tab of tape to the rubberband to help reposition or remove the rubberband later.
- Palpate the anterior fontanel and avoid this area.
- Shave a small area (5 × 5 cm) of scalp hair to allow for taping the catheter to the scalp.

- Confirm that a vessel is a vein by palpation. If pulsations are present, it is an artery.
- You should have the infant held supine with an attendant holding the head securely (See Figure 20-16, page 267).
- After shaving the selected area, don sterile gloves and prepare the area with an alcohol pad and allow it to dry.
- Flush normal saline through a 23-gauge butterfly scalp needle, filling the tubing without air bubbles.
- Insert the needle, bevel up, at an angle near parallel to the skin aiming toward the forehead or ear (See Figure 20-18, page 268).
- Begin 1 cm away from the vein to anchor the needle in the skin.
- Advance the needle slowly into the vein until blood return is noted in the tubing.
- Tape a 2-cm strip of tape over the needle onto the scalp (See Intravenous Infusions, Hand, page 277). Continue to hold the needle securely.
- Have an assistant protect the infant's eyes while you cut off the rubberband.
- Attach a flushed T-connector and syringe to the butterfly tubing and slowly infuse normal saline into the vein.
- Check visually and by palpation for signs of infiltration. The line should flush easily.

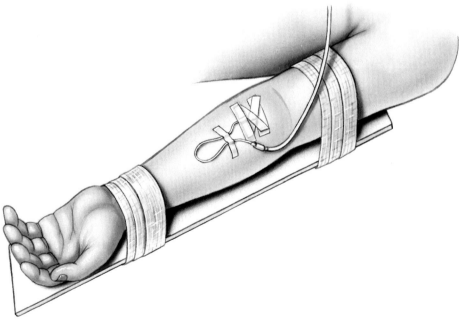

Figure 21-5.
Intravenous infusions—Antecubital fossa. Technique.

• When placement is verified, continue taping into place. A 5-cm strip of tape, adhesive side up, is placed beneath the needle and crisscrossed above the needle, anchored on the butterfly grips (Figure 21-6). A 2-cm strip of tape is placed perpendicular to the needle over the butterfly grips.

• A 2 × 2-inch gauze pad can be folded beneath the butterfly grips to stabilize the position at the needle.

• A sterile conforming gauze bandage can be wrapped around the head, or a medicine cup can be placed over the needle to keep it from being dislodged (Figure 21-6).

• All connections should be taped.

e. External jugular:

This site should be reserved for experienced clinicians. It should be used only in emergencies or when no other sites are available.

The external jugular vein crosses perpendicular to the sternocleidomastoid muscle in a line between the angle of the mandible and the middle of the clavicle (See Figures 20-19 and 20-20, pages 268 and 269). The vein runs superficial and lateral to the carotid artery, which should be located by palpation and avoided.

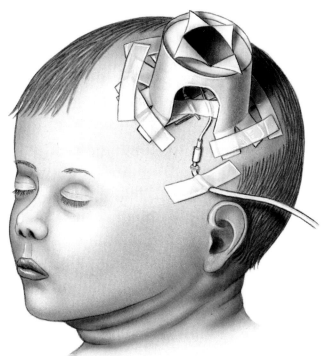

Figure 21-6.
Intravenous infusions—Scalp. Technique.

• You should have the child lying supine with a roll beneath the shoulders to help extend the neck (See Figure 20-19, page 268). Alternatively, place an infant supine with the head slightly over the end of the examination table (See Figure 20-20, page 269).

• You *must* have the head immobilized by an assistant (See Figure 20-20, page 269).

• Identify the vein and prepare it with an alcohol swab.

• Stretch the surrounding skin taut.

• Introduce the needle of an intravenous catheter in a direction from the jaw toward the clavicle, immediately above the vein, and at an angle nearly parallel to the skin (See Figure 20-19, page 268).

• When blood return occurs, advance the plastic catheter, remove the needle, and immediately attach the flushed T-connector and syringe to the hub (See Figure 21-4, page 279).

• Infuse normal saline to check for line placement.

• When the line is infusing easily, tape the hub to the skin with a 2-cm length of tape, placed perpendicular to the catheter.

• Slip a longer strip of tape, adhesive side up, below the hub.

• Crisscross the tape over the hub on to the skin to anchor the hub.

• Use transparent catheter dressing over the crisscrossed tape, hub and entry site.

• Place another 2-cm length of tape perpendicular to the catheter, over the hub.

• You need not immobilize the neck.

5. Side Effects and Complications: Hematoma, extravasation of intravenous fluid, and infection are the major complications of intravenous line placement.

Special care should be taken *not* to accidentally introduce air into the system when inserting lines in children with congenital heart disease involving a right-to-left shunt. Special filters are indicated for the infusion tubing in these cases.

B. Intraosseous Infusions

1. Purpose: The anterior tibial intraosseous route is used in life-threatening situations when an intravenous line cannot be established. If there is no intravenous access within 5 minutes of a resuscitative effort, an intraosseous line should be inserted. Fluid and electrolyte solutions and most resuscitative medications may be infused through an intraosseous line.

2. Selection of Patients:

a. Indications: Intraosseous access is used in life-threatening ("code") situations.

b. Contraindications and Precautions: There are no contraindications to line placement. Certain medications such as calcium and hypertonic saline (3%) are caustic to the soft tissues and can cause extensive tissue injury if they extravasate.

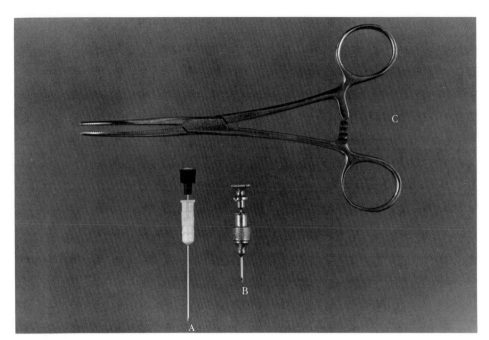

Figure 21-7.
Intraosseous infusions. Equipment and supplies: **A,** 19-gauge spinal needle; **B,** Bone marrow needle; **C,** Kelly clamp.

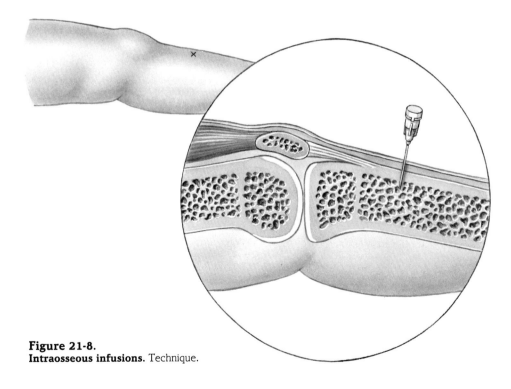

Figure 21-8.
Intraosseous infusions. Technique.

3. Equipment and Supplies (See Appendix for equipment and supplies manufacturers and suppliers. Appendix is keyed to italicized words in the equipment and supplies lists):

- Povidone-iodine *pad*
- Alcohol *pad*
- 19-gauge spinal *needle* or bone marrow *needle* (Figure 21-7)
- Curved Kelly *clamp* (Figure 21-7), to stabilize the needle
- Normal saline *solution,* for flushing
- 2 × 2-inch gauze *pads*

4. Description of Procedure:

- Hold the leg securely.
- Palpate the flat surface of the tibia in an area clearly distal to the knee joint. You should place the line below the level of growth plate (1–3 cm below the tibial tuberosity) (Figure 21-8).
- Prepare the skin with povidone-iodine and alcohol.
- Introduce the selected needle perpendicular to the skin surface and directly through the skin and periosteum (Figure 21-8).
- You may or may not encounter a release of resistance when the marrow has been entered.
- Place an empty 5-mL syringe on the inserted needle.
- Pull back on the syringe. A small amount of blood and marrow should enter the syringe.
- Secure the needle in place by holding it with a curved Kelly clamp near the skin surface (Figure 21-9). You can place a stack of 2 × 2 sponges between the skin and the clamp and tape them to anchor the clamp and needle in place.
- Remove the syringe and place a normal saline flush on the needle and infuse. Fluid should flow easily without superficial signs of extravasation.
- Infuse fluids or medications, checking frequently for the functional status of the line.
- As soon as an adequate intravenous line is available, the intraosseus needle can usually be removed.

5. Side Effects and Complications: Damage to the growth plate can occur if the needle is incorrectly placed in this area. Infection, bleeding, and extravasation of fluid can result after placement of an intraosseous line.

II. Administration of Blood Products

Modern blood banking techniques provide blood components specific for various transfusion needs. It is the clinician's responsibility to be familiar with different blood products to provide the most appropriate therapy for the patient and to conserve blood resources.

The purpose of most transfusion therapy is to correct anemia. However, unless cardiac function is threatened by

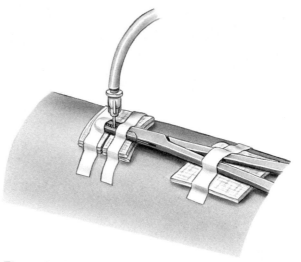

Figure 21-9.
Intraosseous infusions. Technique.

the degree of anemia and the patient is symptomatic, transfusion is usually not indicated as the first choice of therapy. Chronic transfusion programs are used to suppress the patient's own red cells in conditions such as severe sickle cell anemia and thalassemia, preventing sickle cell crises and hemolysis.

Blood products are also used to replace platelets and coagulation factors in various bleeding disorders.

A. Selection of Blood Products

See Table 21-2 for dosage and administration.

1. Blood Groups and Compatibility

In most situations every unit of blood should be of the recipient's ABO and Rh blood group and cross-matched to ensure compatibility before transfusion. The cross-match is done by testing the recipient's serum against the donor's red cells for evidence of unexpected antibodies in the recipient's serum. The blood also may be cross-matched by testing recipient blood cells against donor serum. Even with a completely compatible cross-match, there is the possibility of a hemolytic reaction after transfusion; not all unexpected antibodies are detectable.

With every unit of blood transfused there is the possibility of stimulating antibody formation; therefore, a cross-match is necessary even on previously matched blood if the patient has been receiving repeated transfusions. At critical times when transfusion must be done without waiting the hour or more for complete cross-matching, or when type-specific blood is unavailable, there are alternatives (Table 21-2).

2. Whole blood is indicated to replace massive blood loss and treat accompanying hemorrhagic shock. Fresh whole

Table 21-2. Administration of Blood Products

Blood Component	Content	Major Indications	Dosage	Administration	Complications (see text)	Comments
Whole blood	Red cells Plasma Few platelets or coagulation factors Cell breakdown products Donor proteins	Major blood loss Exchange transfusion	As necessary to replace volume and treat shock	IV with blood filter	Transfusion reaction Infection Sensitization to donor antibodies	
Packed red cells (PRBC)	Red cells (Hematocrit = 70%) Plasma Few white cells and platelets	Most transfusion situations Chronic anemias Suppress patient's erythropoiesis in severe sickle cell disease or thalassemia	Patient weight (kg) × desired increment in hematocrit Usually 10 mL/kg Do not exceed 30 mL/kg per 24 hours	IV with blood filter over 1–3 hours	Transfusion reactions Less chance of volume overload	Severely anemic patient with hemoglobin < 5 g. Use 5 mL/kg PRBC to prevent volume overload
Frozen red cells or leukocyte-poor red cells	Red cells suspended in saline Virtually no white cells or platelets No plasma	Frequently transfused patients who have severe febrile reactions to antileukocyte antibodies in plasma Stockpile rare blood types Autotransfusion	Same as packed red cells	Same as packed red cells	Same as packed red cells	
Fresh frozen plasma (FFP)	Plasma Few cells All coagulation factors No platelets	Treatment of all coagulation deficiencies	Variable, depending on factor deficiency Usually 10 mL/kg q 12 hours	IV with blood filter over 1–3 hours	Volume overload	1 mL FFP contains 1 unit of coagulant activity

Product	Composition	Indications	Dosage/Effect	Administration	Complications	Special Considerations
Platelet concentrate	Platelets Plasma Red cells, white cells	Thrombocytopenia due to decreased platelet production Qualitative platelet disorders and bleeding Glanzmann's disease Bernard-Soulier syndrome	1 unit will raise platelet count by 10,000–20,000/m²	Rapidly through standard blood administration set with an appropriate filter	Infection Allergic reactions Alloimmunization Fever, platelet antibodies Splenomegaly Active bleeding may prevent expected increment in platelets	
Irradiated blood products	Unaltered blood product with inactivation of any lymphocytes present	Prevention of graft-vs.-host disease in neonates and immunocompromised patients				
Cryoprecipitate	Plasma Factor VIII complex (usually 80–90 U/bag) Fibrinogen Factor XIII	Hemophilia A (Factor VIII deficiency) von Willebrand's disease Hypofibrinogenemia	Factor VIII deficiency—1 U Factor VIII/kg raises level by 2% Other disorders (1 bag/10 kg)	IV push with blood filter	Infrequent allergic or febrile reactions Infection transmission	Follow clinical bleeding; PTT, fibrinogen, and Factor VIII level for therapeutic effect in individual patients
Factor VIII concentrate	Lyophilized Factor VIII coagulant	Factor VIII deficiency Not effective for von Willebrand's disease	1 U/kg raises Factor VIII by 2% Factor VIII level of 50% is hemostatic in most circumstances	IV push. Prepare according to package insert Do not shake the vial	Pooled from large number of donors. Infection transmission—especially non-A, non-B hepatitis	Concentrates are heat-treated to prevent transmission of HIV
Prothrombin complex concentrate	Lyophilized Factor II, VII, IX, X	Hemophilia B (Factor IX deficiency) Some instances of Factor VIII deficiency with Factor VIII inhibitor	1 U/kg raises Factor IX level by 1%	IV push as per package insert Do not shake the vial	Pooled from large number of donors. Infection transmission—especially non-A, non-B hepatitis Occasional flushing with rapid infusion	Concentrates are heat-treated to prevent transmission of HIV

blood is also used for exchange transfusion. Blood components are preferred in most other situations. Whole blood more than a few days old does not contain significant levels of the labile coagulation factors or numbers of platelets, and transfusion with other blood components is more efficient and of greater benefit to the patient.

3. Packed red blood cells are prepared by separation of plasma from whole blood. The resulting red cells have a hematocrit of about 70% in a volume of 250 to 300 cc. Packed red cells are used for most transfusion therapy, such as treatment of anemias caused by bone marrow suppression with chemotherapy, severe iron deficiency, and transfusion-dependent chronic anemias—aplastic anemia or pure red cell aplasia.

4. Frozen red cells and leukocyte poor red cells are prepared by freezing glycerolized red blood cells. When thawed and washed to remove the glycerol, the red cells are suspended in saline for transfusion. Frozen cells may be stored for several years. This process removes plasma, white blood cells, and platelets and eliminates most leukocyte antibodies that cause febrile reactions.

The major indications are for use in frequently transfused patients who have had febrile reactions to the presence of antileukocyte antibodies or antibodies to IgA. Cryopreservation also allows stockpiling of rare blood groups and storage of blood for autotransfusion. Frozen cells may be stored for several years, but must be transfused within 24 hours after thawing.

5. Platelet concentrates are prepared from single units of whole blood or by cytopheresis of donors. Platelet transfusion is indicated for bleeding in patients with thrombocytopenia due to decreased platelet production, i.e., aplastic anemia and bone marrow suppression; or in patients with abnormal platelets. Prophylactic platelet transfusions for thrombocytopenic patients who are not bleeding are usually of little value and can cause development of platelet antibodies.

Platelet transfusion may not raise the circulating platelet count in conditions such as presence of platelet antibody (ITP), splenomegaly, active bleeding, and disseminated intravascular coagulopathies.

ABO type-specific and HLA-matched platelets may be useful when the patient is refractory to platelet transfusion because of circulating platelet antibodies.

6. Blood products for treatment of coagulation defects:

a. Fresh frozen plasma (FFP) contains all the known clotting proteins and is useful for treatment of any bleeding caused by coagulation factor deficiencies. It is a single-donor product with minimal likelihood of transmitting infection. The major disadvantage is volume overload, as large amounts of FFP are required for factor replacement.

b. Cryoprecipitate is prepared from FFP and contains Factor VIII complex, including Factor VIII coagulant and von Wille-brand's factor, fibrinogen, and Factor XIII. Cryoprecipitate is used in the treatment of Hemophilia A, von Willebrand's disease, and hypofibrinogenemia. There is no Factor IX in cryoprecipitate; therefore, it is not used to treat patients with Hemophilia B (Christmas Disease). Each bag of cryoprecipitate is prepared from a single donor, and usually several bags of cryoprecipitate are needed for each treatment. The volume is 10 to 25 mL per bag. The Factor VIII content is usually 80 to 90 units per bag of cryoprecipitate, varying with each blood bank's preparation technique.

c. Factor VIII concentrate is a lyophilized (freeze-dried) product containing almost pure Factor VIII prepared from the pooling of thousands of donors for each lot of concentrate. The actual number of units of Factor VIII varies with each lot and is printed on each vial. There is a high risk of transmission of non-A, non-B hepatitis. Each lot of concentrate is tested for the presence of hepatitis B virus and human immunodeficiency virus. Since 1984, the product has also been low-heat–treated, which has virtually eliminated the transmission of human immunodeficiency virus. Factor VIII concentrate is not useful in the management of von Willebrand's disease.

d. Prothrombin concentrates are also lyophilized and contain factor IX and small amounts of Factors II, VII, and X. These are used to treat Factor IX deficiency (Hemophilia B, Christmas Disease).

B. Hazards of Blood Transfusion

Blood transfusion is associated with many risks from acute hemolytic reactions to delayed complications seen weeks after the transfusion. The risks and benefits must be considered carefully. Obtaining informed consent before the administration of any blood product is now standard procedure in most clinics.

1. Hemolytic transfusion reactions are usually caused by the combination of an antibody in the recipient against an antigen present on the donor red cells. The most severe reactions are usually immediate. A delayed hemolysis may occur from 2 days to 3 weeks after transfusion and is usually mild. Most errors in mismatched blood are clerical, involving mistakes in identification of a patient or mislabeling of specimens. The single most important aspect in prevention of serious transfusion reactions is absolute, unequivocal identification of the patient and unit of blood to be given. Signs and symptoms of acute hemolytic reactions usually begin shortly after transfusion is started. There is a sudden onset of:

- Burning along the vein
- Flushing
- Headache
- Lower back pain
- Fever, chills—shock

· Abnormal bleeding
· Renal failure

Any unusual symptom during transfusion requires investigation. When a hemolytic reaction is suspected, stop the transfusion immediately.

· Support the patient with hydration and diuresis using furosemide to increase renal cortical perfusion.
· Report the reaction to the blood bank and follow the blood bank's procedure for transfusion reactions.

2. Allergic reactions are seen in 1% to 3% of all transfusions. Usually the symptoms are manifested as hives, rarely as asthma or pulmonary edema.

· Stop the transfusion and use an antihistamine.
· Prophylactic antihistamines should be used with subsequent transfusions.

3. Febrile reactions are caused by recipient antibodies to donor leukocyte antigens. The reaction is characterized by chills and fever beginning an hour or so after starting a transfusion. It is sometimes difficult to distinguish immediately between a febrile reaction and hemolytic reaction. Usually a hemolytic reaction is more immediate and accompanied by other symptoms.

Stop the transfusion immediately and use symptomatic treatment with antipyretics. These reactions may be prevented by using washed red cells for patients known to have febrile reactions and requiring frequent transfusion.

4. Disease transmission in blood components has become a major concern in recent years. Transfusion-related viral illnesses include those associated with hepatitis A, B, and non-A, non-B viruses; Epstein–Barr virus; cytomegalovirus (CMV), and human immunodeficiency virus (HIV).

Bacteria may be transmitted if blood is contaminated during storage or transfusion. Parasites, such as those causing malaria, are also carried in blood. To prevent transfusion-related disease, testing for viruses is done on donors as well as the blood products. Donors are screened for hepatitis B and HIV. Blood components are also tested for the presence of CMV and HIV before transfusions. Before isolation of the human immunodeficiency virus, acquired immunodeficiency syndrome was frequently transmitted in blood, particularly in coagulation factor concentrates from a large pool of donors. Now these products are heat treated, which has been proven to destroy the virus. Non-A, non-B hepatitis is still a problem in blood transfusion, as there is no readily available test for its presence. Heat treatment has decreased the incidence of this form of hepatitis in pooled blood products.

Chapter 22

Hematologic Procedures

Karen A. Bringelsen

I. Diagnostic Procedures

A. Bleeding Time

The bleeding time is a very useful screening test for assessing platelet function. It is a very sensitive test and will be abnormal in the vast majority of patients with any clinically significant platelet disorder. It is most useful when there is a history of bleeding and the patient has a normal prothrombin time (PT) and partial thromboplastin time (PTT). There are several methods for performing a bleeding time. The preferred one for children is the template version of the bleeding time, using the forearm.

1. Purpose: A bleeding time is performed to assess platelet function and platelet–vessel interaction.

2. Selection of Patients:

a. Indications: The bleeding time is prolonged in conditions affecting platelet aggregation or capillary integrity. As a screening test of coagulation, the bleeding time should be done in conjunction with a platelet count, a smear for evaluation of platelet morphology, and a PT and PTT. The bleeding time will be abnormal in a variety of instances:

　(1) von Willebrand's Disease

　(2) Aspirin ingestion and therapeutic aspirin administration

　(3) Thrombocytopenia

　(4) Uremia

　(5) Vasculitis

　(6) A variety of rare qualitative platelet disorders causing nonthrombocytopenia purpura and petechiae:

　Glanzmann's disease (thrombasthenia), storage pool defects, congenital absence of platelet factor III, Bernard-Soulier syndrome.

b. Contraindications and Precautions: Thrombocytopenia (platelet count of fewer than 50,000 per mL^3) will produce a prolonged bleeding time simply because of the reduced numbers of platelets. The resulting bleeding may be difficult to stop and a bleeding time should not be done.

The ear lobe should not be used as the site for a bleeding time. If the patient has a coagulation disorder, it can be very difficult to control the bleeding at this site.

Performance of an accurate bleeding time is difficult in children under 4 or 5 years of age. The technique must be precise and cannot be done in an uncooperative toddler.

The bleeding time cannot be interpreted in the presence of aspirin or nonsteroidal anti-inflammatory drugs.

3. Equipment and Supplies (See Appendix for equipment and supplies manufacturers and suppliers. Appendix is keyed to italicized words in the equipment and supplies lists):

- Blood pressure cuff
- Alcohol *pads*
- Disposable bleeding time *device* (Figure 22-1)
- Stopwatch
- Filter *papers*
- Sterile adhesive bandage *strip*
- 2 × 2-inch sterile gauze *pads*
- Sterile skin closure *strips*

4. Description of Procedure:

- Perform a bleeding time on the ventral aspect of the forearm.

- Apply a blood pressure cuff to the upper arm and pump it up to a pressure of 40 mm Hg. Maintain this pressure throughout the procedure.
- Prepare the site with alcohol pads and allow it to dry.
- Holding the skin of the forearm taut but not stretched, place the bleeding time device against the skin and press the button. This releases two small blades, making identical, precise 1-mm × 10-mm incisions.
- Start the stopwatch as the incisions are made.
- Carefully blot drops of blood on the filter paper every 10 seconds, being careful not to touch the edge of the wound with the filter paper (Figure 22-2).
- Continue blotting and timing until the bleeding stops.
- Stop the watch and note the time.
- If bleeding continues beyond 15 minutes, stop the test and record the result as "greater than 15 minutes."
- When bleeding stops, simply apply a sterile bandage strip. If the test is terminated while the wounds are still bleeding, apply pressure with dry, sterile gauze until the bleeding stops. Then close the wound with sterile skin closure strips.

5. Side Effects and Complications: Problems are minimal even in patients with von Willebrand's Disease. Prolonged bleeding usually responds to direct pressure over the wound for 10 minutes, followed by application of skin closure strips

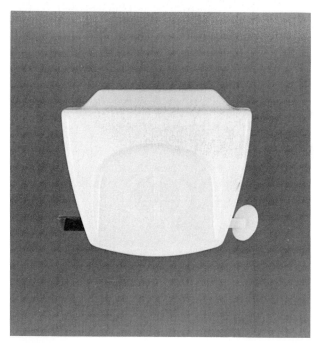

Figure 22-1.
Bleeding time. Equipment and supplies: Disposable bleeding time device.

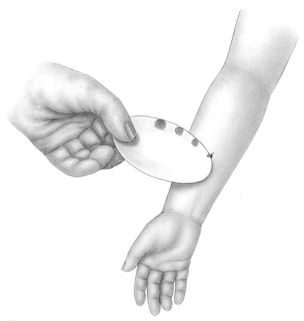

Figure 22-2.
Bleeding time. Technique.

and a pressure dressing. Small scars are common whether or not the bleeding time is abnormal.

6. Interpretation: A normal bleeding time is from 1 to 8 minutes. Prolongation greater than 15 minutes is abnormal and indicates platelet dysfunction. For definitive diagnosis, more specific tests of platelet function are required. Equivocal results of 9 to 15 minutes are difficult to interpret. If the clinical history is suggestive of a bleeding disorder, further evaluation should be done with specific platelet studies. If the clinical history is also equivocal, repeating the bleeding time will often produce a normal test result.

B. Bone Marrow Aspiration

Examination of the bone marrow is often helpful in the diagnosis of hematologic or malignant disease. Bone marrow aspiration is not done often in a general pediatric setting, but the procedure is not difficult to learn. It is somewhat painful and requires practice to develop skill in doing the procedure as quickly as possible while still obtaining an adequate sample. Marrow is usually examined to confirm a suggested diagnosis. There are very few situations when marrow must be obtained as an emergency. Therefore, whenever a bone marrow aspirate is done, the patient's management should be discussed with a hematologist or pathologist to be certain an adequate sample is obtained and processed correctly.

1. Purpose: A sample of bone marrow is obtained to aid in the diagnosis of hematologic abnormalities.

2. Selection of Patients:

a. Indications: Examination of the marrow is indicated in a variety of conditions:

(1) Leukemias

(2) Solid tumors such as lymphomas, neuroblastoma, or Ewing's sarcoma, which metastasize to the bone marrow

(3) Pancytopenia—depletion of red cells, white cells, and platelets

(4) Thrombocytopenia

(5) Suggested aplastic anemia

(6) Evaluation of fever of unknown origin

(7) Suggested storage disease

b. Contraindications and Precautions: There are no absolute contraindications to the procedure. Coagulation abnormalities associated with hemophilia and other known bleeding disorders should be corrected before the procedure. If the platelet count is fewer than 20,000 per milliliter during the procedure, a pressure dressing should be applied afterward to minimize bleeding.

3. Equipment and Supplies (See Appendix for equipment and supplies manufacturers and suppliers. Appendix is keyed to italicized words in the equipment and supplies lists):

Disposable pre-packaged kits containing all the necessary equipment are available. A sterile tray is more economical, however, and may be easily assembled:

- Sterile *gloves*
- Povidone-iodine *solution* or swabs
- 4 × 4-inch sterile gauze *pads*
- *Drape* with a window
- *Lidocaine* (1%)
- 25-gauge *needle* (See Figure 20-7, page 262) and 3.0-mL *syringe* (See Figure 20-7, page 262), for local anesthetic
- No. 11 scalpel *blade* (Figure 22-3)
- Bone marrow *needle*—many varieties are available, each with a minor difference in design. A basic needle, called an Osgood, is a 1½- to 3-inch, 11 to 13-gauge straight needle with a sharp stylet (Figure 22-4). A short 20-gauge needle with a flange at the hub can be used for an infant.
- 10-mL plastic *syringes* (See Figure 20-7, page 262), for marrow aspiration
- Heparin *solution* (1:1000)
- Sterile bandage *strip* or pressure dressing
- 10- to 19-gauge *needle* (See Figure 20-7, page 262)
- Glass microscope *slides*
- 23-gauge *needle* (See Figure 20-7, page 262) on a 3.0-mL *syringe* (See Figure 20-7, page 262), for preparation of marrow smears
- Other necessary equipment depends on the purpose of the procedure and may include culture tubes or extra syringes. "Heparinized" syringes may be needed if extra marrow is to be aspirated for immunologic or cytogenetic studies for suggested leukemia. Syringes are "heparinized" by drawing 0.2 mL of heparin into a syringe, holding the syringe upright, pulling the plunger back so that the inside walls of the syringe are wet with heparin, and expressing the air from the syringe while not allowing the heparin to be expressed.

4. Description of Procedure:

Discuss the procedure with a hematologist or pathologist to be certain proper samples are obtained.

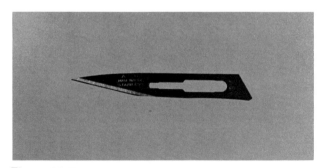

Figure 22-3.
Bone marrow aspiration. Equipment and supplies: No. 11 scalpel blade.

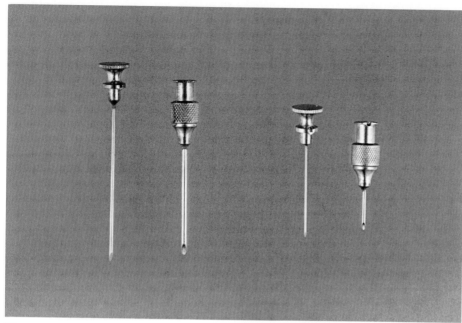

Figure 22-4.
Bone marrow aspiration. Equipment and supplies: Osgood needles and stylets.

a. Site selection:

The posterior iliac crest is the preferred site for most patients. It is easily accessible, easily stabilized, and distant from vital structures.

The anterior iliac crest is also easily accessible, especially in obese patients. However, it is closer to the vital structures of the abdominal cavity and the procedure is more painful at this site.

The anterior tibial tuberosity may be used in the newborn patients and in infants up to age 6 months. Entering at the tuberosity will insure the needle is well below the growth plate of the tibia.

Aspiration from the sternum is contraindicated in children because of the thinness of the bone and proximity to the mediastinum. It is not a preferred site at any age.

The marrow aspiration procedure will be described using the posterior iliac crest.

b. Patient position:
  · Place the child face down on a firm surface.
  · A rolled towel beneath the abdomen will make the hips more prominent (Figure 22-5).
  · If necessary, a parent or assistant may restrain the child's arms and shoulders by pressing the shoulders firmly to the examination table surface and holding the arms above the child's head (Figure 22-5).

· The legs may be held or wrapped in a small sheet for restraint.

· The patient may be sedated with morphine or midazolam (See Table 18-2, page 219) but this is not usually necessary. The procedure is uncomfortable, but it is also quick.

c. Site preparation:
  · Palpate the area to locate the most prominent point on the iliac crest (Figure 22-6).
  · Using sterile technique, including sterile gloves, prepare the site using povidone iodine solution and 4 × 4-inch gauze or presoaked swabs.
  · Drape the area, with the drape window over the site.
  · With a 25-gauge needle on a 3-mL syringe, infiltrate the skin with a small amount of lidocaine and then slowly infiltrate approximately 0.5 mL in the deeper tissue down to but not touching the bone.
  · When the child cannot feel a needle prick on the skin, use a second needle and syringe with lidocaine to anesthetize the periosteum by gently tapping the needle on the bone while injecting 0.5 mL of the lidocaine. This will anesthetize the periosteum and aid in locating a stable site on the bone for the marrow needle. The child will feel a sharp prickly sensation while the lidocaine is injected.

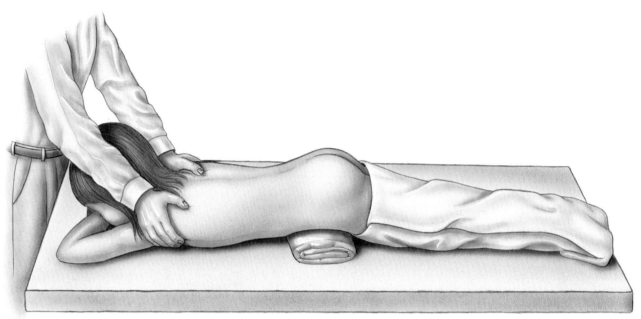

Figure 22-5.
Bone marrow aspiration. Patient restraint.

d. Marrow puncture:
  · Puncture the skin with the no. 11 scalpel blade to allow easier insertion of the marrow needle (optional).
  · With the stylet in place, insert the marrow needle perpendicular to the bone and advance it until it touches the bones.
  · Tap the needle on the bone and locate a spot that is well anesthetized, flat, and perpendicular to the needle. The patient should feel a dull tap, but no sharp pain.
  · Hold the needle firmly between the thumb and forefinger with the hub resting against the palm or base of the first finger. This grip is best for control of the needle.
  · With firm, steady pressure and a rotating motion, push the needle through the bone cortex (Figure 22-7). The child should feel a hard pushing sensation with some sharpness as the needle enters the bone.
  · Continue to advance the needle until it feels firmly "seated" and does not wobble when released. There is no feeling of a "give" when the marrow space is entered.
  · Unless the needle is well controlled and the child is still, the needle may slip off the bone as an attempt is made to enter the marrow space. When this happens there is a sudden "give" and no further resistance is felt. It is not dangerous to have the needle slip from the posterior iliac crest, but it is uncomfortable and prolongs the procedure.

e. Marrow aspiration:
  · Remove the stylet and attach a 10-mL plastic syringe.
  · With a steady pull, draw the plunger back to about the 8.0-mL mark on the syringe barrel while maintaining suction.
  · When marrow appears in the barrel, immediately release the suction and remove the syringe.
  · For marrow smears, 0.5 mL is sufficient, and collecting more than this amount usually dilutes the specimen, making interpretation difficult.
    Aspiration is the most painful part of the procedure and is described as similar to a severe toothache, but lasting only seconds.
  · If *extra marrow* is needed for culture, attach a second syringe and draw an additional few milliliters.
  · *Heparinized marrow* samples may be required when special stains and immunologic studies are used to diagnose and classify leukemia. After the initial 0.5-mL aspirate is obtained, attach the "heparinized" syringe. Usually two samples of 5 to 10 mL of marrow are drawn, but it is best to discuss the situation with a pathologist, because procedures vary among different laboratories. It may be helpful to rotate the needle in 90-degree increments between samples to increase the yield.
  · You may find aspiration difficult because of poor positioning of the needle. A "dry tap" can be associated

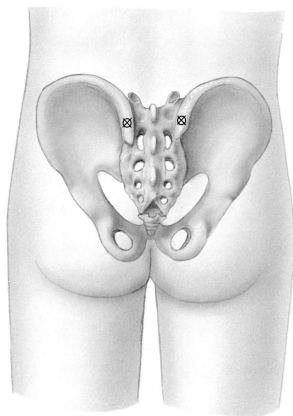

Figure 22-6.
Bone marrow aspiration. Site for aspiration from the iliac crest.

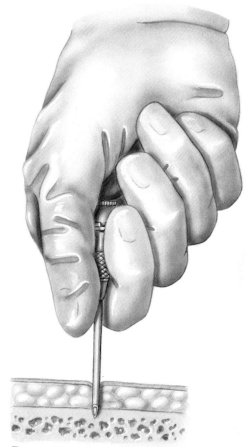

Figure 22-7.
Bone marrow aspiration. Technique.

with leukemic infiltration of the marrow or aplastic anemia. Applying more suction using a 30-mL syringe or repositioning of the needle, usually medially and caudally, will often help in these circumstances. Whenever the needle is repositioned, be sure the stylet is in place to prevent blockage of the needle by bony fragments.

f. Marrow smear preparation:

· Replace the stylet and leave the needle in place while an assistant makes a smear to be sure the sample is adequate.

· You should see small dots of bony spicules on the slide if a proper sample has been obtained (Figure 22-8).

· If the sample is adequate, quickly withdraw the needle with a pulling and rotating motion and apply firm pressure to the site.

· When the platelet count is fewer than 20,000 per milliliter, apply a pressure dressing for 24 hours to help

minimize bleeding. Otherwise use a sterile bandage strip.

· There are many ways to prepare marrow smears using slides or cover slips, depending on the preferences of the hematologist or pathologist in different institutions. The described method is simple and adequate for any evaluation of a marrow aspirate.

(a) Working rapidly before the sample has clotted, attach a 19-gauge needle to the syringe and place a 3- to 4-mm (diameter) drop of marrow toward one end of the upper sides of 8 to 10 clean glass slides (Figure 22-9).

(b) Carefully aspirate any excess blood to leave a concentrated drop of marrow on each slide.

(c) Similar to the commonly used technique for making a blood smear, hold a second slide at a 30-degree

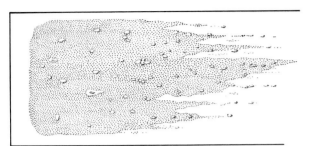

Figure 22-8.
Bone marrow aspiration. Spicules on slide of fresh bone marrow smear.

angle to the slide with the drop of marrow, and gently move the leading edge of the second slide against the drop of marrow (Figure 22-9).

(d) Allow the marrow to spread across the leading edge of the second slide, then push the slide forward, making a thin film of marrow.

(e) Repeat the process to prepare additional slides.

(f) Allow the slides to air dry.

5. Side Effects and Complications: When the posterior iliac crest is used, there are almost no complications. For a few hours, there may be discomfort associated with sitting. The

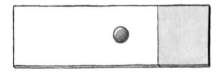

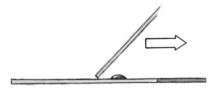

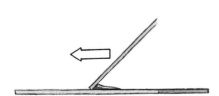

Figure 22-9.
Bone marrow aspiration. Marrow smear preparation.

child often does not even complain of residual soreness the next day. Bruising, or even a hematoma, may occur when the platelet count is low.

6. Interpretation: Slides are sent to the laboratory for staining and are usually interpreted by a hematologist or pathologist.

C. Bone Marrow Biopsy

A marrow biopsy may be done alone, or more commonly, at the same time that a marrow aspirate is done. It is technically more difficult to perform and more painful than a marrow aspiration. Whenever a bone marrow examination is considered, it is best to discuss the procedure with a pathologist or hematologist to determine whether or not a biopsy is necessary.

1. Purpose: A marrow biopsy is done to obtain a core of bone marrow with the architecture and cell distribution undisturbed.

2. Selection of Patients:

a. Indications: There are only a few situations in which a bone marrow biopsy is required. It may be necessary when an aspirate cannot be obtained. For example, the marrow is often difficult to aspirate when it has been replaced by leukemic cells. A biopsy is also required for the diagnosis of aplastic anemia and to exclude solid tumor metastasis to the marrow. A marrow biopsy is not indicated in more common situations such as the diagnosis of idiopathic thrombocytopenic purpura or the evaluation of anemias.

b. Contraindications and Precautions: A platelet count of fewer than 20,000 per milliliter may result in bleeding from the site. Coagulation abnormalities should be corrected before the biopsy. A marrow biopsy should not be performed from the sternum or tibia.

3. Equipment and Supplies (See Appendix for equipment and supplies manufacturers and suppliers. Appendix is keyed to italicized words in the equipment and supplies lists):

Prepackaged disposable bone marrow biopsy *kits* are available with all necessary equipment including the biopsy needle. Alternatively, a sterile tray may be easily assembled:

· See Bone Marrow Aspiration, Equipment and Supplies, page 290

· Bone biopsy *needle:* The Jamshidi needle (Figure 22-10) is the most commonly used. It is a long 11- or 13-gauge needle with a sharp stylet and tapered point. The advantage of a Jamshidi needle is that an aspirate can be obtained with the same needle just before the biopsy. With other types of biopsy needles, a separate puncture is required for marrow aspiration.

· Small bottle of formalin *solution*

· 23-gauge *needle* (See Figure 20-7, page 262), for making "touch preps"

4. Description of Procedure:

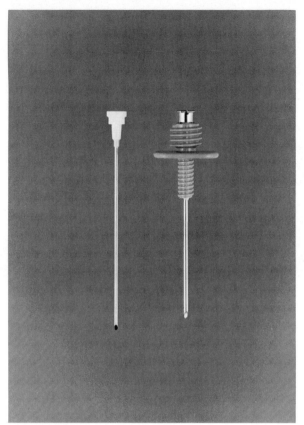

Figure 22-10.
Bone marrow biopsy. Equipment and supplies: Jamshidi needle and stylet.

a. Site selection:
  · The posterior iliac crest (See Figure 22-6, page 293) is the preferred site.
  · The anterior iliac crest may be used.
  · A marrow biopsy should not be attempted from the tibia and certainly not from the sternum.
b. Patient position (See Bone Marrow Aspiration, Patient position, page 291):
c. Site preparation (See Bone Marrow Aspiration, Site preparation, page 291):
d. Marrow puncture:
  · Puncture the skin with a no. 11 blade to allow easier insertion of the biopsy needle.
  · Hold the needle with the hub in the palm and the index finger down the shaft of the needle for the best control and stability (Figure 22-11).
  · With the stylet in place, insert the needle perpendicular to the bone and advance it until it touches the bone.

· Use the same technique as in a marrow aspiration to advance the needle into the marrow cavity (See Bone Marrow Aspiration, Marrow puncture, page 292).
· When the needle is firmly "seated," remove the stylet and aspirate a small amount of marrow for smears.
e. Marrow biopsy:
  · Leaving the stylet out, advance the needle a few millimeters with a clockwise, rotating motion.
  · Reposition the needle, slightly changing the angle, and firmly advance it a few more millimeters.
  · Again reposition the needle slightly and advance it once more. This procedure will pack a marrow core tightly into the shaft of the needle.
  · Without pressure, rock the needle back and forth and side to side and twist counterclockwise to release the marrow core from the surrounding bone.

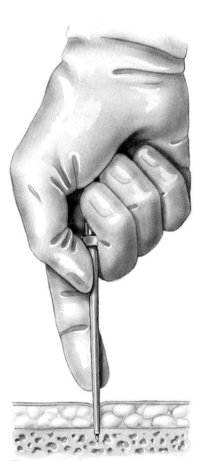

Figure 22-11.
Bone marrow biopsy. Technique.

• Slowly and gently withdraw the needle; a rapid removal is likely to dislodge the biopsy core.

• Manually apply firm pressure to the site with a 4 × 4-inch gauze.

Because obtaining a biopsy is more difficult than performing an aspiration, it often requires two or more attempts. The core of marrow often slips from the needle shaft as the needle is removed. Carefully rocking and rotating the needle before removing it helps break the biopsy specimen from the marrow and allow its release. When a second attempt is necessary, repositioning the needle in the same site usually does not help. It is better to insert the needle in the same skin puncture, but enter the bone at a more medial site.

• To remove the biopsy specimen, insert the straight wire into the needle end of the biopsy needle and push the core out the top of the needle onto a glass slide.

• Using forceps or a needle, gently lift the core and touch it to several areas on a slide, thus making imprints or "touch preps" to be stained.

• The core is then placed in the fixative (formalin) for processing.

5. Side Effects and Complications: There are very few complications when a biopsy is done from the iliac crest. The procedure is more painful than an aspiration, and there may be moderate soreness and discomfort for a few hours after the biopsy. Bruising or a hematoma may result when the platelet count is abnormally low.

6. Interpretation: The slides and biopsy specimen are sent to the laboratory for staining and processing. The marrow is usually examined and interpreted by a hematologist or pathologist.

Chapter 23

Outpatient Toxicologic Procedures

Richard A. Christoph

The majority of poisonings in the United States involve children. Many accidental exposures may result from the natural curiosity of children younger than 5 years of age. However, recent surveillance studies indicate a correlation between child poisonings and a variety of factors associated with parental and familial stress, e.g., families with a history of physical and psychological illness. Aggressive or impulsive child behaviors, overactivity, and poor self-esteem have been noted with increased frequency in children who ingest poisons, especially in those who repeatedly ingest poisons.

The substances involved in childhood poisonings include a wide range of plants, household products, medications intended for internal and external use, paints and hydrocarbons, insecticides and pesticides, and others. The various routes of exposure include skin, eye, inhalation, and envenomation, but poisoning by ingestion accounts for the majority of exposures in all age groups.

Intentional poisonings (self-injury acts, suicide attempts, attention-seeking behaviors) also occur in the pediatric age group. Such intentional exposures represent only 10% to 15% of all poisonings and are quite rare in children younger than 5 years of age. Patients with intentional poisonings represent a cohort more likely to require intensive support, and the substances involved are more likely to be medications intended for internal use.

The procedures outlined in this chapter primarily address issues related to ingestion; however, management of dermal exposures will be discussed briefly. The management of eye exposures is discussed elsewhere (See Eye Procedures, page 69).

I. Procedures to Effect Gastric Emptying

A. Administration of Syrup of Ipecac

1. Purpose: The purpose of this procedure is to empty the stomach of ingested poisons or toxins by inducing emesis. The emetic qualities of syrup of ipecac are due to a local irritant effect on the gastric and intestinal mucosa and due to an effect on the medullary chemoreceptor trigger zone (CTZ). Most studies of syrup of ipecac suggest that it will empty the stomach of about 30% to 60% of its contents.

2. Selection of Patients:

a. Indications: Syrup of ipecac is an especially appropriate means of gastric emptying for the preadolescent before the child's arrival in the emergency department. To minimize the risk of aspiration of vomitus, however, the child should be old enough to maintain a sitting posture and possess adequate head control.

b. Contraindications and Precautions: Induced emesis is contraindicated after the ingestion of a caustic (strong alkali), because the returned caustic would further injure the esophageal mucosa. Induced emesis is also inappropriate in the obtunded or comatose patient or in the patient with seizures, because of the attendant risk of aspiration. The ingestion of simple petroleum distillates usually should not be managed with induced emesis. However, if the petroleum distillate is a vehicle for a more toxic compound such as an insecticide, carbon tetrachloride, or one of the aromatic hydrocarbons (e.g., benzene or toluene), gastric emptying should be induced.

In general, routine gastric emptying is of minimal benefit for the patient whose ingestion occurred several hours before presentation.

Caution should be exercised when inducing emesis in patients who have ingested compounds that characteristically cause dramatic and rapid deterioration in mental status (e.g., tricyclic antidepressants). Emesis may occur after the patient has become obtunded or lost control of his gag reflex, resulting in an increased risk of aspiration.

Make sure that *syrup* of ipecac is used and *not* ipecac *fluid-extract,* which is 14 times more potent and may be fatal.

3. Equipment and Supplies (See Appendix for equipment and supplies manufacturers and suppliers. Appendix is keyed to italicized words in the equipment and supplies lists):
- Syrup of *ipecac*
- Liquid, for oral intake (water, milk, or clear carbonated beverage)
- Emesis *basin*
- Sterile urine *cup,* for collection of emesis specimen for toxicologic analysis

4. Description of Procedure:
- Administer *syrup* of ipecac at a dosage of:

(1) 30 mL by mouth for patients 12 years of age or older

(2) 15 mL by mouth for patients 1 to 12 years of age

(3) 10 mL by mouth for infants 6 to 12 months of age

- Offer 2 to 10 ounces of fluid orally after the syrup of ipecac is taken (water, milk, or a clear carbonated beverage would be equally effective).
- Maintain the child in a sitting posture with the trunk and head leaning slightly forward such that when sudden emesis occurs, the risk of aspiration will be minimized. If the child cannot be maintained in this posture because of central nervous system depression, do not induce emesis.
- Collect emesis for toxicologic analysis if the nature of the ingestion is uncertain. Use a sterile urine cup to collect 60 to 75 mL of emesis.
- Repeat the procedure once if the child has not vomited in 20 to 30 minutes.
- If the child has not vomited within 20 to 30 minutes of the second dose of syrup of ipecac, empty the gastric contents by gastric lavage (See below).

5. Side Effects and Complications: Aspiration is the most frequent complication. Ipecac toxicity is unlikely with the dosage recommended for induction of emesis. Potential toxic effects are due to the presence of emetine, which can affect the peripheral cardiovascular system and heart, the central nervous system, and the gastrointestinal tract.

B. Gastric Lavage

1. Purpose: The purpose of this procedure is to empty the stomach of ingested poisons or toxins. Lavage will empty the stomach of 50% to 60% of its contents.

2. Selection of Patients:

a. Indications: The procedure is appropriate for emptying the stomach of a patient with depressed mental status, obtundation, coma or seizures; however, the effectiveness of gastric lavage in such a patient whose ingestion occurred more than 1 hour before presentation has been recently questioned. Gastric lavage may be indicated in the case of an alert patient who adamantly refuses to cooperate with the administration of syrup of ipecac.

b. Contraindications and Precautions: The procedure is contraindicated after the ingestion of a caustic or corrosive substance. A *relative* contraindication to lavage may be an inability to orotracheally intubate the patient before the lavage. Orotracheal intubation protects the airway from aspiration of vomitus.

3. Equipment and Supplies (See Appendix for equipment and supplies manufacturers and suppliers. Appendix is keyed to italicized words in the equipment and supplies lists):

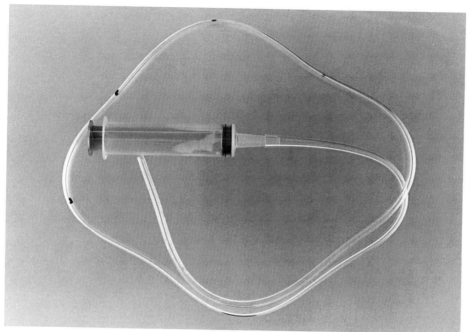

Figure 23-1.
Gastric lavage. Equipment and supplies: Nasogastric tube attached to Toomey syringe.

- Nasogastric *tubes* (Figure 23-1)
- Orogastric lavage *tubes* (Figure 23-2)
- Water-soluble lubricant *jelly*
- 60-mL *syringe* (Figure 23-2), for lavage
- 0.45 normal saline *solution:* 2 to 3 liters
- All equipment listed for endotracheal intubation (See Pulmonary and Cardiac Resuscitation Procedures, page 305) including *suction* equipment and cuffed endotracheal *tubes* (sized 5.0 to 7.5, if available)
- Sterile specimen *cup*
- Elbow *restraint*
- Wrist and ankle *restraints*

4. Description of Procedure:

- Because the use of lavage in the pediatric age group is primarily suggested for the patient exhibiting central nervous system depression, the risk of aspiration must be minimized. Therefore, before the insertion of an orogastric lavage tube, perform endotracheal intubation with an appropriate size endotracheal tube (cuffed if available) (See Pulmonary and Cardiac Resuscitation Procedures, page 305). This may be the only indication for the temporary use of cuffed endotracheal tubes in the pediatric population.
- If the patient is alert and refusing ipecac or is alert and combative, you may need to apply physical restraints

to accomplish gastric emptying by lavage. Physical restraint of the upper extremities is best accomplished by a combination of properly fitted, commercially available elbow restraints and wrist restraints (Figure 23-3). The rigid elbow restraints prevent flexion at that joint. Wrist restraints of "lamb's wool" lining do not pinch or irritate sensitive skin and are fastened at the wrist with either a Velcro® system, (for young children and infants) or an adjustable buckle, depending on the model. The restraint device is connected to cloth straps that are tied to the stretcher to restrain the child's arms by his side.

The lower extremities are secured by use of ankle restraints tied to the "foot-end" of the stretcher. Commercially available ankle restraints, similar in function and application to the above-mentioned wrist restraints, are ideal.

- Immediately before the insertion of the gastric decontamination tube, assure suction is available, so as to remove any regurgitated stomach contents from the airway. An assistant is frequently necessary to maintain the child's head and neck in proper and stable position, slightly flexed at the neck (Figure 23-3).
- Choose the largest diameter lavage tube that can be passed comfortably (Table 23-1). This will maximize pill fragment retrieval. Usually the orogastric route is appro-

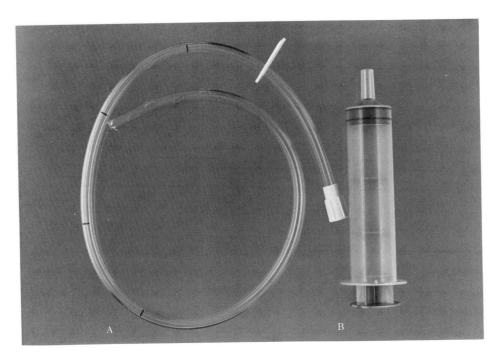

Figure 23-2.
Gastric lavage. Equipment and supplies: **A,** Orogastric lavage tube; **B,** 60-mL Toomey syringe.

priate for the poisoned child with a depressed level of consciousness, especially if the child has already been orotracheally intubated as noted above. For orogastric lavage, a 34-French orogastric lavage tube is usually used in the teenager, whereas even a preschooler can tolerate a 14- to 18-French nasogastric tube inserted by the orogastric route. If a nasogastric introduction is preferred, an 8-French nasogastric tube is used in a 1-year-old child, and a teenager can tolerate an 18-French nasogastric tube. When nasogastric lavage is used, it is less necessary for you to intubate the trachea before the lavage. Gagging, vomiting, and aspiration may still occur, however.

· Determine the length of tube to be inserted by measuring from the nares (nasogastric introduction) or from the lips (orogastric introduction) to the xiphoid and adding 8 to 10 cm (Figure 23-4).

· Position the patient on his left side to reduce the risk of aspiration. Some suggest placing the patient in the Trendelenburg position.

· Pass the tube into the stomach by the orogastric route (orogastric lavage is preferred when feasible) (See Gastrointestinal Procedures, page 126). If a nasogastric introduction is used, be careful to lubricate the tube and follow the floor of the nose during insertion. Try to avoid lacerating the inferior turbinate.

· Check the position of the tube by listening for borborygmus with a stethoscope over the stomach while rapidly introducing 20 to 30 mL of air into the tube by means of an air-filled syringe.

· Have an assistant maintain the tube position by hand, so that the tube location may be adjusted during the lavage. Adjustment may be necessary to optimize lavage return.

· Instill 10 to 15 mL/kg of lavage fluid with a 60-mL syringe. Half-normal (0.45 N) saline would be a satisfactory lavage fluid.

· Using the lavage syringe, remove the fluid. Save the

Table 23-1. Appropriate Gastric Lavage Tube Sizes for Different Age Groups

	Nasogastric Tube Size	Orogastric Tube Size
Infant	8 French	12–14 French
Child	10–16 French	14–18 French
Adolescent	18 French	34 French

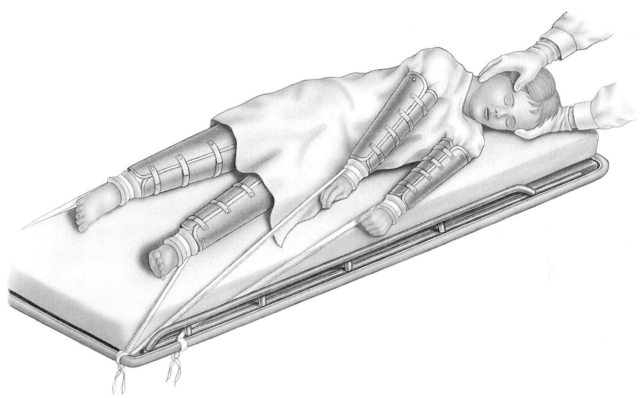

Figure 23-3.
Gastric lavage. Restraint of patient.

first return of lavage fluid for toxicologic analysis whenever the nature of the ingestion is uncertain. A total of 60 to 75 mL of lavage fluid can be collected in a sterile urine cap for this purpose.

· Repeat the lavage procedure until the lavage return is clear and a total of 2 to 3 liters of lavage fluid have been used.

5. Side Effects and Complications: The greatest risk in performing gastric lavage is aspiration. It is appropriate to protect the airway by endotracheal intubation before orogastric lavage. Nasogastric tube insertion may result in minor bleeding from nares as the tube is passed between the floor of the nose and the inferior turbinate.

II. Procedures to Reduce Absorption

A. Administration of Activated Charcoal

1. Purpose: The purpose of this procedure is to absorb large nonpolar toxic compounds to prevent intestinal absorption.

2. Selection of Patients:

a. Indications: Use activated charcoal when syrup of ipecac is contraindicated (caustics, corrosives, hydrocarbons, etc.). Activated charcoal is always used in conjunction with a cathartic (See below). The charcoal may be mixed as a slurry with the cathartic solution itself, or may be mixed with water, to be followed by administration of a cathartic. Use activated charcoal if enough time has elapsed since the ingestion to have allowed substantial quantities of the poison or toxin to pass from the stomach into the intestine. Use activated charcoal if a large volume of poison or toxin has been ingested. Multiple dosages of activated charcoal should be used in cases where enterohepatic recirculation of the ingested compound occurs (e.g., tricyclics, barbiturates). Activated charcoal given enterally is useful in accelerating the elimination of several medications, even when those medications are administered *parenterally* (e.g., lead, theophylline, nortriptyline).

b. Contraindications and Precautions: Contraindications include bowel perforation and persistent emesis (patient will vomit the charcoal).

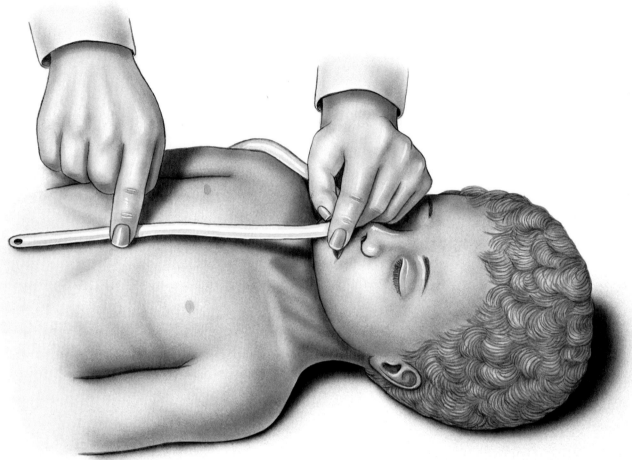

Figure 23-4.
Gastric lavage. Estimation of appropriate tube length.

3. Equipment and Supplies (See Appendix for equipment and supplies manufacturers and suppliers. Appendix is keyed to italicized words in the equipment and supplies lists):
 · Gowns
 · Activated *charcoal*
 · Slurry vehicle: Activated charcoal is often used with one of the cathartics serving as the vehicle for the slurry. However, sterile water or normal saline *solution* may also be used
 · Cup, if activated charcoal slurry is to be administered orally
 · Nasogastric or orogastric *tube,* if that route is preferred (See Figures 23-1 and 23-2, pages 299 and 300)
 · Water-soluble lubricant *jelly*

 · 60-mL *syringe* if nasogastric or orogastric tube is used (See Figure 23-2, page 300)
4. Description of Procedure:
 · The operator and all assistants should wear gowns; activated charcoal is invariably messy!
 · Mix activated charcoal as a slurry with a cathartic (See below). The dosage of activated charcoal is 1 mg/kg of the child's body weight.
 · Administer the charcoal–cathartic slurry orally after the patient has ceased vomiting.
 · If multiple doses are indicated, repeat the dose in 4 hours and every 4 hours thereafter for four doses, or until charcoal is seen in the stools.
 · If a child cannot or will not tolerate activated charcoal

orally because of its consistency, the material may be given through a nasogastric tube, even if gastric emptying was originally accomplished by emesis. If the gastric lavage was performed and if activated charcoal is indicated, administer the charcoal before withdrawal of the lavage tube:

· Connect the 60-mL syringe (without plunger) to the gastric tube.

· Pour 15 to 20 mL of the charcoal–cathartic slurry into the syringe and allow the slurry to gravity-drain into the stomach. Do not use the plunger to force the slurry into the stomach, because the patient may vomit.

· Repeat the above step until the entire dosage of charcoal–cathartic slurry has been administered.

5. Side Effects and Complications: Aspiration of charcoal can occur during emesis. Repeated doses of charcoal carry a risk of bowel obstruction. Repeated doses of cathartic carry a risk of fluid and electrolyte disturbances.

B. Administration of a Cathartic

1. Purpose: The purpose of this procedure is to reduce intestinal transit time, thus decreasing intestinal absorption of a poison or toxin and increasing stool elimination.

2. Selection of Patients:

a. Indications: Indications include ingestions requiring the use of activated charcoal and ingestions of substances requiring an increase in bowel elimination.

b. Contraindications and Precautions: Concurrent diarrhea may make the use of cathartics unnecessary. Bowel perforation is a contraindication to their use.

3. Equipment and Supplies (See Appendix for equipment and supplies manufacturers and suppliers. Appendix is keyed to italicized words in the equipment and supplies lists):

· Cathartic Solutions:
Magnesium citrate: 0.5 mL/kg to a maximum of 200 mL.
Magnesium sulfate (10% solution): 2.5 mL/kg or 250 mg/kg, to a maximum of 20 g.
Sodium sulfate (10% solution): 2.5 mL/kg or 250 mg/kg, to a maximum of 20 g.
Sorbitol (70% solution): 2.8 mL/kg or 2.0 g/kg, to a maximum of 150 g.

4. Description of Procedure:

· Administer the cathartic orally or by nasogastric or orogastric tube. If a gastric tube is used to administer the cathartic, follow the steps for placement of a nasogastric tube or orogastric tube (See Enteral Intubation, page 133) as well as the steps for administration of a charcoal–cathartic slurry (See page 301).

5. Side Effects and Complications: Sorbitol is the most rapidly acting cathartic. A potential disadvantage to its use is the frequent development of abdominal cramps and diarrhea.

Recently there have been reports of hypernatremic dehydration and neurologic deterioration in small children and infants who received constant infusions of activated charcoal in 70% sorbitol. Therefore, the use of 70% sorbitol in this age group should be accompanied by extreme caution.

Sorbitol is metabolized to fructose and should not be given to patients intolerant of fructose.

Saline cathartics such as magnesium citrate, magnesium sulfate, and sodium sulfate can induce electrolyte disturbances and hypermagnesemia. They are slower acting than sorbitol.

III. Dermal Exposures

Many medications and most liquid industrial and agricultural chemicals can be easily absorbed transdermally, a classic example being organophosphate insecticides.

1. Purpose: The purpose of this procedure is to reduce systemic absorption of a toxin by removing the material from the skin as quickly as possible.

2. Selection of Patients:

a. Indications: Patients exposed to a potentially injurious dose of toxin or chemical in which transdermal absorption of the material may occur could benefit from this procedure.

b. Contraindications and Precautions: Nursing and physician personnel should meticulously avoid contamination while tending to the poisoned patient. Protective clothing (long-sleeved gowns and gloves, and, in certain circumstances, goggles) should be worn.

3. Equipment and Supplies (See Appendix for equipment and supplies manufacturers and suppliers. Appendix is keyed to italicized words in the equipment and supplies lists):

· Mild soap (e.g., "Ivory," Nutragena, others)
· Copious water for irrigation
· Long-sleeved gowns and gloves for the personnel
· *Goggles* (for certain exposures, e.g., organophosphates)

4. Description of Procedure:

· If the skin is intact, thorough washing with soap and warm water should be followed by rinsing and repeated washing with soap and water.

· If the skin has been burned or has open denuded areas, irrigate with generous amounts of sterile water or sterile saline if available.

· The length of time spent irrigating the affected skin and the volume of irrigation fluid used may vary depending on the nature of the exposure. Deeply penetrating caustics such as alkalis may require irrigation for 30 to 45 minutes or more, using dozens of liters of irrigant. Some suggest prolonged rinsing of such alkali burns under a forceful water stream from a faucet.

5. Side Effects and Complications: Thorough washing and irrigation of affected skin may be painful for the child, especially in the case of burned or denuded skin. Analgesia may be necessary.

A major concern should exist regarding careless or inadequate irrigation of skin, especially in the case of alkaline caustic exposures. Thorough cleansing of skin cannot be overemphasized.

IV. Eye Exposures (See Eye Procedures, page 69)

Chapter 24

Pulmonary and Cardiac Resuscitation Procedures

Richard A. Christoph

Most cardiopulmonary arrests in the pediatric age group are secondary to a respiratory cause. It follows that most successful resuscitative efforts in this age group result from expert and efficient management of airway and ventilation. Airway management and ventilation therefore must be the preeminent focus of therapy in the initial management of the pediatric arrest victim.

Because of their age, size, and family reactions, most pediatric arrest victims, as compared with adult victims, arrive at a medical care facility with far fewer field interventions having been performed by rescue personnel. The physicians and nurses must often "start from scratch." Extreme efficiency is required in this often tense scene. The "code leader," who should be identified from the outset, must remain globally aware of the patient's overall situation on a minute-to-minute basis. Although ongoing discussions between participants may be appropriate, this "code leader" should remain in firm control of the care being provided.

Technical difficulties can be associated with pediatric resuscitation for a number of reasons (e.g., difficulty in obtaining intravenous access, inexperience in dealing with pediatric patients). Differences in the anatomy and physiology of the pediatric patient become important factors during pediatric resuscitations.

The procedures in this chapter are organized in order of priority, the "ABC's" of resuscitation. The airway ("A") is the first priority. Without an open and patent airway, attempts to provide assisted breathing will fail. Similarly, if the apneic child's breathing ("B") is not assisted, then attempts to provide circulatory support ("C") will be fruitless.

During an actual resuscitative effort, one should conserve time and resources in such a way as to intervene effectively in each "A," "B," and "C." Once the airway has been effectively managed, *immediately* address the issue of breathing. From there, attentions are directed to circulation.

An attempt is made to sequence each procedure within the "ABC" framework in order of priority and in order of increasing intervention. In a given resuscitation, certain of the procedures will be unnecessary. Use only those procedures necessary to accomplish the goals of establishing, with certainty, the integrity of airway, breathing, and circulation.

A knowledge of the anatomy of the airway of infants and children is crucial to the provision of successful resuscitation. The infant is an obligate nasal breather until about the third month of life. Coupled with the small anatomic size of the neonatal and young infant's nares, this contributes to the relatively greater respiratory distress at this age from otherwise benign nasal mucosal congestion and mucoid rhinorrhea.

The adenoids and tonsils of a child are relatively larger than those of the adult. Being vascular and somewhat friable structures, this size differential may interfere with nasopharyngeal suctioning or placement of a nasopharyngeal airway or a nasotracheal tube.

The soft tissues of the child's oropharynx, larynx, and neck are more pliable. They are more likely to obstruct the airway if the neck is flexed or hyperextended to an extreme degree. These factors impact on head and neck positioning measures to optimize the child's airway.

The child's larynx is directed more cephalad and more anteriorly than the larynx of the adult. This may make visualization of the larynx with a laryngoscope more difficult.

The narrowest part of the pediatric airway is the subglottic trachea, whereas the adult airway is narrowest at the glottis. As a result, the child is more prone to croup symptoms. Also, this narrowness serves as a physiologic "cuff" for any endotracheal tubes that are placed. Cuffed endotracheal tubes are contraindicated in children less than 7 to 8 years of age, because of the increased risk of tracheal wall ischemia associated with the presence of the cuff. The consequences of such ischemia might include the development of subglottic scarring and subglottic stenosis. An exception to this prohibition is the temporary use of cuffed endotracheal tubes

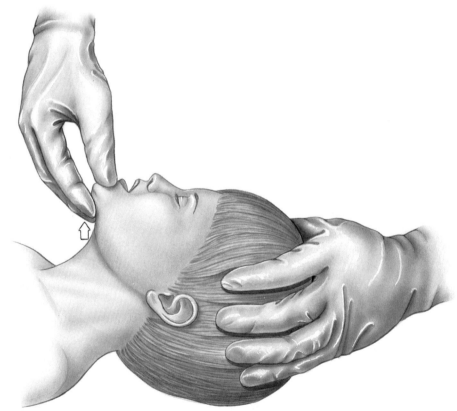

Figure 24-1.
Airway management procedures: Positioning of the head and neck—Chin Lift.
Technique.

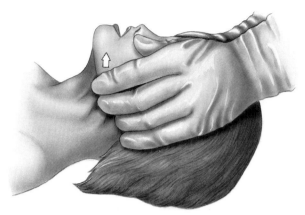

Figure 24-2.
Airway management procedures: Positioning of the head and neck—Jaw thrust. Technique.

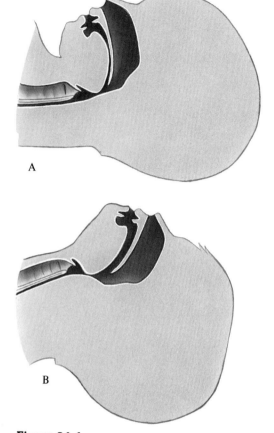

Figure 24-4.
Airway management procedures: Positioning of the head and neck. A, Excessive neck flexion. **B,** Excessive neck extension.

for the purpose of airway protection during orogastric lavage.

I. Airway Management Procedures

A. Positioning of the Head and Neck

1. Purpose: Correct head and neck positioning will manipulate the child's airway anatomy so as to maximize the patency of the airway.

2. Selection of Patients:

a. Indications: Proper positioning is the first step in the management of a child of any age with significant signs or symptoms of upper airway compromise such as marked retractions, dyspnea, stridor, cyanosis, or excessive secretions.

b. Contraindications and Precautions: There are no contraindications to proper head and neck positioning except for a possible cervical spine injury, which may be a potential contraindication to the use of the "sniffing position" (See below). In this case, chin lifts and jaw thrust may be used safely.

3. Equipment and Supplies: None

4. Description of Procedure:

 • *Chin lift:* Grasp the patient's submental chin with your thumb and index finger and gently pull anteriorly (Figure 24-1).

 • *Jaw thrust:* Locate the angles of the mandible with the fingerpads of both index fingers and pull anteriorly (Figure 24-2).

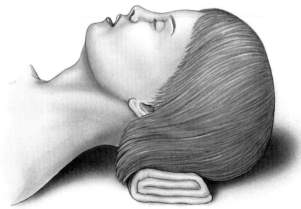

Figure 24-3.
Airway management procedures: Positioning of the head and neck—Sniffing position. Technique.

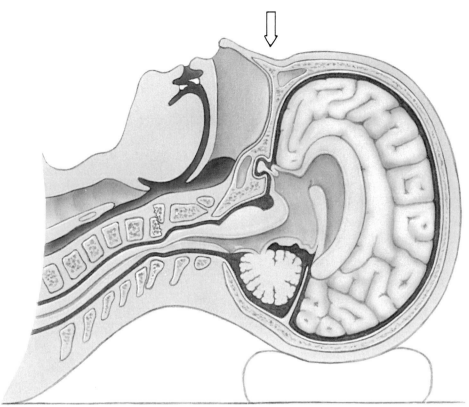

Figure 24-5.
Airway management procedures: Positioning of the head and neck. Sniffing position resulting in an aggravated spinal cord injury in a patient with an unstable cervical spine injury.

· *Sniffing position:* Place several thicknesses of towel under the patient's occiput so as to gently flex the neck at the shoulders while extending the neck gently at the occiput (Figure 24-3).

5. Side Effects and Complications: As a result of pliability of the child's airway soft tissues, *excessive* neck flexion (Figure 24-4A) or extension (Figure 24-4B) may result in further airway compromise.

The "sniffing position" may result in an aggravated spinal cord injury in the patient with an unstable cervical spine injury (Figure 24-5).

B. Management of an Obstructed Airway Due to a Foreign Body in Infants Under 1 Year of Age

1. Purpose: These maneuvers are used to remove a foreign body lodged in the oropharynx or glottis and restore a patent airway.

2. Selection of Patients:

a. Indications: This procedure is reserved for the infant less than 1 year of age with a witnessed or strongly suspected aspirated foreign body resulting in airway embarrassment. Before performing this procedure, proper head and neck positioning should be attempted and followed by assisted ventilation (See page 327). If assisted ventilation is unsuccessful because of a totally or partially occluded upper airway, then proceed with these obstructed airway procedures.

b. Contraindications and Precautions: For children older than 1 year the procedures differ somewhat. (See Management of an Obstructed Airway Due to a Foreign Body in Children Older Than 1 Year of Age, page 310).

3. Equipment and Supplies (See Appendix for equipment and supplies manufacturers and suppliers. Appendix is keyed to italicized words in the equipment and supplies lists):

· *Suction* machine (wall-mounted or portable)

· Assorted suction *catheters* (Yankauer and flexible) (Figure 24-6)

· Laryngoscope *handle* and assorted *blades* (Figure 24-7)

· Magill *forceps* (child) (Figure 24-8)

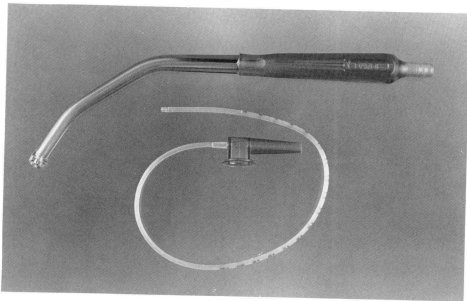

Figure 24-6.
Airway management procedures: Management of an obstructed airway due to a foreign body in infants under 1 year of age. Equipment and supplies: **A,** Yankauer suction catheter; **B,** Flexible suction catheter.

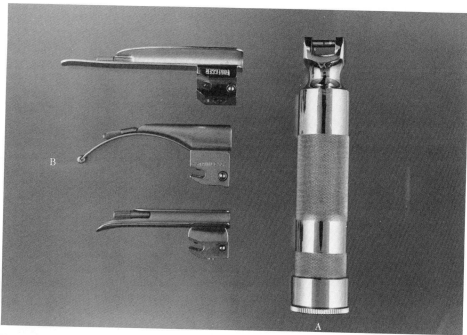

Figure 24-7.
Airway management procedures: Management of an obstructed airway due to a foreign body in infants under 1 year of age. Equipment and supplies: **A,** Laryngoscope handle; **B,** Laryngoscope blades (1. Miller, for older child, 2. MacIntosh, 3. Miller, for younger child or infant).

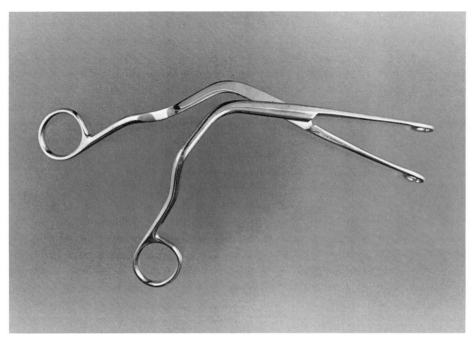

Figure 24-8.
Airway management procedures: Management of an obstructed airway due to a foreign body in infants under 1 year of age. Equipment and supplies: Magill forceps.

4. Description of Procedure:

If the choking infant can breathe and is able to cough, allow the infant to cough without interference. The child's natural cough mechanism is more effective at foreign body retrieval than extraneous measures of assistance.

If the infant is not breathing and cannot cough, reposition the head and neck.

Assist ventilations (See page 327); if unsuccessful:
  • Support the head in a head-down and prone position and administer four sharp back blows with the heel of your palm directed toward the infant's midthoracic spine (Figure 24-9).
  • If a foreign body is visualized, remove it manually. If no foreign body is visible, do not perform a "blind finger sweep."

Reattempt assisted ventilation; if unsuccessful:
  • Support the head in head-down and supine position and administer four chest thrusts (Figure 24-10).
  • If a foreign body is visualized, remove it manually. Do not perform a "blind finger sweep."

Reattempt assisted ventilation; if unsuccessful:
  • Use direct laryngoscopy in an attempt to retrieve the foreign body with the Magill forceps (Figure 24-11). (See Orotracheal Intubation, page 317).

  • If you are successful in removing the foreign body, suction secretions and assist with ventilations using 100% oxygen.
  • If you are unsuccessful in removing the foreign body, consider a needle cricothyroidotomy (See Needle Cricothyroidotomy, page 321).

5. Side Effects and Complications: To prevent displacement of the foreign body more distally into the trachea, insure that the head is directed downward when performing back blows or chest thrusts.

C. Management of an Obstructed Airway Due to a Foreign Body in Children Older than 1 Year of Age

1. Purpose: These maneuvers are used to remove a foreign body and restore the patient's airway.

2. Selection of Patients:

a. Indications: This procedure is reserved for the child older than 1 year of age or the adolescent with a witnessed or strongly suspected aspirated foreign body that is resulting in airway embarrassment. Before performing this procedure, proper head and neck positioning should be attempted, followed by assisted ventilation. If assisted ventilation is unsuc-

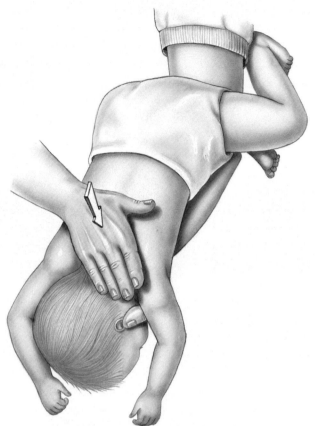

Figure 24-9.
Airway management procedures: Management of an obstructed airway due to a foreign body in infants under 1 year of age—Back blows. Technique.

cessful because of a totally or partially occluded upper airway, then proceed with these obstructed airway procedures.
b. Contraindications and Precautions: The Heimlich maneuver should not be performed on victims of near drowning unless an aspirated solid foreign body is strongly implicated as a precipitating factor in the near drowning.
3. Equipment and Supplies (See Appendix for equipment and supplies manufacturers and suppliers. Appendix is keyed to italicized words in the equipment and supplies lists):
  · *Suction* machine (wall-mounted or portable)
  · Assorted suction *catheters* (Yankauer and flexible) (See Figure 24-6, page 309)
  · Laryngoscope *handle* and assorted *blades* (See Figure 24-7, page 309)
  · Magill *forceps* (child and adult) (See Figure 24-8, page 310)

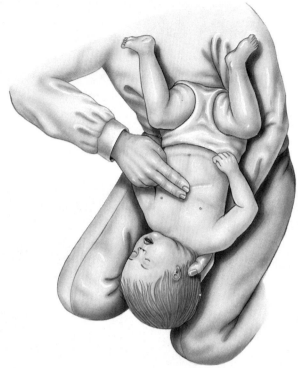

Figure 24-10.
Airway management procedures: Management of an obstructed airway due to a foreign body in infants under 1 year of age—Chest thrusts. Technique.

4. Description of Procedure:
  · If the choking child can breathe and is able to speak or cough, allow the child to cough without interference. The child's natural cough mechanism is more effective at foreign body retrieval than extraneous measures of assistance.
  · If the child is not breathing and cannot speak or cough, reposition the child's head and neck (See Figures 24-1, 24-2, and 24-3, pages 306 and 307).
  · Assist ventilations; if unsuccessful, perform the Heimlich maneuver for the *conscious* child:
    — Position yourself behind the child.
    — Wrap both of your arms around the child's waist (Figure 24-12).
    — Make a fist with one hand, and place the thumb side against the child's abdomen in the midline slightly above the navel.
    — Grasp the fist with your other hand.
    — Press into the child's abdomen with quick, distinct, and sharp upward thrusts.
    — Repeat until the foreign body is expelled or until

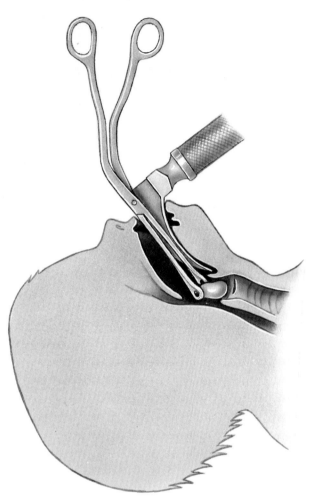

Figure 24-11.
Airway management procedures: Management of an obstructed airway due to a foreign body in infants under 1 year of age—Removal of the foreign body with Magill forceps. Technique.

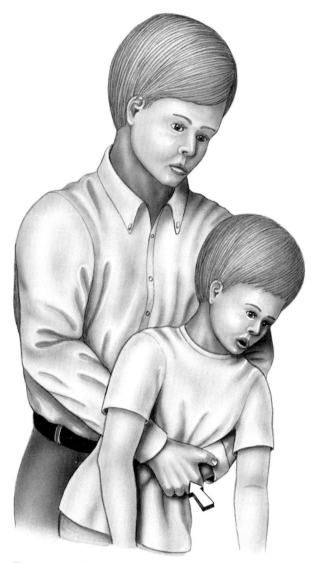

Figure 24-12.
Airway management procedures: Management of an obstructed airway due to a foreign body in children older than 1 year of age—Heimlich maneuver for the *conscious* child. Technique.

the victim becomes unconscious. If the child becomes unconscious, place the child supine on the ground and proceed with the Heimlich maneuver for the *unconscious* child:

(a) Kneel astride the victim's thighs and place the heel of one hand over the midline abdomen between the umbilicus and xiphoid (Figure 24-13). Place your second hand on top of the first.

(b) Press into the abdomen with quick, upward (cephalad-directed) thrusts.

(c) Repeat for 6 to 10 thrusts.

— If the Heimlich maneuvers are not successful in expelling the foreign body, repeat the maneuvers until

the foreign body is expelled. If repeated Heimlich maneuvers fail to restore the airway, consider an emergency cricothyroidotomy (See Needle Cricothyroidotomy, page 321).

— If the Heimlich maneuver is successful in expelling the foreign body, reattempt ventilations.

— If assisted ventilations are successful:

(a) Suction secretions.

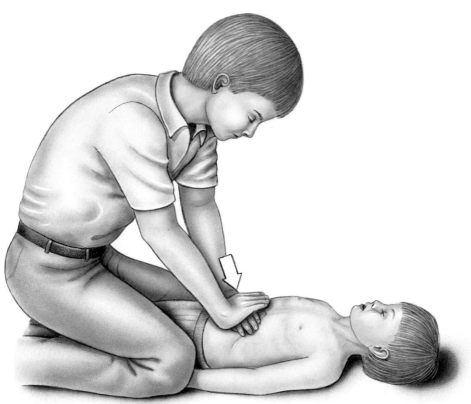

Figure 24-13.
Airway management procedures: Management of an obstructed airway due to a foreign body in children older than 1 year of age—Heimlich maneuver for the *unconscious* **child.** Technique.

(b) Provide 100% oxygen and assist ventilations as necessary.

— If ventilations are unsuccessful:

(a) Properly reposition the child's head and neck.

(b) Repeat the Heimlich procedures.

(c) Consider an emergency cricothyroidotomy (See Needle Cricothyroidotomy, page 321 and Surgical Cricothyroidotomy, page 323).

5. Side Effects and Complications: These procedures are advisable only if aspiration of a foreign body is witnessed or strongly suggested. Airway obstruction due to infection (epiglottitis, croup) or due to angioedema may be worsened by these procedures (back blows or the Heimlich maneuver).

D. Suctioning Procedures

1. Purpose: Suctioning removes accumulated or improperly mobilized secretions to optimize the patient's airway. These secretions may include saliva, mucous, sputum, blood, or vomitus.

2. Selection of Patients:

a. Indications: A child of any age may demonstrate a significant degree of dyspnea or stridor due to oropharyngeal or nasopharyngeal secretions. A characteristic gurgling or rattling sound will occur. Such secretions should be suctioned when present. Be prepared to suction the child with an inadequate cough or gag reflex due to trauma, central nervous system depression, or inadequate pulmonary toilet due to acute or chronic illnesses.

b. Contraindications and Precautions: Be cautious about nasopharyngeal suctioning in cases of *severe* maxillofacial trauma. There are reported cases of intracranial placement of nasogastric tubes and nasopharyngeal suction catheters in such situations. Hemorrhage from the nose may occur if the flexible catheter causes lacerations or abrasions to the inferior turbinate or adenoids. Familiarize yourself with the anatomy of the turbinates so as to ease passage of the catheter tip into the nasopharynx.

3. Equipment and Supplies (See Appendix for equipment

and supplies manufacturers and suppliers. Appendix is keyed to italicized words in the equipment and supplies lists):

- Wall-mounted suction apparatus (preferred) or portable *suction* machine with suction *tubing*
- Sterile water
- Yankauer suction *catheter* (used for vomitus or thick or tenacious secretions) (See Figure 24-6, page 309)
- Flexible *catheters* (sizes 6, 8, 10, 12, and 14 French) (for mucous, blood or saliva) (See Figure 24-6, page 309)

4. Description of Procedure:

- Attach a suction catheter (Yankauer or flexible catheter) of choice to the wall-mounted or portable suction unit. Use a Yankauer suction catheter for vomitus and particularly tenacious or globular material, such as oropharyngeal blood clots. The Yankauer suction catheter is exclusively for oropharyngeal suctioning. With the suction unit "on," insert the Yankauer suction catheter well into the child's oropharynx and remove all the material. Cleanse the suction catheter by inserting it into a cup of sterile water.
- If a flexible suction catheter is used, lubricate the flexible catheter by rinsing in sterile water. Insert the tip of the flexible suction catheter into the sterile water and occlude the side part with your fingertip for a few sec-

onds. The suction action will be initiated. Release the side part to discontinue suction action.

- Insert the catheter into the patient's mouth and oropharynx with the suction action "off." When the catheter tip is correctly positioned in the posterior oropharynx, activate suction by occluding the side port with your finger. Withdraw the catheter slowly over a period of 3 to 5 seconds with the suction activated.
- Rinse the catheter as noted above. Repeat oropharyngeal suctioning as needed and rinse the catheter after each suctioning pass.
- Insert the catheter into each nares and gently advance it to the posterior nasopharynx. Be sure to advance the catheter tip between the inferior turbinate and the floor of the nose. Activate the suction action and slowly withdraw the catheter over a period of 3 to 5 seconds.
- Rinse the catheter in sterile water as mentioned above. Repeat the suctioning as indicated.

5. Side Effects and Complications: Hemorrhage is the most common complication.

E. Insertion of a Nasopharyngeal Airway

1. Purpose: This is an excellent way to maintain a patent airway in a patient who is semiconscious or who has a partial

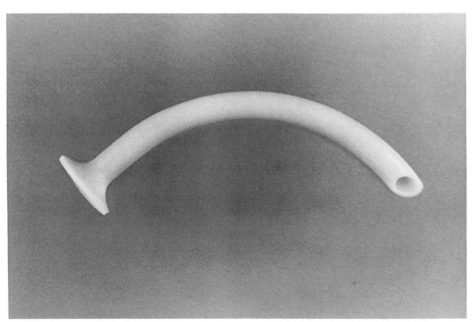

Figure 24-14.
Airway management procedures: Insertion of a nasopharyngeal airway.
Equipment and supplies: Nasopharyngeal airway.

gag reflex, or in a patient who cannot or will not tolerate an oropharyngeal airway.

2. Selection of Patients:

a. Indications: The child should be older than 2 to 3 years of age and have a need for a protected airway, but should have a partially intact gag reflex. A nasopharyngeal airway is often used in the case of a child who cannot or will not tolerate an oropharyngeal airway, but who is in need of airway assistance.

b. Contraindications and Precautions: A nasopharyngeal airway should not be used in the child less than 2 years of age or in the child with massive maxillofacial trauma. In such cases, a possible intracranial placement of the nasopharyngeal airway through a cribriform plate fracture could lead to devastating sequelae.

3. Equipment and Supplies (See Appendix for equipment and supplies manufacturers and suppliers. Appendix is keyed to italicized words in the equipment and supplies lists):

· Nasopharyngeal *airway* (Figure 24-14)
· Water-soluble *lubricant*

4. Description of Procedure:

· Select a proper size nasopharyngeal airway. The diameter of the airway should be sized according to the internal diameter of the nares. The length should be estimated by placing the airway on the side of the patient's face (Figure 24-15). The flange should be at the nares, while the tip of the airway should align itself with the angle of the mandible. In this way, the airway tip will reside behind the tongue when it is properly placed.

· Lubricate the nasopharyngeal airway with lubricant.

· With a slight gentle twisting motion, insert the nasopharyngeal airway into the nose beneath the inferior turbinate until the flange rests against the nares (Figure 24-16).

5. Side Effects and Complications: The passage of the nasopharyngeal airway may abrade the turbinates, nasal mucosa, or adenoids, resulting in minor epistaxis, which usually can be managed with suction.

If the nasopharyngeal airway is too short, the tongue may fall against the oropharynx and obstruct the airway.

The nasopharyngeal airway that is too long may induce gagging or wretching.

F. Insertion of an Oropharyngeal Airway

1. Purpose: The oropharyngeal airway is used in the patient without a gag reflex to lift the mandibular block of soft tissues

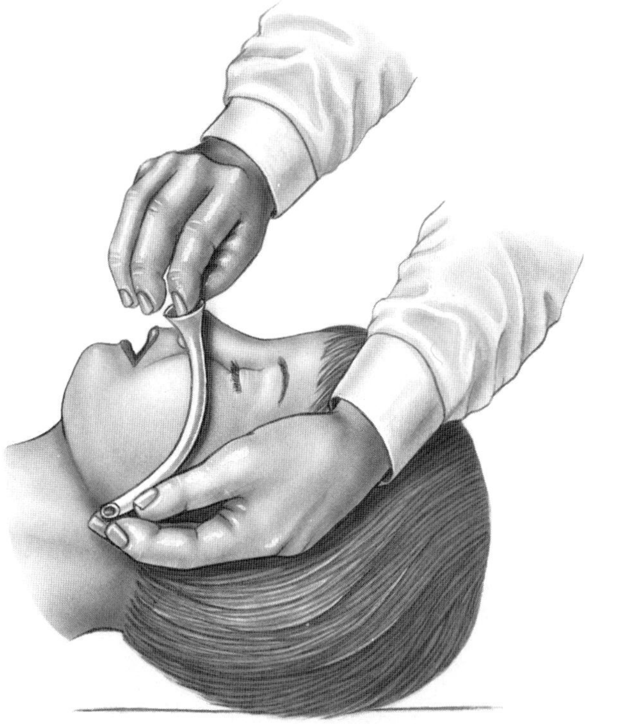

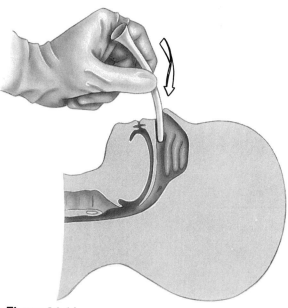

Figure 24-15.
Airway management procedures: Insertion of a nasopharyngeal airway—Estimation of appropriate length of airway. Technique.

Figure 24-16.
Airway management procedures: Insertion of a nasopharyngeal airway. Technique for insertion.

away from the posterior pharyngeal wall. This procedure should provide an adequate upper airway. Additionally, this device provides a "teeth-block" to prevent biting of oral soft tissues, orotracheal tubes, or suction catheters.

2. Selection of Patients:

a. Indications: The oropharyngeal airway can be used in any aged child as long as a properly fitting airway is available. The primary indication for its use is the need for upper airway assistance as evidenced by sonorous inspiratory stridor or gurgling sounds. It may also be used as a "teeth-block" for a patient with seizures, with an orotracheal tube in place, or requiring frequent oral suctioning. The patient should have an absent gag reflex.

b. Contraindications and Precautions: The oropharyngeal airway should not be used in an awake patient who has an intact gag reflex. The patient will likely vomit. An improperly sized oropharyngeal airway can create worse upper airway obstruction than existed previously.

3. Equipment and Supplies (See Appendix for equipment and supplies manufacturers and suppliers. Appendix is keyed to italicized words in the equipment and supplies lists):

- Tongue *blade* (Figure 24-17)
- Oropharyngeal *airways* (Figure 24-17)

4. Description of Procedure:
- Select a proper size oropharyngeal airway. An oropharyngeal airway is sized by comparing the airway with the distance from the mouth to the angle of the mandible (Figure 24-18).
- The preferred method for insertion in a *young child* involves the use of a tongue blade to depress and anteriorly displace the tongue away from the posterior pharyngeal wall (Figure 24-19).
- Then insert the oropharyngeal airway "right side up" so that the curvature of the device conforms to the curve of the tongue.
- Advance the airway completely until the flange or "bite block" rests against the incisors.
- Withdraw the tongue blade.
- The airway should maintain its proper position.
- An alternative method for the *older child* or adolescent may eliminate the need for a tongue blade:
  — Place the airway in the child's mouth "upside down" so that the curvature of the device is opposite to the natural curve of the tongue.
  — Advance the airway until it is about two thirds of the way in, then rotate the airway 180 degrees and

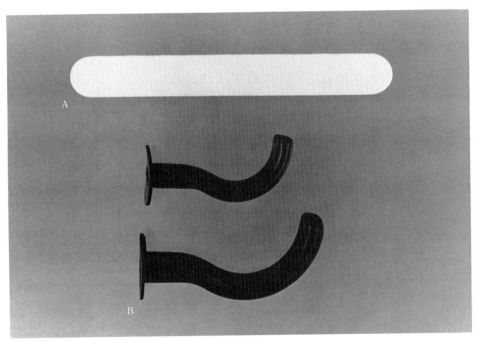

Figure 24-17.
Airway management procedures: Insertion of an oropharyngeal airway.
Equipment and supplies: **A,** Tongue depressor; **B,** Oropharyngeal airways.

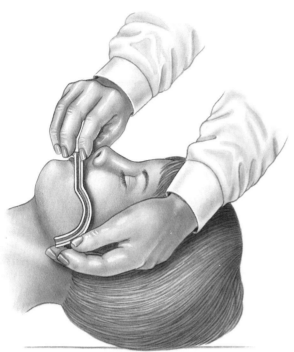

Figure 24-18.
Airway management procedures: Insertion of an oropharyngeal airway—Estimation of appropriate length of airway. Technique.

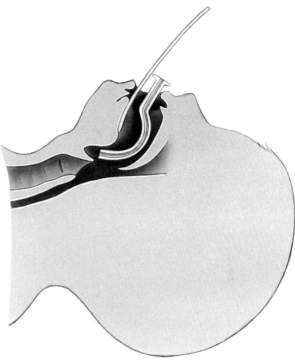

Figure 24-19.
Airway management procedures: Insertion of an oropharyngeal airway. Technique for insertion in a young child.

continue to advance it until the flange (or "bite block") rests against the incisors.

5. Side Effects and Complications: Improper placement of the oropharyngeal airway may result in "pinching" of the tongue against the posterior pharynx, thus further occluding the patient's airway.

Laryngospasm may result if the tip of the oropharyngeal airway presses against the larynx itself. Proper sizing before insertion should prevent this complication.

Lacerations or abrasions to the oral mucosa and tongue or broken teeth may result from overly aggressive or careless insertion. The preferred method, using the tongue depressor, should help prevent these complications.

The child with an intact gag reflex may not tolerate an oropharyngeal airway, because of gagging and vomiting. In such cases, consider placing a nasopharyngeal airway (See page 314).

G. Orotracheal Intubation—the Definitive Airway

1. Purpose: Orotracheal intubation is the definitive method of securing the airway of a child, adolescent, or adult.

2. Selection of Patients:

a. Indications: Orotracheal intubation is indicated in any aged patient who is in need of a secure airway. The patient's airway may have been compromised as a result of

- Trauma;
- Central nervous system depression;
- The actual or imminent aspiration of vomitus, blood or other secretions; or
- Supraglottic and glottic edema resulting from angioedema or infection (e.g., epiglottitis, croup).

Additionally, a child in need of mechanical assisted ventilation (cardiopulmonary resuscitation or respiratory failure with hypoxemia) will require intubation.

b. Contraindications and Precautions: It may be necessary to avoid orotracheal intubation in cases of potentially unstable cervical spine injury. In such situations, strict neutrality of the cervical spine is essential. Maintaining cervical neutrality is difficult during orotracheal intubation, and requires an assistant for this role in addition to the laryngoscope operator. Alternatives include nasotracheal intubation, needle cricothyroidotomy, or surgical cricothyroidotomy.

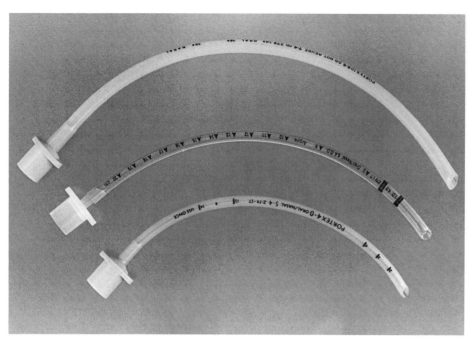

Figure 24-20.
Airway management procedures: Orotracheal intubation. Equipment and supplies:
Uncuffed orotracheal or endotracheal tubes.

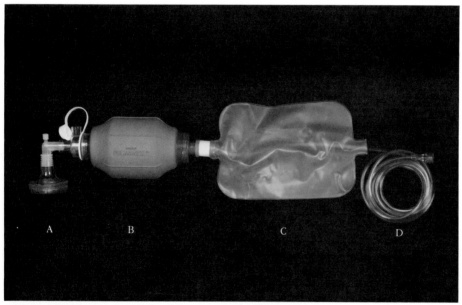

Figure 24-21.
Airway management procedures: Orotracheal intubation. Equipment and supplies:
A, Face mask; **B,** Ventilator bag; **C,** Reservoir bag; **D,** Oxygen tubing.

3. Equipment and Supplies (See Appendix for equipment and supplies manufacturers and suppliers. Appendix is keyed to italicized words in the equipment and supplies lists):
- Laryngoscope *handle* (See Figure 24-7, page 309) (extra batteries and extra light bulbs should be immediately accessible)
- Laryngoscope *blades* (See Figure 24-7, page 309). Become familiar with one style of blade (preferably Miller) and a few sizes.
- Uncuffed orotracheal or endotracheal *tubes* (Figure 24-20)
- *Stylet* (rarely necessary but can be used if desired)
- Oxygen source
- Oxygen administration *tubing* and ventilator *bag* with oxygen reservoir, for oxygenation and assisted ventilation before insertion of an endotracheal tube (Figure 24-21)
- *Suction* machine (wall-mounted or portable)
- Suction device (Yankauer and flexible *catheters*) (See Figure 24-6, page 309)
- 1-inch *tape*
- Stethoscope

4. Description of Procedure:
- Do not perform this procedure precipitously. Make sure all equipment and personnel are ready.
- Preoxygenate the patient with 100% oxygen and assist with ventilations if necessary for at least 1 to 3 minutes or until cyanosis clears (See Breathing, Oxygen Administration, page xxxx).
- Select an appropriate size endotracheal tube according to the formula:

$$\frac{\text{Age (years)} + 16}{4}$$

Have available one endotracheal tube of the calculated size plus one smaller and one larger.
- Insure a functional light source and the availability of all equipment, including suction.
- Tape should be cut to appropriate sizes (See Taping/Securing an Endotracheal Tube, page 321).
- Position the patient in a "sniffing position."
- Stand at the patient's head.
- Hold the handle of the laryngoscope with your left hand. Attach the appropriate sized laryngoscope blade (Miller blade preferred) to the handle.
- Open the mouth of the patient with the thumb and index finger of your right hand using the "scissors movement" (Figure 24-22).
- Insert the blade of the laryngoscope into the right side of the mouth; and, as the laryngoscope blade is advanced toward the glottis, sweep the tongue toward the left out

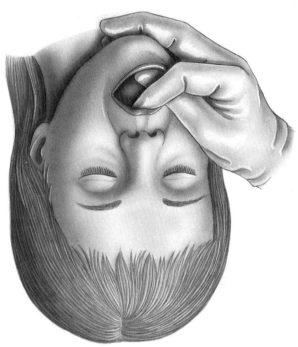

Figure 24-22.
Airway management procedures: Orotracheal intubation—"scissors movement." Technique.

of the field of vision (Figure 24-23A). The tip of the smaller Miller blade has a gentle curve (See Figure 24-7C, page 309). Many operators find it useful to take advantage of this gentle curve in placing the blade tip in the vallecula when intubating children younger than 1 year of age. In doing so, the blade tip is being used in a manner similar to the curved (or MacIntosh) blade. In children older than 1 year of age, however, the tip of the Miller blade is optimally placed *under* the epiglottis. In this way, the blade tip directly lifts the epiglottis up and away from the view of the true vocal cords.
- Elevate the mandibular tissue block by exerting force along the axis of the laryngoscope handle (Figure 24-23B). Do not use the alveolar ridge or teeth as a fulcrum or lever to assist in laryngeal visualization.
- Observe the anatomy of the airway as the blade tip is advanced. Locate the epiglottis, vallecula, arytenoids, esophagus, and the true cords (Figure 24-23C). Identification of the airway anatomy in a systematic fashion will help you avoid getting "lost" and will reduce the chances of malintubation.
- An assistant may provide cricoid pressure by applying gentle pressure on the cricoid cartilage with the thumb

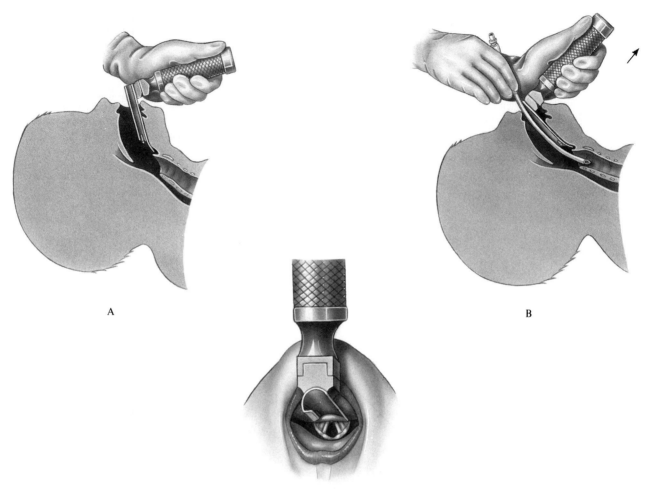

Figure 24-23.
Airway management procedures: Orotracheal intubation. A, Technique for
insertion of the laryngoscope blade (in a patient less than 1 year of age); **B,** Technique
for elevating the mandibular tissue block; **C,** Technique for visualizing the epiglottis,
vallecula, arytenoids, and true cords.

and index finger (Selleck maneuver). This maneuver
may assist with visualization and will reduce the chance
of emesis and aspiration.

· With the right hand, pass the endotracheal tube
through the true cords (glottis) and advance the tube
into the trachea approximately 2 to 3 cm. Watch the tube
as it passes through the cords. Some endotracheal tubes
have a marker on the tube that, when passed to the level
of the cords, will ensure proper positioning.

· Attach the endotracheal tube adaptor to the ventilator
source (See Breathing, Assisted Ventilation, page 327),
such as a bag–valve apparatus.

· Provide a series of assisted breaths.

· Auscult the breath sounds over both anterior chest
walls, over both axillae, and over the stomach.

· If the endotracheal tube position is satisfactory by
auscultation, tape the tube into secure position (See
Taping/Securing an Endotracheal Tube, page 321) and
continue to assist with ventilations as needed.

· Confirm the endotracheal tube position with an anteroposterior chest radiograph when possible. The endotracheal tube tip should be located at the second
thoracic vertebra.

5. Side Effects and Complications:

a. Hypoxemia—Preoxygenate with 100% oxygen for at least
1 to 3 minutes or until cyanosis clears. Limit any single intu-

bation attempt to 30 seconds from the last assisted breath to the first breath with the endotracheal tube.

b. Broken teeth—Avoid using the teeth and the alveolar ridge as a fulcrum to facilitate visualization of laryngeal structures. Elevate the mandibular tissue block by exerting force along the axis of the laryngoscope *handle*.

c. Aspiration of vomitus—The risk can be minimized by having ready suction available and by having an assistant provide cricoid pressure to occlude the esophagus.

d. Esophageal placement of the endotracheal tube—Observe the endotracheal tube as it passes through the glottis. Avoid blindly inserting the tube. Listen for adequate breath sounds as the appropriate locations over the chest, axillae, and stomach. Remember that an endotracheal tube placed in the esophagus may offer a transmitted gurgling sound when the "breath sounds" are auscultated over the chest. Be sure you are hearing true breath sounds rather than sounds from the esophagus or stomach. Confirm the endotracheal tube position with an anteroposterior chest radiograph.

e. Malposition of an endotracheal within the trachea—Take care not to advance the endotracheal tube too far once it passes the glottis (2–3 cm for small child or 3–5 for a teenager). Listen for equal and true breath sounds. Confirm the position of the endotracheal tube (tip at the body of the second thoracic vertebra) by an anteroposterior chest radiograph.

f. Accidental extubation—Take caution in moving your patient from one location to another. Securely tape the endotracheal tube in place (See Taping/Securing Endotracheal Tubes, below).

g. Biting of the endotracheal tube by the patient—Use an appropriate sized oropharyngeal airway as a teethblock.

H. Taping/Securing an Endotracheal Tube

1. Purpose: Once placed, the endotracheal tube must be securely taped to maintain its original position. Accidental extubation or inadvertent advancement of the tube to a bronchial position can be avoided by properly securing the tube.

2. Selection of Patients:

a. Indications: The patient with an endotracheal tube in place requires securing of the tube.

b. Contraindications and Precautions: None

3. Equipment and Supplies (See Appendix for equipment and supplies manufacturers and suppliers. Appendix is keyed to italicized words in the equipment and supplies lists):

- 1-inch cloth *tape*
- Tincture of *benzoin*

4. Description of Procedure:

- Cut two 8- to 12-cm (depending on the patient's size) pieces of tape.
- Tear one end of each piece of tape down the center of its length to a point midway between its ends (Figure 24-24A).

- Dry any mucous or secretions from the lips and face.
- Apply tincture of benzoin to both cheeks and the upper lip.
- Bring the endotracheal tube over to one side of the mouth to enhance its stability.
- Note the centimeter marker indicated on the endotracheal tube at the level of the lips.
- Apply the tape as illustrated (Figure 24-24B and C). Starting on the side of the cheek nearest the endotracheal tube, fix the wider (uncut) end of the tape onto the skin of the cheek to which benzoin has been applied. Position the tape so that the upper of the two lengthwise-cut "tails" will be applied across the upper lip and so that the crux between the two "tails" lines up adjacent to the endotracheal tube at the corner of the mouth. In a spiral fashion, wrap the lower "tail" around the endotracheal tube, maximizing the amount of tape in contact with the endotracheal tube, thus reducing chances of slippage. Apply the second piece of tape to the other cheek, upper lip, and endotracheal tube in a mirror-reverse fashion.
- Auscult again over the chest, both axillae, and stomach to insure proper tube position.

5. Side Effects and Complications: Accidental extubation or malpositioning of the endotracheal tube may occur during the taping sequence. Reassess the tube's position after the tube has been secured with tape.

I. Needle Cricothyroidotomy with Jet Insufflation Technique for Assisted Ventilation

1. Purpose: This nearly "last resort" technique may be used to provide a temporary airway. It can provide oxygenation and assisted ventilation for up to 30 to 45 minutes until a more definitive airway (e.g., endotracheal tube, surgical tracheostomy) can be secured.

2. Selection of Patients:

a. Indications: This technique can be used in children less than 12 years of age. It is potentially useful when conditions such as edema of the glottis (angioedema, epiglottitis), laryngeal foreign body, laryngeal fracture, or severe oropharyngeal hemorrhage make orotracheal intubation impossible.

b. Contraindications and Precautions: In children greater than 12 years of age, a surgical cricothyroidotomy would be preferable to the needle cricothyroidotomy (See Surgical Cricothyroidotomy, page 323). A needle cricothyroidotomy should *not* be used in children for whom an adequate nonsurgical airway can be achieved.

(1) The child can only be adequately oxygenated and ventilated by this technique for 30 to 45 minutes. Hypercarbia is inevitable, as complete exhalation is inadequate. The ensuing acidosis will eventually become problematic.

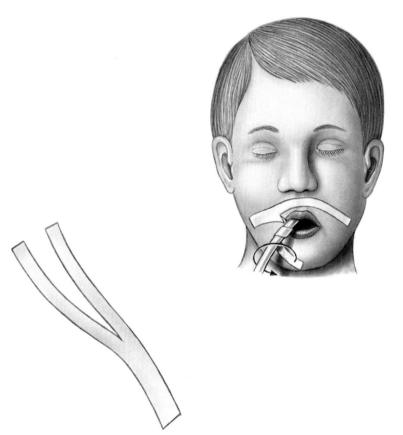
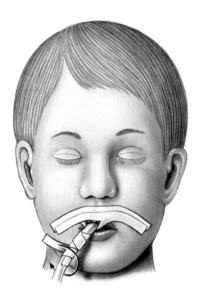

Figure 24-24.
Airway management procedures: Orotracheal intubation. Technique for taping an
endotracheal tube in place.

(2) Be alert to the possibility of pneumothorax or other air leak due to the increased intrathoracic pressures.

3. Equipment and Supplies (See Appendix for equipment and supplies manufacturers and suppliers. Appendix is keyed to italicized words in the equipment and supplies lists):

· 14-gauge plastic *cannula* over a steel needle
· Intravenous connector *tubing,* cut to a length of 3 to 4 inches (including the male adapter)
· Oxygen tubing with a "whistle hole" out in the side near the end
· Wall oxygen source
· 1-inch cloth *tape*

4. Description of Procedure:

· Insert the 14-gauge "angiocath" through the child's cricothyroid membrane into the trachea. If possible, insert the plastic cannula into the trachea distal to any airway obstruction that may be present. A foreign body

obstructing the airway may be dislodged by the increased intrathoracic pressures resulting from this technique. If this occurs, remove the foreign body, suction secretions, and endotracheally intubate the patient as soon as possible. Hyperventilate the patient using the endotracheal tube to correct any preexisting hypercarbia. If endotracheal intubation is successful, remove the plastic cricothyroidotomy cannula.

· Once the plastic cannula is within the trachea lumen, remove the steel stylet and advance the plastic cannula toward the carina.

· Care must be taken to insure proper positioning of the plastic cannula and to avoid leaking of the cannula. Maintenance of the proper position should be done by hand. Do not attempt to tape the cricothyroidotomy cannula to the neck.

· Connect the plastic cannula to a 3- to 4-inch piece of

intravenous connector tubing. The male adapter of the tubing will insert into the hub of the plastic cannula.

· Firmly lodge the cut end of the intravenous connector tubing into the end of the oxygen tubing nearest the "whistle hole." Seal the junction with 1-inch cloth tape.

· Attach the other end of the oxygen tubing to the wall oxygen source. Turn on the wall oxygen source to provide a flow of 15 liters per minute.

· Provide intermittent ventilation by alternately occluding and releasing the "whistle hole" in the side of the oxygen tubing with your index finger. Occlude for 1 second (inspiration), then release for 4 seconds (expiration). Repeat this rhythmic process to ventilate and oxygenate the patient.

· Immediately arrange for a more definitive airway.

5. Side Effects and Complications: Hypercarbia and respiratory acidosis are inevitable.

Tracheobronchial air leak (subcutaneous emphysema, pneumomediastinum, pneumopericardium, pneumothorax) may result from excessive ventilatory pressures.

Laceration of the cricothyroid cartilage may result from the cannula insertion.

Hemorrhage or hemoptysis can occur around the incision site or at a point where the cannula traumatizes the tracheal mucosa.

Kinking of the cricothyroidotomy cannula may result in further compromise of air exchange.

An air leak in the intravenous connector tubing–oxygen tubing system may result in inadequate oxygenation and ventilation.

J. Surgical Cricothyroidotomy

1. Purpose: Surgical cricothyroidotomy is a technique used to provide a secure airway for a patient older than 12 years of age in whom endotracheal intubation is not possible.

2. Selection of Patients:

a. Indications: Candidates for the procedure are children older than 12 years of age who cannot be orotracheally intubated because of edema of the glottis (angioedema, epiglottitis), an irretrievable foreign body in the glottis, a laryngeal fracture, severe oropharyngeal hemorrhage, or severe maxillofacial trauma in the setting of a potentially unstable cervical spine injury.

b. Contraindications and Precautions: Children who are less than 12 years of age do not yet have fully developed cricothyroid cartilage and may suffer permanent tracheal damage from this procedure. Children in this age group should undergo temporary needle cricothyroidotomy (See page 321) instead of surgical cricothyroidotomy.

Surgical cricothyroidotomy should *not* be used in children

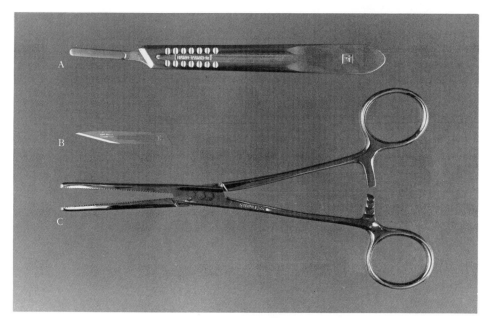

Figure 24-25.
Airway management procedures: Surgical cricothyroidotomy. Equipment and supplies: **A,** Scalpel handle; **B,** No. 11 scalpel blade; **C,** Curved hemostat.

in whom an adequate nonsurgical airway can be achieved, using any of the previously described techniques (except needle cricothyroidotomy).

3. Equipment and Supplies (See Appendix for equipment and supplies manufacturers and suppliers. Appendix is keyed to italicized words in the equipment and supplies lists):

· No. 11 scalpel *blade,* with or without a *handle* (Figure 24-25)

· Curved *hemostat* (Figure 24-25)

· Tracheostomy cannula (5.0–7.0-mm internal diameter (See Figure 24-36, page 332)

· Orotracheal *tube* (5.0–7.0) (See Figure 24-20, page 318)

4. Description of Procedure:

· Using a no. 11 scalpel blade, make a "stab"-like puncture incision through the skin and the underlying cricothyroid membrane (Figure 24-26A). The width of the incision should approximate the width of the widest part

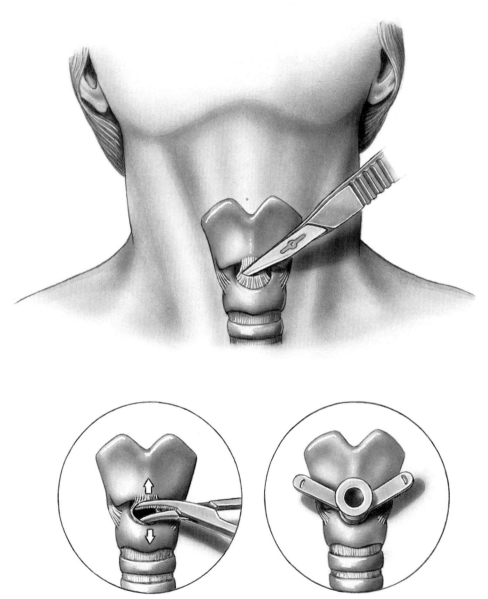

Figure 24-26.
Airway management procedures: Surgical cricothyroidotomy. Technique.

of the scalpel blade. Too wide an incision may cause hemorrhage, result in an unacceptable air leak, and impair stabilization of the tube.

· With the curved hemostat, dilate the incision opening just enough to accommodate the orotracheal tube selected (Figure 24-26B).

· Insert the tracheostomy cannula or orotracheal tube into the opening and direct the tube to its proper position (Figure 24-26C). The tip of the tube should rest in the midtrachea well above the carina.

· If an orotracheal tube is used, obtain an anteroposterior radiograph of the chest to confirm proper tube placement.

5. Side Effects and Complications: Malposition of the orotracheal tube can easily occur.

Damage to the cricothyroid cartilage may result from overly aggressive extension of the incision.

Hemorrhage from the incision site is usually minimal, but excessive hemorrhage into the airway can compromise ventilation.

II. Breathing

A. Oxygen Administration

1. Purpose: Supplemental oxygen is a necessity in cardiopulmonary resuscitation (CPR); other cases of hypoxemia and dyspnea may also require supplemental oxygen.

2. Selection of Patients:

a. Indications: Children requiring CPR must be given supplemental oxygen at the highest concentration available. Patients with dyspnea from a wide range of causes will benefit from supplemental oxygen. Oxygen is indicated for nearly all cases of major trauma and traumatic shock.

b. Contraindications and precautions: Certain patients with chronic obstructive pulmonary diseases (such as cystic fibrosis, bronchopulmonary dysplasia, and severe asthma) may retain carbon dioxide. As a result, they may theoretically depend on a relative hypoxemia to stimulate spontaneous respirations. The addition of supplemental oxygen to some of these patients *may* result in a loss of respiratory drive or apnea.

3. Equipment and Supplies (See Appendix for equipment and supplies manufacturers and suppliers. Appendix is keyed to italicized words in the equipment and supplies lists):

· Oxygen source
· Nasal *cannulae* (Figure 24-27)
· Masks:
    · Simple face *masks:* used to provide an imprecise 21% to 40% inspired oxygen concentration, depending on the oxygen flow rate
    · Venturi *masks:* used to provide precise oxygen concentrations of 25%, 28%, 32%, or 40%
    · Non-rebreathing *masks:* used to provide up to 100% oxygen concentration
· Oxygen *hoods*

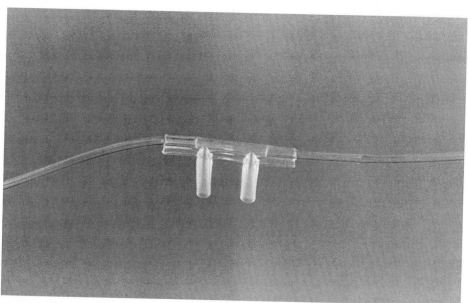

Figure 24-27.
Breathing: Oxygen administration. Equipment and supplies: Nasal cannula.

- Oxygen *tents*
- Oxygen *tubing* (See Figure 24-28, page 318)
- *Oximeter* (for measuring ambient oxygen concentrations within an oxygen hood or oxygen tent)

4. Description of Procedure:
- Nasal cannulae are well tolerated by older children.
   — The two nasal prongs are gently inserted approximately 1 cm into both nares.
   — The cannula tubing is brought around each ear and secured by sliding the plastic cinch ring snugly under the chin.
   — The other end of the nasal cannula tubing is connected to a wall oxygen source or to a portable oxygen cylinder, and the flow is adjusted to meet the needs of the patient.

   — The communicative child may complain of a drying effect on the nasal mucosa. Moisture can be added to the oxygen by bubbling it through sterile water as it leaves the oxygen source.

- A variety of *simple face masks* are available to supply the oxygen concentrations noted above. All are held in place by an elastic strap brought around the head, and are connected to the oxygen source by oxygen tubing. The alert infant or toddler may not tolerate the elastic strap used to hold the mask in place, but may be more cooperative if a parent or assistant holds the mask near the child's face.

- A *Venturi mask* differs from a simple face mask by the presence of a plastic oxygen–air mixture adapter placed between the mask and the oxygen tubing (Figure 24-

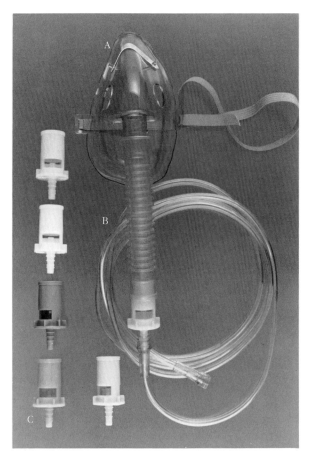

Figure 24-28.
Breathing: Oxygen administration. Equipment and supplies: **A,** Venturi mask; **B,** Oxygen tubing; **C,** Oxygen–air mixture adaptors.

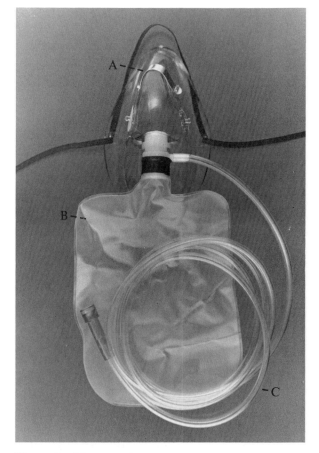

Figure 24-29.
Breathing: Oxygen administration. Equipment and supplies: **A,** Non-rebreathing mask; **B,** Oxygen reservoir; **C,** Oxygen tubing.

28). Four such adapters are available in each Venturi mask set-up. Indicated on each is the flow rate (in liters per minute) necessary to provide a specific oxygen concentration.

· After determining the oxygen concentration needed for your patient, connect the appropriate adapter and adjust the flow rate from the oxygen source.

· *Non-rebreathing masks* are designed to supply oxygen in high concentrations (Figure 24-29). They use an oxygen reservoir bag that must be filled for the mask to be effective, requiring an oxygen flow of 12 to 15 liters per minute.

· Oxygen *hoods and tents* are used less frequently than in the past. Hoods are useful for neonates and small infants. An oximeter is needed to monitor the ambient oxygen concentration. Tents provide a very humid environment, which many clinicians find useful in the management of laryngotracheobronchitis (croup).

5. Side Effects and Complications: Drying of nasal mucosa can occur if adequate moisture is not provided.

Some children feel claustrophobic when a face mask is applied directly to the face.

Sudden hyperoxemia may affect the respiratory drive in some patients with chronic carbon dioxide retention and chronic hypoxia.

B. Assisted Ventilation

1. Purpose: Temporary ventilatory assistance can maintain air exchange when spontaneous respiratory efforts are absent or are functionally inadequate.

2. Selection of Patients:

a. Indications: Assisted ventilation is indicated for patients with cardiopulmonary arrest, apnea, or respiratory failure due to any cause and immediately after endotracheal tube insertion.

b. Contraindications and Precautions: When using any bag–valve mask to assist ventilations in infants, be sure that the third, fourth, and fifth fingers are grasping the patient's mandible and not the submandibular soft tissues. Compressions of the soft tissues could lead to airway obstruction.

3. Equipment and Supplies (See Appendix for equipment and supplies manufacturers and suppliers. Appendix is keyed to italicized words in the equipment and supplies lists):

· Ventilation masks:
  · Fitted *masks* (Figure 24-30)
  · Circular infant *masks* (Figure 24-31)

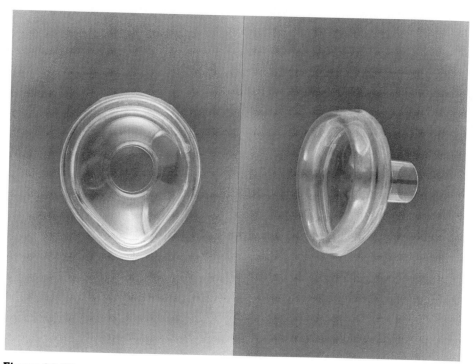

Figure 24-30.
Breathing: Assisted ventilation. Equipment and supplies: Fitted mask (two views).

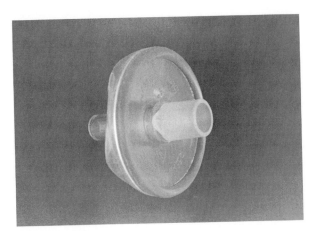

Figure 24-31.
Breathing: Assisted ventilation. Equipment and supplies;
Circular infant mask.

· "Pocket" *masks* (Figure 24-32)
· Ventilator bags:
  · Self-inflation *bags* (preferred) (See Figure 24-21, page 318)

· Anesthesia *bags* (Figure 24-33)
· Oxygen reservoirs (a necessity if oxygen concentrations of greater than 40% to 50% are needed)

4. Description of Procedure:
· Ventilation techniques such as *mouth-to-mouth, mouth-to-nose, mouth-to-mouth and nose, mouth-to-tracheostomy,* or *mouth-to-endotracheal tube* can be used when ventilator equipment is unavailable.
· With the patient in the supine position, open the airway using the techniques previously described in this chapter.
· If the patient is an infant, place your mouth over the patient's nose and mouth (Figure 24-34). If the patient is older, place your mouth over the child's mouth while pinching the nares with one hand so as to prevent escape of air through the nose (Figure 24-35).
· Form a tight seal.
· Offer four quick but gentle breaths.
· Make sure the chest expands (reflecting air entry into the lungs).
· Remove your mouth between breaths and watch, and listen for exhalation.
· Continue to assist breathing at the rate noted in Table 24-1.

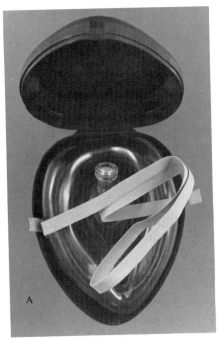

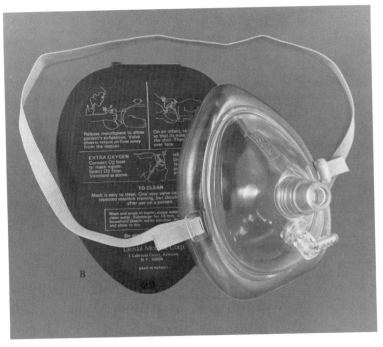

Figure 24-32.
Breathing: Assisted ventilation. Equipment and supplies: "Pocket" mask (**A,** Mask in case, **B,** Mask removed from case and everted for use).

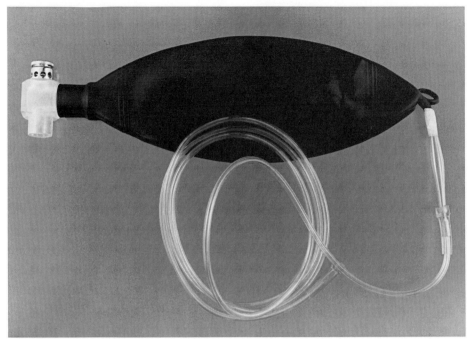

Figure 24-33.
Breathing: Assisted ventilation. Equipment and supplies: Anesthesia bag with oxygen tubing.

- If the child has a tracheostomy or endotracheal tube in place, ventilate through that orifice as noted above.
- *Self-inflating bag–valve–masks* require a reservoir to deliver 100% oxygen. Expertise can only be acquired through practice.
- Position the face mask over the mouth and nose of the patient. Firmly hold the mask in place with the thumb and index finger of your left hand, while using your third, fourth, and fifth fingers to grasp the patient's mandible. In doing so, you simultaneously accomplish a chin lift, stabilization of your hand as well as the patient's face, and a tight seal between the mask and the face.
- Use the right hand to compress the ventilation bag.
- Watch for a symmetric chest rise. Auscult over the anterior chest and both axillae to assure the adequacy of air exchange as well as the symmetry and quality of the breath sounds.
- Ventilation effectiveness may be limited by:
  — The lack of a tight seal between the mask and the child's face.
  — Inadequate head and neck positioning. The child ideally should be maintained in the "sniffing position."
  — An inadequate airway. Use chin lift, jaw thrust, and possibly an oropharyngeal or nasopharyngeal airway to facilitate air exchange.
  — Gastric distention. Offering breaths gently and in a steady, even fashion will reduce the chance of air entry into stomach. Be prepared to decompress the stomach of swallowed air by inserting a nasogastric tube.
- *Anesthesia bag–mask* ventilation requires a high level of experience and expertise. Inflation of the bag is dependent on oxygen flow. The pressure within the bag, which is transmitted to the child's tracheobronchial tree, is adjusted by means of a release valve on the mask casting.
- There are suggested ventilation rates for various age groups (Table 24-1).

5. Side Effects and Complications: Inadequate air exchange may result from a lack of a tight seal between the resuscitator's mouth or the ventilation mask and the patient's face, inadequate head and neck positioning, lack of an oropharyngeal airway or nasopharyngeal airway, and inadequate minute volume due to a low rate of assisted ventilations or inadequate tidal volume.

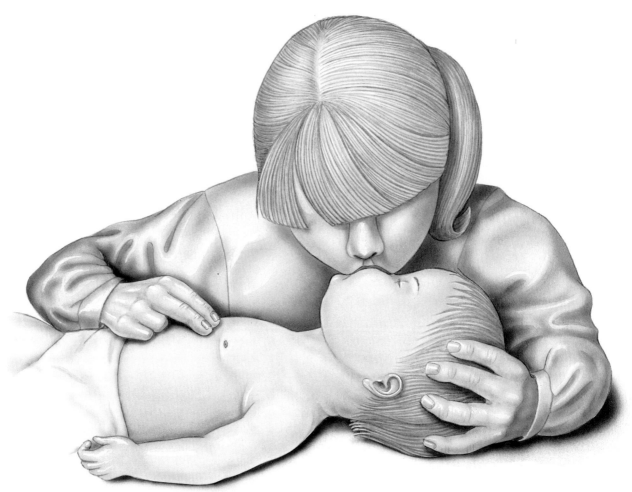

Figure 24-34.
Breathing: Assisted ventilation—Mouth-to-mouth and nose ventilation. Technique.

Introduction of air into the stomach deprives the lungs of needed tidal volume and may distend the stomach, impending diaphragmatic excursion.

Tracheobronchial air leaks (pneumothorax, pneumomediastinum, subcutaneous emphysema) usually result from inappropriately high airway pressures. The pressure within the ventilation bag may be too high or the tidal volume of each assisted breath may be too large.

C. Tracheostomy Care: (Preexistent Tracheostomy)

1. Purpose: A preexistent tracheostomy may be compromised by accumulated secretions, which can progress to occlusion of the airway. These secretions must be effectively suctioned or the tracheostomy cannula should be replaced.

2. Selection of Patients:

a. Indications: Obstruction secondary to secretions, hemorrhage, mucous plug, or foreign body; accidental dislodgment; inability to replace the cannula during home tracheotomy care are indications for the procedure.

b. Contraindications and Precautions: None

3. Equipment and Supplies (See Appendix for equipment and supplies manufacturers and suppliers. Appendix is keyed to italicized words in the equipment and supplies lists):

- Oxygen and oxygen *tubing*
- Suction equipment (See Figure 24-6, page 309)
- Tracheostomy *cannulae* (Figure 24-36)
  - A cannula the same diameter as the patient's cannula
  - A cannula one size smaller than the patient's cannula
- Bandage *scissors*

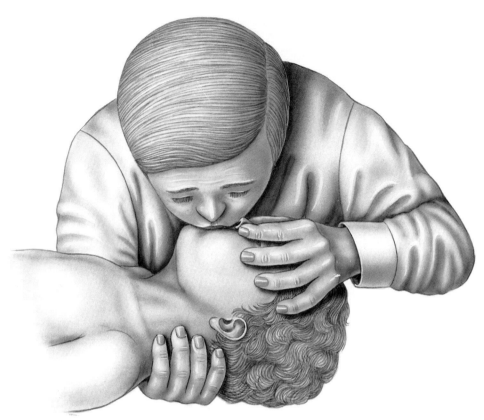

Figure 24-35.
Breathing: Assisted ventilation—Mouth-to-mouth ventilation. Technique.

· Tracheostomy twill *tape* (Figure 24-36)
· An endotracheal *tube* sized equal to or slightly smaller than patient's tracheostomy cannula (See Figure 24-20, page 318)
· Self-inflating ventilation bag with reservoir (See Figure 24-21, page 318)
4. Description of Procedure:
a. Suctioning of partially obstructed tracheostomy cannula:

· Ventilate and oxygenate with 100% oxygen through the cannula.
· Place towels under the child's shoulders so as to moderately extend the neck.
· Attempt to pass a suction catheter through the cannula and withdraw as under "Suctioning" (See page 313). If unsuccessful, reventilate with 100% oxygen and repeat the suctioning until the cannula is clear.

Table 24-1. Guidelines for Compressions and Ventilations During Cardiopulmonary Resuscitation

	Infant	Child	Adolescent
Depth of compressions:	½ to 1 inch	1 to 1½ inches	1½ to 2 inches
Rate of compressions:	≥ 100 per minute	80–100 per minute	80–100 per minute
Ratio of compressions to ventilations	5 to 1	5 to 1	5 to 1
Rate of assisted ventilations where a spontaneous pulse is present	15 to 20 per minute*	15 per minute*	12 per minute*

* Rate of assisted ventilations may be faster if hyperventilation is desired.

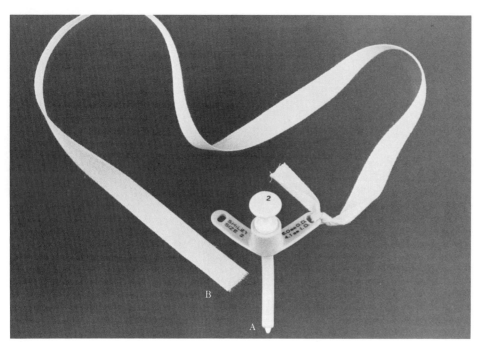

Figure 24-36.
Breathing: Tracheostomy care. Equipment and supplies: **A,** Tracheostomy cannula;
B, Tracheostomy twill tape.

· If the suction catheter cannot pass, replace the tracheostomy cannula immediately.

b. Replacement of obstructed tracheostomy cannula:
   · Carefully cut the twill tape that holds the tracheostomy cannula in place. Avoid cutting the child's neck.
   · Remove the tracheostomy cannula, observing the tracheocutaneous tract left by the cannula.
   · Immediately replace the cannula with a fresh tracheostomy cannula, following the preexisting tract.
   · Gently press the flanges against the neck.
   · Ventilate the child using a self-inflating ventilation bag with 100% oxygen.
   · Auscultate for equal breath sounds.
   · Replace the twill tape and secure the cannula by tying knots to snug the cannula flanges toward the child's neck while the neck is in the flexed position.

c. Replacement of a dislodged trach cannula:
   · Replacement must be immediate.
   · Use of the same tracheostomy cannula may be necessary, even though it might not be sterile.
   · If the stoma has constricted and will not allow replacement:
       (a) Replace with a smaller cannula, or

       (b) Replace with a smaller endotracheal tube, or
       (c) Replace with a length of oxygen tubing, which may be used later as a stylet to guide a new cannula into the trachea. Provide 100% oxygen through the oxygen tubing.
       (d) Immediately obtain a surgery consultation for definitive surgical dilation and cannula replacement.

5. Side Effects and Complications: Hemorrhage can occur as the cannula is suctioned or replaced.

Hypoxemia, hypercarbia, and respiratory/metabolic acidosis may individually or jointly complicate the procedure.

III. Circulation

A. External Cardiac Compression

1. Purpose: External cardiac compression is a technique designed to provide sufficient blood flow to sustain vital organs (brain and myocardium) during periods of inadequate cardiac output. It is also referred to as "closed chest massage."

2. Selection of Patients:

a. Indications: External chest compressions should be instituted immediately after the assessment and restoration of airway and breathing in situations of:

(1) Cardiac arrest (asystole), which in children is usually secondary to respiratory arrest.

(2) Inadequate cardiac output, even if cardiac electrical activity is present.

(3) Adequacy of cardiac output is assessed by checking for the presence and quality of peripheral pulses (femoral, brachial, axillary, carotid), the color of the skin, nails, and mucous membranes, and capillary refill.

b. Contraindications and Precautions: External chest compressions are not necessary when cardiac activity is present with the generation of a pulse. An electrocardiogram should be performed *after* the airway has been secured *and* the child has been assisted with ventilations (using 100% oxygen when available).

3. Equipment and Supplies (See Appendix for equipment and supplies manufacturers and suppliers. Appendix is keyed to italicized words in the equipment and supplies lists):

• Stethoscope and sphygmomanometer (helpful but not required)

• Cardiac monitor (helpful but not required)

4. Description of Procedure:

a. *Two-finger technique* (for neonates and infants):

• Assess for the need for external cardiac compressions.

• Place the infant on a firm backboard.

• If necessary, reduce the dead space between the child's back and the backboard created by the child's prominent occiput. Reduce the dead space by placing several thicknesses of towel between the child's scapulae.

• Apply pressure over the midsternum using your index and third finger (Figure 24-37). The pads of the tips of your two fingers should be located in the midline just below an imaginary line drawn between the nipples.

• See Table 24-1 for the depth of compressions, the rate of compressions per minute, and the ratio of compressions to ventilations in each age group.

• Compression and release times should be equal.

• Assist with ventilations according to the table.

• An assistant should check for the presence of a femoral or brachial pulse during chest compressions to confirm effectiveness.

b. *Thaler technique* (for *neonates* and *small infants*):

• Assess the need for external cardiac compressions.

• A backboard is not necessary as it is with the two-fingered technique.

• Link the fingers of both hands posteriorly over the infant's thoracic spine while the thumbs compress the mid sternum (Figure 24-38). Avoid compressing the chest wall rather than the sternum.

• The rates for the compressions, the depths of the compressions, and the ratios of compressions to ventilations are identical to those used with the two-fingered technique (See Table 24-1, page 331).

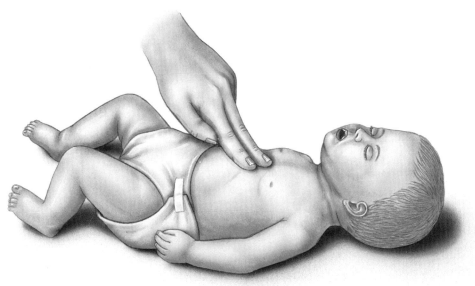

Figure 24-37.
Circulation: External cardiac compression—Two-finger compression. Technique.

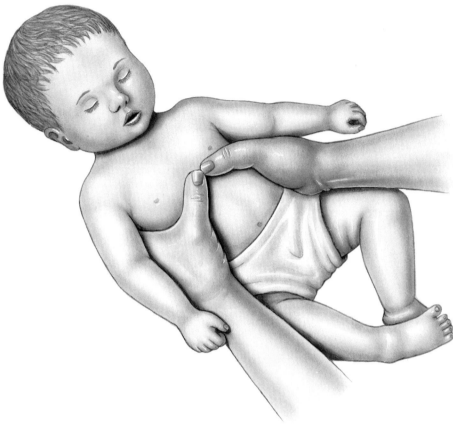

Figure 24-38.
Circulation: External cardiac compression—Thalar method. Technique.

• Assist with ventilations according to Table 24-1.
• An assistant should check for the presence of a pulse with each chest compression. This should preferably be done at the brachial pulse (See Figure 2-8, page 16), although the femoral pulse (See Figure 2-1, page 11) can be an alternative.

c. External cardiac compressions for children older than 1 year:

• Assess the need for external cardiac compressions.
• Place the child in the supine position on a firm backboard or on the floor.
• Locate the lower half of sternum.
• Place the heel of one hand over the midline of the lower half of the sternum. Be sure to avoid pressure on the xiphoid, as lacerations to the liver may occur during chest compressions.
• If the patient is a *smaller child,* only one hand is used (Figure 24-39). In this case, use your free hand to maintain proper head and neck positioning.

• In the *larger child,* place the heel of your other hand directly on top of the first (Figure 24-40).
• Lift your fingertips off of the child's chest wall, compressing only with the heel of the hand.
• Begin chest compressions, using a smooth and continuous rhythm. The compression and release times should be equal.
• See Table 24-1, page 331, for depth and rate of compressions for the child and for the proper chest-compression-to-ventilation ratio.
• Assist with ventilations according to Table 24-1.
• An assistant should check for the presence of a pulse with each chest compression. This can be done at the brachial (See Figure 2-8, page 16), carotid (See Figure 2-3, page 11), or femoral (See Figure 2-1, page 11) artery pulse site.

5. Side Effects and Complications: Rib fractures and sternal fractures are less common in children than in adults, but can occur. Chest wall fractures can result in lacerations to the

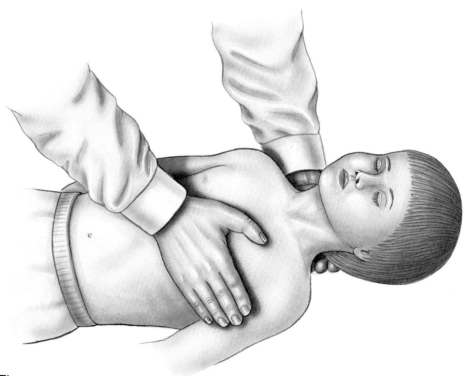

Figure 24-39.
Circulation: External cardiac compression—For the smaller child. Technique.

liver, spleen, lungs, or intercostal vessals. Liver lacerations and tears in large abdominal veins (portal vein, inferior vena cava) have been reported in the absence of rib fractures. They may have resulted from compressions over the xiphoid.

Bronchopulmonary air leak (pneumothorax, pneumomediastinum, and subcutaneous emphysema) may result from excessively increased intrathoracic pressures.

Generation of inadequate peripheral pulse may be due to severe hypovolemia, tension pneumothorax, cardiac tamponade, or improper technique.

B. Cardiac Monitoring

1. Purpose: Cardiac monitoring allows the practitioner to assess visually and interpret the child's cardiac electrical activity on a continuous basis.

2. Selection of Patients:

a. Indications: Monitoring is indicated for hypotension, pulselessness, asystole, bradyarrhythmias, and tachyarrhythmias of any cause. Cardiac monitoring is strongly advised during the intravenous administration of certain medications, such as aminophylline, diphenylhydantoin, diazepam, digoxin, and phenobarbital, as well as other vasoactive drugs. "Blind" defibrillation or cardioversion is not recommended; therefore, a cardiac monitor should be in place before performing these procedures.

b. Contraindications and Precautions: None

3. Equipment and Supplies (See Appendix for equipment and supplies manufacturers and suppliers. Appendix is keyed to italicized words in the equipment and supplies lists):

- Cardiac monitor
- Monitor electrode patches

4. Description of Procedure:

- Affix the monitor electrodes in the standard fashion:
  (1) *White:* right anterior shoulder ("white-on-the-right")
  (2) *Black:* Left anterior shoulder
  (3) *Red or Green:* Lower abdomen
- Turn the power to "On."
- Choose the desired "lead" on the monitor. Most mon-

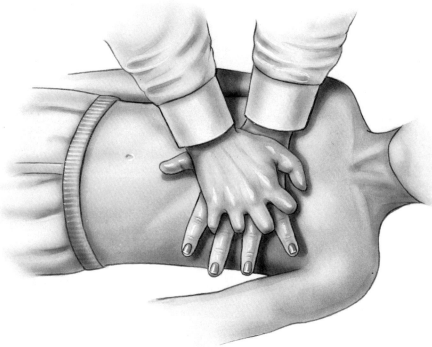

Figure 24-40.
Circulation: External cardiac compression—For the larger child. Technique.

itors offer at least leads I, II, and III; others offer all six limb leads. Usually lead II or lead III offers a satisfactory waveform.
· Adjust the monitor gain to optimize the QRS wave form.
· Interpret the cardiac rhythm on the oscilloscope or on a rhythm strip.
5. Side Effects and Complications: Placement of electrodes over the midportion of both anterior hemithoraces will interfere with interpretation of chest radiographs, so keep the electrodes over the anterior shoulders.

C. Defibrillation

1. Purpose: This technique is meant to transform ventricular fibrillation into a stable, cardiac rhythm that generates a pulse and blood pressure.
2. Selection of Patients:
a. Indications: Defibrillation is indicated in the presence of monitored ventricular fibrillation.
b. Contraindications and Precautions: Unmonitored (or presumed) ventricular fibrillation should not be defibrillated "blindly."

3. Equipment and Supplies (See Appendix for equipment and supplies manufacturers and suppliers. Appendix is keyed to italicized words in the equipment and supplies lists):
· Cardiac *monitor*
· *Defibrillator* with correct size (4.5-cm diameter for neonates and infants and 8.0-cm diameter for older children) *paddles* (Figure 24-41).
· Electrode *gel*
4. Description of Procedure:
· Recognize ventricular fibrillation on the monitor.
· Prepare the paddles with a generous application of electrode gel to insure proper contact and to prevent an electrical burn.
· Turn the defibrillator power to "On."
· Insure that the synchronous cardioversion mode is "Off."
· Set the defibrillator to the desired energy level (2 Joules/kg).
· Charge the defibrillator.
· Place the paddles in the proper location on the patient's chest wall (Figure 24-41). Apply firm pressure.
· Insure that all personnel, including yourself, are "all clear" of direct contact with the patient.

- Discharge energy by simultaneously pressing the discharge buttons on both paddles.
- Check the monitor for a change in rhythm.
- Check the patient for the presence of a peripheral pulse.
- If necessary, repeat the above sequence using 4 J/kg of discharge energy.
- Once the arrhythmia is corrected, address any concurrent metabolic disarray.

5. Side Effects and Complications: Skin burns and subcutaneous burns occasionally occur from direct contact with the paddles. Myocardial injury due to multiple energy discharges may complicate the procedure. An electrical "arc" may electrocute you or your assistants between the patient and a human contact. Failure to discharge energy may result from failure to turn off the synchronous cardioversion mode on the defibrillator or failure to turn the defibrillator "On," select energy level, charge the paddles, or simultaneously press the discharge buttons (in this order). Metabolic disarray such as hypoxemia or metabolic acidosis usually are present as a result of cardiac dysfunction.

D. Direct-Current Synchronous Cardioversion

1. Purpose: Direct-current synchronous cardioversion is used to convert ventricular tachycardia (VT) or paroxysmal supraventricular tachycardia (PSVT) into a sinus rhythm, generating a more effective cardiac output.
2. Selection of Patients:
a. Indications: The procedure is indicated for ventricular tachycardia associated with severe hypotension and paroxysmal supraventricular tachycardias (PSVT), including atrial fibrillation and atrial flutter, associated with profound hypotension and shock, or associated with *severe* congestive heart failure.
b. Contraindications and Precautions: Patients with tachyarrhythmias who are normotensive or mildly hypotensive should be offered an attempt at pharmacologic cardioversion before the use of direct current synchronous cardioversion. The procedure should not be attempted for patients in ventricular fibrillation, as the synchronous mode will not allow the discharge of energy without sensing a QRS wave form.
3. Equipment and Supplies (See Appendix for equipment and supplies manufacturers and suppliers. Appendix is keyed to italicized words in the equipment and supplies lists):
- Cardiac *monitor*
- *Defibrillator* equipped with synchronous cardioversion mode and correct size (4.5-cm diameter for neonates and infants and 8.0-cm diameter for older children) *paddles* (See Figure 24-41, this page).
- Electrode *gel*

4. Description of Procedure:
- Recognize ventricular tachycardia or paroxysmal su-

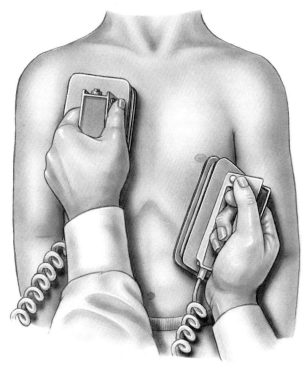

Figure 24-41.
Circulation: Defibrillation. Proper placement of defibrillator paddles.

praventricular tachycardia in a child who is either pulseless or in profound cardiogenic shock secondary to the tachyarrhythmia.
- Prepare the paddles with electrode gel.
- Turn the defibrillator power "On."
- Insure that the synchronous cardioversion mode is "On."
- Set the unit to the desired energy level (2 J/kg).
- Press the designated button to "charge" the unit.
- Place the paddles at the proper location on the patient's chest wall and apply firm pressure (See Figure 24-41, this page).
- Insure that all personnel, including yourself, are "all clear" of contact with the patient.
- Discharge energy by simultaneously pressing both discharge buttons on the paddles. Be prepared for a variable (0.5–2 seconds) delay before the energy is discharged. Keep the discharge buttons pressed until the unit does discharge energy.
- Check the monitor for a change in rhythm.
- Check the patient for the presence of a peripheral pulse. If a pulse is present, obtain a blood pressure reading.

- Repeat the above sequence if rhythm fails to convert to sinus rhythm.

5. Side Effects and Complications: The side effects and complications of the procedure are the same as for Defibrillation (See page 336), except that the operator should insure that the synchronous cardioversion switch is turned "On."

IV. Resuscitative Drug Therapy

A. Essential Resuscitative Drugs

1. Oxygen:

The fundamental goal of resuscitation is to restore oxygenation and cellular nutrition to cerebral and myocardial tissues before the development of irreversible injury.

Oxygen therapy is of preimminent importance during resuscitation efforts. It is also indicated for acute hypoxemia secondary to any cause.

The dosage of oxygen in the arrest situation is 100%.

The only potential complication of oxygen use in the resuscitation process is depression of the respiratory drive in patients with severe obstructive pulmonary disease associated with chronic carbon dioxide retention.

2. Epinephrine:

Epinephrine is the classic alpha- and beta-adrenergic agonist. Its alpha-adrenergic effects result in vasoconstriction, causing a rise in systolic and especially diastolic blood pressure. Its beta effects create an increased heart rate, and a mild increase in inotropic tone.

Indications for its use include asystole, ventricular fibrillation, electromechanical dissociation, and hypotension. The usual dosage is 0.1 mL/kg (1:10,000), to a maximum of 5 mL, intravenously or via the endotracheal tube.

Unlike the adult, epinephrine-induced coronary ischemia is rare in the pediatric age group. However, its use may predispose to certain supraventricular arrhythmias.

3. Atropine:

Atropine is the parasympatholytic drug used in resuscitative efforts. Its desired effects include the peripheral "vagolytic" action, which increases heart rate.

Indications for its use include bradycardia associated with hypotension, ventricular ectopy, or symptoms of poor central nervous system or cardiac perfusion. If the bradycardia is resulting from hypoxia or hypoventilation, however, it should be treated with supplemental oxygen and assisted ventilation before the administration of atropine.

The usual dosage of atropine is 0.01 mg/kg intravenously or via the endotracheal tube, with a minimum dose of 0.20 mg. This may be repeated every 5 minutes for a total of four doses or to a maximum dosage of 0.04 mg/kg, whichever is smaller. In organophosphate poisoning, much larger doses of atropine may be necessary.

Atropine may cause drying of secretions, anhidrosis, fever, pupillary dilatation, urinary retention, bronchial mucous plugging, flushing of skin, and major and minor central nervous system disturbances. The older child may complain of blurred vision or photophobia. Generally, all of these potential reactions are not of immediate concern in a resuscitation attempt.

4. Glucose:

Oral or parenteral glucose reverses hypoglycemia. Because infants have decreased glycogen stores compared with adults, hypoglycemia is a factor in a wide range of pathologic processes affecting this age group.

The indication for treatment with intravenous glucose is presumed or confirmed hypoglycemia.

The usual intravenous dosage is 0.5 to 1.0 g/kg (2–4 mL/kg). This may be repeated as needed based on measured glucose results.

Because hyperosmolality and interstitial–intracellular osmolar shifts may occur with parenteral glucose administration, push the glucose slowly when possible.

The blood glucose level should be determined after glucose administration.

5. Sodium Bicarbonate ($NaHCO_3$):

Metabolic acidosis may occur in any resuscitative effort.

Sodium bicarbonate is used for the correction of severe lactic acidosis or other metabolic acidosis. Remember, the byproducts of sodium bicarbonate buffering (carbon dioxide and water) must be eliminated through proper ventilation, so appropriately ventilate or even hyperventilate the patient to assure carbon dioxide excretion from the lungs.

Metabolic acidosis should be confirmed by arterial blood gas analysis before treatment with sodium bicarbonate. The use of sodium bicarbonate for suggested but unconfirmed acidosis is controversial. It is appropriate to treat such instances with hyperventilation until arterial blood gas analysis is available.

The initial dosage is 1 mEq/kg intravenously, by slow push. The solution should be diluted according to the patient's age:

a. Greater than 6 months of age: 1 mEq/mL

b. Less than 6 months of age: 0.5 mEq/mL

Subsequent doses are administered according to arterial blood gas analysis and are calculated by the formula:

$$\text{milliequivalents } NaHCO_3 = 0.3 \times \text{Weight (kilograms)} \times \text{Base Excess}$$

Example: An 8.0-kg infant who is being resuscitated has an initial arterial blood gas analysis as follows:

- pH = 7.10
- PCO_2 = 35 Torr
- PO_2 = 96 Torr
- HCO_3 = 10 mEq/liter
- BE = −18

The calculated initial dosage of NaHCO$_3$ would be:

$$\text{milliequivalents NaHCO}_3 = 0.3 \times 8.0 \times 18$$
$$= 43 \text{ mEq NaHCO}_3$$

Hypernatremia and hyperosmolality may occur after excess or rapid administration of sodium bicarbonate. Sodium bicarbonate may inactivate epinephrine if the two substances are mixed. Sodium bicarbonate may precipitate calcium gluconate or calcium chloride when the two are mixed.

6. Calcium:

The use of calcium during resuscitative efforts remains controversial. Ostensibly, intravenous calcium enhances myocardial contractility and increased conduction velocity through the ventricle. However, there is virtually no clinical study data to support the use of calcium to improve resuscitative outcome in patients who are not known to be hypocalcemic. The American Heart Association has withdrawn support for its use in its Advanced Cardiac Life Support protocols. Therefore, the routine use of calcium is not recommended in a resuscitative effort unless the patient is suffering from documented hypocalcemia.

When it is used, the dosage of calcium is:

a. **Calcium gluconate: 30 mg/kg, slowly intravenously**

b. **Calcium chloride: 10 mg/kg slowly intravenously**

Side effects of calcium infusions include hypercalcemia and precipitation out of solution if calcium infusions are mixed with sodium bicarbonate.

Chapter 25

Radiologic Procedures

Joan McIlhenny

The purpose of this chapter is to provide a brief overview of the radiologic examinations most commonly used in evaluating pediatric outpatients (Table 25-2). This information should help you get the most out of the radiologic studies you request.

It is important for the primary physician to understand exactly what information can be obtained from an examination and what the examination involves for the chid and his family. Ideally, the primary physician should consult with the radiologist before the procedure so that the evaluation can be tailored to the child's presentation and specific preparations and sedation, if necessary, can be discussed. Families want to know the risks and benefits and costs of radiologic studies, and well-informed parents are usually less anxious and better able to help the child in the radiology department.

I. Diagnostic Radiology Modalities

A. X-rays

X-rays are a form of electromagnetic radiation. They are emitted from a vacuum tube when the target anode is hit with a stream of electrons from a heated cathode. Other forms of electromagnetic radiation include ultraviolet light, visible light, infrared light, and television signals. X-rays have a very short wavelength and are able to penetrate the different components of the child's body to form an image on a film. Fluoroscopy and computerized axial tomography are two specialized forms of x-ray examinations.

Fluoroscopy allows the radiologist to view the radiographic image instantaneously on a television screen. Thus, a moving image can be observed and certain examinations such as swallowing in the upper gastrointestinal series can be monitored. The main disadvantage of fluoroscopy is that it increases the radiation exposure to the child.

Computerized axial tomography (CT) uses a rotating fan beam of x-rays and multiple detectors to measure the amount of transmitted radiation. A computer then analyzes the measurements and creates a detailed cross-sectional image of the child. Infants and small children usually need sedation for CT scans. Consult with your radiology department to coordinate this part of the child's care (i.e., designating who will be responsible for giving the sedation and monitoring the child).

B. Scans

Nuclear medicine scans use radioactive labeled substances called radiopharmaceuticals, which predominantly emit gamma rays, to study selected areas of the human body and to obtain physiologic information. The distribution of the radiopharmaceutical in the body is detected and measured by a gamma camera containing a sensitive crystal placed next to the child. The radiopharmaceutical may be given orally, intravenously, or instilled through a catheter in the bladder, depending on the type of study planned. The images take many minutes to acquire; sedation may be necessary for small children because motion causes serious degradation of the image. Because the isotope decays over time, the biologic effect of the radiation from nuclear medicine studies may be less than that from conventional x-ray examinations.

C. Ultrasound

High-frequency sound waves are generated by electrical stimulation of the piezoelectric crystal in the ultrasound transducer. As they pass through the child's body these transmitted sound waves are then reflected, or attenuated, depending on the acoustic properties of the tissues being examined. Because ultrasound waves are reflected by bone and air, an examination may be of limited value if the area of interest is obscured by overlying bowel gas. Body fat attenuates the sound beam, making an obese patient difficult to examine. Children, who typically have less body fat than adults, are ideal ultrasound patients. The examination uses no radiation and has no known harmful effects. Usually children do not need to be sedated for ultrasound exams. The performance of the examination, however, is very dependent on the skill and experience of the ultrasonographer.

D. Magnetic Resonance Imaging (MRI)

When a child is placed in an MRI machine, the hydrogen atoms in her body are influenced by the strong magnetic field of the machine. Typical field strengths for medical imaging are 0.3 Tesla up to 2 Tesla. The earth's gravitational field is 0.5 gauss. One Tesla equals 10,000 gauss. The hydrogen atoms line up like tiny magnets along the long axis of the magnetic field. Radiowaves of a specific frequency are used to alter the direction of the hydrogen atoms. When the radiowaves are turned off, the atoms go back to their original state and energy is released in the form of radiowaves. These waves are detected and a computer generates an image based on the distribution of hydrogen nuclei within the area of the body being imaged. There are no known harmful side effects of clinical MRI. Most suture wires and joint prostheses are made from nonmagnetic metals. Patients with cardiac pacemakers and feromagnetic implants such as aneurysm clips should not be imaged because the magnet could cause malfunction or dislodgment of such an implant. The main advantages of MRI imaging include the ability to image in any plane, no ionizing radiation, and high-contrast resolution. Disadvantages include expense, long imaging times, frequent need for sedation, inability to use metallic monitoring equipment, and claustrophobia experienced by patients in the tunnel-like magnet.

II. Radiation Exposure

The potential harmful effects of ionizing radiation in the low dose range used for medical diagnosis include teratogenesis, carcinogenesis, and mutagenesis. Direct tissue injury, such as skin erythema, does not occur in the low dose range used for medical imaging. In general, the medical benefits of diagnostic radiology far outweigh the potential risks of ionizing radiation for pediatric patients.

A. Teratogenesis

The developing fetus is especially sensitive to radiation injury during the first trimester of pregnancy. The pediatrician should be certain that the adolescent patient is not pregnant when ordering radiologic studies. Electives studies should be scheduled to occur within the first 10 days of the menstrual cycle.

B. Carcinogenesis

Carcinogenesis is one of the potential long-term risks of ionizing radiation for the pediatric patient. The three main cancers linked to high-dose radiation exposure in childhood such as experienced from the atomic bombs in Hiroshima and Nagasaki are leukemia, thyroid cancer, and breast cancer. Even though the doses used in diagnostic radiology are low, the pediatrician should consider carefully the benefits versus the risks of certain examinations if the test involves irradiating the active bone marrow (especially the skull, because a large percentage of the active marrow is located in the skull during early childhood; e.g., skull films and head CT scans), the thyroid (e.g., neck films), or female breast tissue (chest wall; e.g., rib films, scoliosis spine films).[1]

C. Mutagenesis

Mutagenesis is another potential long-term risk of ionizing radiation exposure. Even though the risk of mutagenesis is low in children, the gonads are routinely shielded to avoid genetic damage to descendants.

III. Consultation

1. Consult with a radiologist before you order an examination if you are uncertain of the best test to order. The factors of growth and maturation may influence the selection of examinations.
2. Always include pertinent history, physical examination, and laboratory data on the request.
3. List known allergies and current medications.
4. Do not order "routine" examinations such as preoperative chest films on children unless clinically indicated.
5. Know what the examination involves for your patient so that you can counsel the child and her family. Families usually want to know the details of how the examination is performed, can they stay with their child, what you expect to learn from the test, and the risks of the examination. Frequently asked questions include: "Is there a prep?" "Is the test uncomfortable?" "Does it hurt?" "Does it require fasting?" "Will an IV be started?" "Will the child be sedated or restrained?" "How long does it take?" Answers to these questions vary from institution to institution, so always check with your radiology department.

IV. Patient Preparation for Procedures

A. Oral Intake
In general, food and liquid intake are restricted for radiologic studies in which intravenous or oral contrast is given or when sedation of the child is planned. Studies should be scheduled to be as convenient as possible for the family's and the child's schedule. Usually a child is not fasted longer than her usual feeding schedule safely allows (Table 25-1).

A patient undergoing upper gastrointestinal fluoroscopy should have her oral intake restricted according to Table 25-1; the restriction insures that the child is hungry enough to drink the liquid barium and that the mucosal detail of the gastrointestinal tract is not obscured by food particles.

B. Bowel Preparation
The purpose of a bowel preparation is to insure that the colon is as clean as possible. The only study that requires a preparation is an air-contrast barium enema. Air-contrast barium enemas are performed to evaluate rectal bleeding and inflammatory bowel disease. Retained stool can resemble or hide polyps and obscure mucosal detail.

Unlike adults, children are not given bowel preparations before intravenous pyelography.

Table 25-1. Restriction of Oral Intake Required for Selected Radiographic Procedures

Patient's Age	Duration of Restriction
Newborn	2 hours
Under 1 year	4 hours
1 to 2 years	6 hours
Over 2 years	8 hours

C. Intravenous Access
Intravenous access is necessary for intravenous pyelography, contrast-enhanced computerized tomography, most nuclear medicine scans, and intravenous sedation.

D. Sedation
Computerized tomography and other examinations may require sedation. Sedation protocols vary from hospital to hospital, so check with your radiology department.

Artifacts caused by motion can severely degrade the radiographic image. The goal of sedation for an imaging procedure is "conscious sedation," which is defined by the American Academy of Pediatrics as "a minimally depressed level of consciousness that retains the ability to maintain a patent airway independently and continuously and to respond appropriately to physical stimulation and/or verbal command."

The following points should be emphasized:

1. All children should be evaluated by a physician before sedation.
2. It should be clear which physician is to assume responsibility for ordering and administering the medication and for monitoring the patient after the medication.
3. Sedatives appropriate for radiologic procedures are included in Table 18-2, page 219.

E. Restraints
Immobilization is an important part of many radiographic procedures. It decreases motion artifact on films, minimizes repeat examinations, and decreases radiation dose to the patient by allowing for optimum positioning. Typically, for fluoroscopic exams, Velcro straps are used with a wooden board that has an octagon attached at each end. The child then can be easily rotated into lateral and oblique positions. For CT, the child is swaddled in a sheet.

Reference
1. Hilton SV, Edwards DK, Hilton JW. Practical Pediatric Radiology. Philadelphia: WB Saunders, 1984:575–602.

Table 25-2. Commonly Performed Radiologic Procedures for the Pediatric Outpatient

	Voiding Cystourethrogram (VCUG)	Intravenous Pyelogram (IVP)
Radiologic technique	The bladder is catheterized with an 8-French pediatric feeding tube. A urine specimen is obtained for culture. Bladder filling is monitored fluoroscopically. Spot films of the bladder, urethra (during voiding), and renal areas are obtained by the radiologist.	The child voids completely before the study. A KUB (kidneys, ureters, bladder) scout film is obtained. Low osmolarity nonionic contrast (2 mL/kg) is injected intravenously. Films are taken immediately postinjection and at 10 minutes. Additional films may be requested by the radiologist, depending on the indications for the exam and the findings.
Indications	Documented history of urinary tract infection Vesicoureteral reflux Urethral obstruction (posterior urethral valves) Voiding difficulty Ectopic ureter, ureterocele	Urinary tract infection Vesicoureteral reflux Hematuria Obstruction
Contrast material or imaging agent	18% radiographic contrast (Cystografin, dilute)	Low-osmolarity nonionic contrast (2 mL/kg)
Restriction of oral intake	None	The child should be NPO (See Table 25-1, page 342) to avoid the risk of vomiting and aspiration. The child does not need to be dehydrated.
Bowel preparation	None	No bowel preparation is needed for a pediatric IVP.
IV access	None	Yes
Sedation	None	None
Position	Supine	Supine or prone
Restraint	Necessary for infants and small children	May be necessary for infants and small children
Time required	30 minutes	30 minutes
Approximate cost (1990)	$200	$200

	Radionuclide Renal Scan	Radionuclide Cystography
Radiologic technique	The radionuclide is injected intravenously. Serial images are obtained to assess perfusion, structure, function, and excretion.	The bladder is catheterized and 1.0 mCi of Tc-99m is instilled with saline. The bladder is filled to capacity with saline and then the patient voids.
Indications	History of urinary tract infection Assess renal function Lower urinary tract obstruction Renal transplant assessment	History of urinary tract infection Vesicoureteral reflux Follow-up examinations in children who have had a fluoroscopic VCUG
Contrast material or imaging agent	Tc-99m-DTPA (function, definition of collecting system) Tc-99m Glucoheptonate (structure and function) Tc-99m DMSA (structure, anatomy of cortex)	Tc-99m in saline
Restriction of oral intake	None	None
Bowel preparation	None	None
IV access	Yes	No
Sedation	Not usually required	None
Position	Supine	Supine and sitting
Restraint	May be necessary for infants and small children	May be necessary for infants and small children
Time required	1–2 hours	30 minutes
Approximate cost (1990)	$500	$250

continued on page 344

Table 25-2. Commonly Performed Radiologic Procedures for the Pediatric Outpatient (continued)

	Barium Swallow	Upper Gastrointestinal Series
Radiologic technique	The child drinks barium from a bottle or cup while being observed fluoroscopically. In certain circumstances the radiologist may choose to administer the barium via a nasogastric tube positioned in the midesophagus.	The child drinks barium from a bottle or cup. The esophagus, stomach, and duodenum are monitored fluoroscopically and spot films are obtained by the radiologist. The child is encouraged to drink enough barium to simulate a regular feeding. If the child refuses to drink, the barium is administered via a nasogastric tube.
Indications	Swallowing difficulty; motility disorder Tracheo-esophageal fistula Vascular ring or sling Hiatal hernia Gastroesophageal reflux	Bowel obstruction (malrotation, duodenal web) Vomiting Abdominal pain Gastroesophageal reflux Gastric outlet obstruction Ulcer
Contrast material or imaging agent	Barium Water-soluble contrast if a perforation is suspected	Barium
Restriction of oral intake	NPO (See Table 25-1, page 342)	NPO (See Table 25-1, page 342)
Bowel preparation	None	None
Sedation	None	None
Position	Erect and/or prone or supine	Erect or prone or supine
Restraint	May be necessary for infants and small children	May be necessary for infants and small children
Time required	30 minutes	30 minutes
Approximate cost (1990)	$225	$250

	Small Bowel Follow-Through	Enteroclysis (small bowel enema)
Radiologic technique	The child drinks additional barium after the upper gastrointestinal series is obtained. Serial films are obtained at 15- to 30-minute intervals until the barium column reaches the cecum. Spot films of the terminal ileum are obtained.	Because of the high radiation exposure of this examination, enteroclysis is not routinely ordered on children unless a previous upper gastrointestinal series with a small bowel follow-through has already been performed and there is a strong indication for the test. Under fluoroscopic guidance, a nasogastric tube is advanced to the duodeno-jejunal junction. A barium solution is injected at a fixed rate until the entire small bowel has been studied. Multiple spot films are obtained.
Indications	Abdominal pain Inflammatory bowel disease Partial obstruction	Inflammatory bowel disease Lymphoma Small bowel benign or malignant neoplasm Partial obstruction
Contrast material or imaging agent	Barium	Barium solution and methyl cellulose
Restriction of oral intake	NPO (See Table 25-1, page 342)	NPO (See Table 25-1, page 342)
Bowel preparation	None	None
Sedation	None	None
Position	Lying supine or prone on examining table	Lying supine or prone
Restraint	May be necessary for infants and small children	May be necessary for small children
Time required	Depends on bowel transit time, usually 1–3 hours	Depends on bowel transit time, usually less than 1 hour
Approximate cost (1990)	$180	$350

	Barium Enema (single contrast)	Air-Contrast Barium Enema
Radiologic technique	A red rubber catheter or pediatric enema tip is inserted in the rectum. Under fluoroscopic control, barium is administered from a bag suspended above the patient. Multiple spot films are obtained by the radiologist.	Under fluoroscopic control, the colon is coated with barium and distended with air. Multiple films in different positions are obtained.
Indications	Constipation Hirschsprung's disease Intussusception	Inflammatory bowel disease Rectal bleeding Polyps
Contrast material or imaging agent	Barium	Barium and air
Restriction of oral intake	None	Clear liquid diet for 36 hours before study
Bowel preparation	None	Preparation to cleanse colon: Castor oil (1 mL/kg) administered orally the afternoon before the study. Fleet enema or large-volume saline enema on the evening preceding and on the morning of the study.
Sedation	None	None
Position	Supine or prone	Lying supine, prone, bilateral, decubitus positions
Restraint	Usually required for infants and small children	—
Time required	30 minutes	1 hour
Approximate cost (1990)	$200	$250

	Abdominal Ultrasound	Pelvic Ultrasound
Radiologic technique	Multiple longitudinal, transverse, and oblique scans are performed in the upper abdomen. Particular attention is paid to the liver, gall bladder, pancreas, spleen, and kidneys. The examination is usually directed to answer specific clinical questions.	The child must have a full urinary bladder to act as an acoustic window for evaluating pelvic structures and to push air-filled bowel loops out of the pelvis. Multiple longitudinal oblique and transverse scans are obtained.
Indications	Abdominal pain Abdominal mass or abscess Evaluation for gall stones	Ovarian size Ovarian pathology Intrauterine pregnancy Ectopic pregnancy Pelvic abscess or mass Pelvic inflammatory disease Uterine pathology
Contrast material or imaging agent	None	None
Restriction of oral intake	NPO (See Table 25-1, page 342) to insure distention of gall bladder.	No restriction. The patient is encouraged to drink liquids to have a full urinary bladder.
Bowel preparation	No recent barium studies before examination	No recent barium studies before examination
Sedation	None	None
Position	Supine	Supine
Time required	30 minutes	30 minutes
Approximate cost (1990)	$300	$150

continued on page 346

Table 25-2. Commonly Performed Radiologic Procedures for the Pediatric Outpatient (continued)

	Renal Ultrasound	Head Ultrasound
Radiologic technique	Multiple longitudinal and transverse scans are performed through the kidneys and bladder.	The anterior fontanelle is used as an acoustic window to image the brain. Multiple coronal and parasagittal scans are obtained.
Indications	Urinary tract infection Suspected renal anomalies Renal mass or abscess Urinary tract obstruction Localization for renal biopsy Assessment of renal transplant	Hydrocephalus (assessment of ventricular size) Evaluation and follow-up of germinal matrix-related hemorrhage
Contrast material or imaging agent	None	None
Restriction of oral intake	None	None
Bowel preparation	None	None
Sedation	None	None
Position	Supine	Supine
Time required	30 minutes	15 minutes
Approximate cost (1990)	$250	$250

	Head Computerized Tomography (CT)	Head Magnetic Resonance Imaging (MRI)
Radiologic technique	Axial or coronal scans are obtained with or without intravenous contrast enhancement.	Axial, coronal and sagittal scans with and/or without gadolinium enhancement are obtained.
Indications	Tumor Infection Trauma Hydrocephalus Hemorrhage/vascular disease White matter disease	Tumor Infection Hemorrhage White matter disease Congenital abnormality
Contrast material or imaging agent	If required, low-osmolarity nonionic water-soluble contrast (2 mL/kg) is administered intravenously before scanning.	Gadolinium DTPA may be used, given intravenously
Restriction of oral intake	If sedation or intravenous contrast enhancement is planned, the child should be NPO (See Table 25-1, page 342) to avoid aspiration. If no sedation or contrast is planned, the child may eat and drink before the examination.	If sedation or intravenous contrast enhancement is planned, the child should be NPO (See Table 25-1, page 342) to avoid aspiration. If no sedation or contrast is planned, the child may eat and drink before the examination.
Bowel preparation	None	None
IV access	Necessary for contrast enhancement	Necessary for contrast enhancement
Sedation	May be necessary for infants and small children (See Table 18-2, page 219)	Usually necessary for infants and small children (See Table 18-2, page 219)
Position	Supine	Supine
Time required	Less than 1 hour	1 hour
Approximate cost (1990)	$400 (without contrast)	$900

	Abdominal Computerized Tomography (CT)	Pelvic Computerized Tomography (CT)
Radiologic technique	Serial scans are performed through the upper abdomen to the iliac crests after oral and intravenous contrast administration.	Serial scans are performed from the iliac crests to the symphysis pubis after intravenous and oral contrast administration.
Indications	Abdominal mass, abscess Trauma Metastatic disease evaluation	Pelvic mass or abscess Trauma Congenital anomaly
Contrast material or imaging agent	Dilute oral gastrografin to opacify bowel loops. Intravenous low-osmolarity nonionic contrast to opacify blood vessels and cause contrast enhancement (2 mL/kg).	Dilute oral gastrografin to opacify bowel loops. Intravenous low-osmolarity nonionic contrast to opacify blood vessels and bladder and cause contrast enhancement (2 mL/kg).
Restriction of oral intake	NPO (See Table 25-1, page 342) to insure that child will drink an adequate amount of oral contrast material administered by radiology department.	NPO (See Table 25-1, page 342) to insure that child will drink an adequate amount of oral contrast material administered by radiology department.
Bowel preparation	No recent barium studies before examination	No recent barium studies before examination
IV access	Yes	Yes
Sedation	May be required for infants and small children. Sedation (See Table 18-2, page 219) should be given after intravenous access has been obtained and after oral contrast has been given.	May be required for infants and small children. Sedation (See Table 18-2, page 219) should be given after intravenous access has been obtained and after oral contrast has been given.
Position	Supine	Supine
Time required	1 hour	1 hour
Approximate cost (1990)	$900	$900

	Chest Computerized Tomography (CT)	Radionuclide Bone Scan
Radiologic technique	Serial 1-cm scans are performed through the chest with or without contrast administration. Contrast is usually given when the mediastinum is the area of interest and if an inflammatory process is being evaluated.	After intravenous administration of Tc-99m MDP, immediate flow images are obtained over the area of primary interest. Blood pool images of this area are then obtained approximately 15 minutes later. Two-hour delayed bone images of the entire skeleton are then acquired.
Indications	Mediastinal mass Lung abscess Empyema Metastatic disease	Bone pain Osteomyelitis Septic arthritis Metastatic disease Avascular necrosis Stress fracture Child abuse
Contrast material or imaging agent	Intravenous low-osmolarity nonionic contrast may be given (2 mL/kg)	Tc-99m MDP
Restriction of oral intake	NPO (See Table 25-1, page 342) if contrast administration or sedation is planned	None
Bowel preparation	None	None
IV access	If intravenous contrast is planned	Yes
Sedation	May be required for infants and small children (See Table 18-2, page 219)	May be required for infants and small children (See Table 18-2, page 219)
Position	Supine	Supine
Time required	1 hour	3 hours
Approximate cost (1990)	$900 (with contrast)	$550

continued on page 348

347

Table 25-2. Commonly Performed Radiologic Procedures for the Pediatric Outpatient (continued)

	Skull Films	Paranasal Sinuses
Radiologic technique	Four routine views: Caldwell (15° occipitofrontal), lateral, Towne's (30° frontooccipital), and basal projections	Three routine views: Caldwell (15° occipitofrontal), lateral, and Water's (occipitomental) projections
Indications	Fracture Evaluation of sella turcica Premature closure of sutures Deformity Localization of ventricular shunt Osteomyelitis Foreign body Calvarial neoplasm	Infection (sinusitis, osteomyelitis) Chronic nasal obstruction
Contrast material or imaging agent	None	None
Restriction of oral intake	None	None
Bowel preparation	None	None
Sedation	None	None
Position	Supine	Erect
Time required	30 minutes	30 minutes
Approximate cost (1990)	$150	$140

	Cervical Spine	Extremity
Radiologic technique	Five routine views: anteroposterior, lateral, right and left obliques, odontoid	Anteroposterior and lateral view, oblique if necessary.
Indications	Trauma Arthritis Neck pain	Trauma Infection Neoplasm
Contrast material or imaging agent	None	None
Restriction of oral intake	None	None
Bowel preparation	None	None
Sedation	None	None
Position	Supine	Supine
Time required	30 minutes	30 minutes
Approximate cost (1990)	$125	$75

	Chest	Abdomen
Radiologic technique	Anteroposterior and lateral	Supine and erect or left lateral decubitus abdomen, erect chest
Indications	Infection	Abdominal pain
	Neoplasm	Bowel obstruction
	Trauma	Mass
	Chest pain	Bowel perforation
		Evaluation of ventriculoperitoneal shunt
Contrast material or imaging agent	None	None
Restriction of oral intake	None	None
Bowel preparation	None	None
Sedation	None	None
Position	Erect or supine	Supine and sitting or standing
Time required	30 minutes	30 minutes
Approximate cost (1990)	$75	$100

Appendix

Prepared by:

Lisa W. Morris
Susan T. Campbell
Carolyn B. Southall
Martha L. Criss, LPN
Elizabeth L. Lawton, RN, PNP

Equipment and Supplies Manufacturers

Description	Trade Name	Manufacturer or Supplier
Airway, Nasopharyngeal	Nasopharyngeal Airway	Portex, Inc. Wilmington, MA 01887
Airway, Oropharyngeal	Oropharyngeal Airway	Portex, Inc. Wilmington, MA 01887
Alcohol, Isopropyl	Isopropyl Rubbing Alcohol	Halsey Drug Co., Inc. Brooklyn, NY 11233
Angiocatheter	I.V. Catheter Placement Unit	Johnson & Johnson Critikon Tampa, FL 33607
Applicator, Calcium Alginate-Tipped	Calgiswab	Spectrum Diagnostics, Inc. Glenwood, IL 60425
Applicator, Cotton-Tipped	Medi-Pak Sterile Cotton-tipped Applicator	Whittaker General Medical Richmond, VA 23228
Applicator, Dacron-Tipped	Puritain	Hardwood Products, Inc. Guilford, ME 04443
Applicator, Fiber-Tipped	Cotton-tipped Applicator	Whittaker General Medical Richmond, VA 23228
Applicator, Metal with Roughened Tip	Lathbury Applicator	Storz Instrument Company St. Louis, MO 63122
Applicator, Sigmoidoscopic Cotton-tipped	Scopettes, Proctosigmoidoscopic	Birchwood Labs, Inc. Eden Prairie, MN 55344
Applicator, Silver Nitrate	Silver Nitrate Applicators	Graham-Field Inc. Hauppauge, NY 11788
Armboard	Armboard, Disposable, 9 × 3.5 inches	Medline Disposamed Medline Industries Mundelein, IL 60060
Aspirator, Rubber Bulb	Ear Syringe	Storz Instrument Company St. Louis, MO 63122
Bacitracin	Bacitracin Ointment, USP	Henry Schein Inc. Port Washington, NY 11050
Bag, Anesthesia	Anesthesia Ventilator Bag	Ohmeda Medical Madison, WI 53707
Bag, Enema	Cleansing Enema Set	American Hospital Supply Div. of American Hospital Supply Corp. McGaw Park, IL 60085
Bag, Self-Inflating	Self-inflating Ventilator Bag	Ohmeda Medical Madison, WI 53707
Bag, Urine Collection	Pediatric Urine Collector	Seamless Hospital Products Co. Div. of Dart Industries, Inc. Wallingford, CT 06492
Bag, Ventilator, Self-inflating, Anesthesia	Ventilator/Anesthesia/Self-inflating Bag	Ohmeda Medical Madison, WI 53707
Bandage, Elastic	Tensor Attached Clip Elastic Bandage	Becton-Dickinson and Co. Rochelle Park, NJ 07662

Equipment and Supplies Manufacturers *(continued)*

Description	Trade Name	Manufacturer or Supplier
Bandage, Kerlix Gauze	Kerlix, 6-ply, Stretched Gauze, 4.5 in. × 4.1 yd.	Kendall Healthcare Products Co. Mansfield, MA 02048
Bandage, Kling (Cotton, 3 or 4 inches)	Kling, Conforming Gauze Bandage, 3 in. × 5 yd., Sterile	Johnson & Johnson Products, Inc. New Brunswick, NJ 08903
Bandage, Muslin	Triangular Muslin Bandage, Unbleached	Parke-Davis & Co. Detroit, MI 48232
Bandage, Plaster	Specialist Plaster Bandage, Fast-setting, 3 in. × 3 yd.	Johnson & Johnson Products, Inc. New Brunswick, NJ 08903
Bandage, Sterile Conforming Gauze	Kendall Kerlix Roll	Kendall Co. Boston, MA 02101
Basin, Emesis	Autoclavable Emesis Basin	Medline Dynacor Div. of Medline Industries, Inc. Mundelein, IL 60060
Basin, Kidney-Shaped	Basin	Baxter Healthcare Corp. American Hospital Div. Virginia Beach, VA 23452
Batting, Red Cross Cotton (6 to 8 inches)	Red-Cross Cotton, Sterile, Absorbent	Johnson & Johnson Products, Inc. New Brunswick, NJ 08903
Benzoin, Tincture of	Tincture Benzoin Compound	Barre National, Inc. Baltimore, MD 21207
Blade, Laryngoscope	Laryngoscope Blade Miller: 0, 1, 2, 3 McIntosh: 2, 3, 4	Blue Ridge Anesthesia & Critical Care, Inc. Lynchburg, VA 24502
Blade, Scalpel, #11	Steri-Sharps Sterile Stainless Steel Surgical Blade #11	Seamless Hospital Products Co. Div. of Dart Industries, Inc. Wallingford, CT 06492
Blade, Scalpel, #15	Personna Surgical Blade #15	Owens and Minor, Inc. Richmond, VA 23230
Blade, Tongue	Tongue Depressor	Whittaker General Medical Richmond, VA 23228
Block, Bite	Disposable Jaw Locks	Halbrand, Inc. Willoughby, OH 44094
Board, Restraint	Papoose Board	Olympic Medical Company Seattle, WA 98109
Bottle, Enema	Sodium Phosphate and Biphosphate Enema	C.B. Fleet Co. Lynchburg, VA 24501
Brush, Cytology	Cytobrush Cell Collector	International Cytobrush, Inc. Hollywood, FL 33081
Brush, Soft	Scrub-Sponge Brush	Anchor Brush Company Aurora, IL 60507
Bulb, Enema	Pediatric Enema Bulb	C.B. Fleet Co. Lynchburg, VA 24501
Bulb, Rubber	Insufflator Bulb	Welch Allyn Skaneateles Falls, NY 13153

Equipment and Supplies Manufacturers *(continued)*

Description	Trade Name	Manufacturer or Supplier
Cannula, Intravenous	IV Cannula	Travenol Laboratories, Inc. Deerfield, IL 60015
Cannula, Nasal	Pediatric Nasal Cannula	Salter Laboratories Arvin, CA 93203
Cannula, Plastic	IV Placement Unit	Johnson & Johnson Co. Critikon Tampa, FL 33630
Cannula, Tracheostomy	Disposable Low Pressure Tracheostomy Tube	Shiley, Inc. Irvine, CA 92714
Cap, Plastic (for heparin lock)	PRN Adapter	Deseret Medical, Inc. Parke Davis and Co. Sandy, UT 84070
Capsule, Enteral	Multipurpose Suction Biopsy Tube	Quinton Instrument Co. Seattle, WA 98121
Catheter, Suction	Suction Catheter with Vacuum Control	Vicra Division of Travenol Laboratories Dallas, TX 75220
Catheter, Suction, Flexible	Suction Catheter with Vacuum Control	Travenol Laboratories, Inc. Deerfield, IL 60015
Catheter, Suction, Rectal	Disposable Sigmoidoscopic Suction Instrument	Busse Hospital Disposables Great Neck, NY 11021
Catheter, Suction, Rigid Tip	Yankauer Suction Instrument	Davol, Inc. Sub. of CR Bard, Inc. Cranston, RI 02920
Catheter, Urinary	Urethral Catheter	Henry Schein, Inc. Port Washington, NY 11050
Cellulose, Oxidized	Surgicel	Johnson & Johnson Hospital Services New Brunswick, NJ 08903
Charcoal, Activated	Charcoaid	Owens and Minor, Inc. Richmond, VA 23230
Chart, Visual Acuity	Eye Test Chart	Bernell Corporation South Bend, IN 46634
Clamp, Bell Circumcision	Gomco Clamp	American V. Mueller American Hospital Supply Corp. Chicago, IL 60648
Clamp, Fine Curved	Fine Curved Clamp	Baxter Healthcare Corp. V. Mueller Division McGaw Park, IL 60085
Clamp, Kelly	Forceps, Curved, 6.25 inches (Kelly)	Surgical Specialties, Inc. Crofton, MD 21114
Clamp, Mosquito	Herwig Mosquito Forceps Curved/ Straight	General Medical Corp. Richmond, VA 23228
Clamp, Straight	Straight Clamp	Surgicot, Inc. Smithtown, NY 11787

Equipment and Supplies Manufacturers *(continued)*

Description	Trade Name	Manufacturer or Supplier
Clipper, Fingernail	Scissors, Straight Iris, 4.5 inch	McCoy Surgical Supplies Maryland Heights, MO 63043
Collars, Soft	Soft, Foam, Emergency Padded Clavical Splint	Orthomedic Jefferson City, TN 37760
Connector, "T"	Extension Set with "T"	Abbott Laboratories Inc. North Chicago, IL 60064
Container, Sterile	Collector, Urine Specimen, Pediatric, Sterile	Hollister, Inc. Libertyville, IL 60048
Cover Slips	Coverglass #1½ 22 × 22 millimeter	Baxter Healthcare Corp. Columbia, MD 21045
Cream, Estrogen Containing	Premarin Vaginal Cream	Ayerst Div. of American Home Products Corp. New York, NY 10017
Crutches	Adjustable Wooden or Aluminum Axillary Crutches	Guardian Products, Inc. Sun Valley, CA 91352
Cube, 1 Inch	Cubical Counting Block	Constructive Playthings Grandview, MO 64030
Cup, Sterile Plastic, with Lid	Sterile Urine Specimen Collector	Hollister, Inc. Libertyville, IL 60048
Cup, Tin	Stainless Steel Camper's Cup	Campmoor Paramus, NJ 07653
Curet, Bone	Bone Curet	Zimmer, Inc. Warsaw, IN 46580
Curet, Ear, Plastic	Flex Loop Ear Curet	Bionix Corporation Toledo, OH 43614
Curet, Skin	Cannon Curet	George Tiemann and Co. Plainview, NY 11803
Curve, Height Velocity	Height Velocity Charts	Serono Laboratories, Inc. Randolph, MA 02368
Curve, Physical Growth	Growth Charts	Ross Laboratories Columbus, OH 43216
Cutters, Wire	Wire Cutters	Zimmer, Inc. Warsaw, IN 46580
Defibrillator	Defibrillator	Biomedical Specialties Crofton, MD 21114
Device, Disposable, Bleeding Time	Bleeding Time Device	Organon Teknika Corp. Durham, NC 27704
Device, Measuring	Harpenden Infantometer	Siber Hegner and Co., Inc. Carlstadt, NJ 07072
Dish, Petri	Sterilized Disposable Plastic Petri Dishes	Fisher Scientific Fair Lawn, NJ 07410
Drain, Latex Rubber	Penrose Drain Tube	Southeastern Hospital Supply Richmond, VA 23228

Equipment and Supplies Manufacturers *(continued)*

Description	Trade Name	Manufacturer or Supplier
Drape, Window	Fenestrated Drape	Baxter Healthcare Corp. Virginia Beach, VA 23452
Dressing, Figure Eight	Figure Eight Dressing	Florida Orthopedics Opa-Locka, FL 33054
Dressing, Transparent Catheter	OpSite #4575	Smith & Nephew Medical Massillon, OH 44646
Dropper, Eye, Glass/Plastic	Dropper Bottles	Baxter Healthcare Corp. Columbia, MD 21045
Electrodes with Rubber Straps	Electrode Set for 3700 Inducer	Wescor, Inc. Logan, UT 84321
Ephedrine	L-ephedrine Sulfate Powder, 1 oz.	City Chemical Corp. New York, NY 10011
Extractor, Comedone	Schamberg Expressor	George Tiemann and Co. Plainview, NY 11803
Extracts, Allergen	Extracts	Greer Laboratories, Inc. Lenoir, NC 28645
Extracts, Commercial	Inhalant, Food, Venom, or Drug Allergens	Hollister-Stier Div. of Miles Laboratories, Inc. Spokane, WA 99220
Felt, Orthopedic (½-inch thick)	Orthopaedic Felt	Southern Prosthetics Supply Alpharetta, GA 30201
Filter, Cobalt	Storz E-6862-A	Storz Ophthalmic Instrument Co. St. Louis, MO 63122
Fixative, Pap Smear	95–99% Isopropyl Alcohol	Baxter Healthcare Corp. Scientific Products Div. McGaw Park, IL 60085
Foam, Adhesive-backed (½-inch thick)	Self-Adhering Foam Pads, 7⅞ × 11¾ × ½ inches	3M Company Medical Products Div. St. Paul, MN 55101
Forceps, Alligator	Noyes Ear Forceps	American V. Mueller Div. of American Hospital Supply Corp. Chicago, IL 60648
Forceps, Magill, Child and Adult	Magill Forceps, Adult and Child	SMS, Inc. Columbia, MD 21044
Forceps, with Teeth	Toothed Forceps	Merit Misdome-Frank Corp. New York, NY 10003
Forceps, Tissue	Adson Tissue Pliers	Hu-Friedy Manufacturing Chicago, IL 60618
Gauze, Antibacterial Impregnated	Xeroform	American Hospital Co. American Hospital Supply Corp. McGaw Park, IL 60085
Gauze, Bandage, Sterile Conforming	Kling	Johnson & Johnson Products, Inc. New Brunswick, NJ 08903

Equipment and Supplies Manufacturers *(continued)*

Description	Trade Name	Manufacturer or Supplier
Gauze, Finger Roll	Kendall Kerlix Roll, Narrow	Kendall Co. Boston, MA 02101
Gauze, Iodine Impregnated	NuGauze	Johnson & Johnson Products, Inc. New Brunswick, NJ 08903
Gauze, Iodoform	NuGauze Iodoform Packing Strip	Henry Schein Pharmaceutical Port Washington, NY 11050
Gauze, Petroleum Jelly	Petroleum Gel Gauze	Sherwood Medical Co. St. Louis, MO 63103
Gauze, Roller	Kendall Kerlix Roll, Narrow	Kendall Co. Boston, MA 02101
Gel, Electrode	ECG Gel Pads	3M Co. Medical Products Div. St. Paul, MN 55144
Gloves, Examination (Non-sterile)	Flexam Floor/Exam Latex Gloves	American-Pharmaseal Co. Div. of American Hospital Supply Corp. Valencia, CA 91355
Gloves, Sterile	Neutralon Sterile Brown Surgical Gloves-Hypoallergenic	Surgikos, Inc. (A Johnson & Johnson Co.) Arlington, TX 76010
Goggles	Flexible Cover Goggle	Sellstrom Manufacturing Co. Palatine, IL 60067
Gun, Ear Piercing	Coren Ear Piercing Instrument	New England Medical Specialties Quincy, MA 02169
Hammer, Reflex	Percussion Hammer	Henry Schein, Inc. Port Washington, NY 11050
Handle, Laryngoscope	Laryngoscope Handle	Blue Ridge Anesthesia and Critical Care, Inc. Lynchburg, VA 24502
Handle, Scalpel	Scalpel Knife	Bard Parker Becton-Dickinson and Co. Lincoln Park, NJ 07035
Hemostat, Curved	Kelly Curved Hemostat	Hu-Friedy Manufacturing Chicago, IL 60618
Holder, Needle	Crile Wood Needle Holder	Hu-Friedy Manufacturing Chicago, IL 60618
Hood, Oxygen	Oxygen Hood	Shiley, Inc. Irvine, CA 92716
Hook, Blunt Right-Angled	Right Angle Pick	Storz Instrument Co. St. Louis, MO 63122
Inclinometer	Scoliometer	Orthopedic Systems, Inc. Hayward, CA 94545
Inhaler, Metered Dose (Albuterol)	Proventil Inhaler	Schering Corp. Kenilworth, NJ 07033

Equipment and Supplies Manufacturers *(continued)*

Description	Trade Name	Manufacturer or Supplier
Inhaler, Metered Dose (Beclomethasone Dipropionate)	Beclovent Inhaler	Glaxo, Inc. Research Triangle Park, NC 27709
Inhaler, Metered Dose (Cromolyn)	Intal Inhaler	Fisons Corp. Bedford, MA 01730
Instrument, Doppler Ultrasound	Ultrasound Stethoscope	Medasonics Mountain View, CA 94039
Intravenous Set with Tubing	Intravenous Solution Administration Set	Travenol Laboratories, Inc. Deerfield, IL 60015
Ipecac, Syrup of	Ipecac Syrup, USP Emetic	Pharmaceutical Associates, Inc. Greenville, SC 29605
Jelly, Lubricating	Surgical Lubricant Sterile Bacteriostatic	E. Fougera and Co. Div. of Altana, Inc. Melville, NY 11747
Jelly, Lubricating Water Soluble	K-Y Lubricating Jelly	General Medical Corp. Richmond, VA 23261
Jelly, Lubricating with Lidocaine	Xylocaine (2% Lidocaine HCl) Jelly	Astra Pharmaceutical Products, Inc. Westborough, MA 01581
Jelly, Petroleum	Surgilube	E. Fougera and Co. Div. of Altana, Inc. Melville, NY 11747
Kit, Bone Marrow Biopsy	Monoject Bone Marrow Biopsy Tray	General Medical Corp. Richmond, VA 23261
Kit, Clear Adhesive Tape Test	Diagnostic Tapes	J.B. Roerig Div. Pfizer Pharmaceuticals New York, NY 10017
Kits, Epinephrine Emergency	Anakit	Hollister-Stier Laboratory Div. of Cutter Lab., Inc. Spokane, WA 99207
Kits, Epinephrine Emergency	Epi-Pen	Center Laboratories Div. of EM Industries, Inc. Port Washington, NY 11050
Knife, Myringotomy	Myringotomy Knife	Richards Medical Co. Memphis, TN 38116
Lamp, Alcohol	Alcohol Lamp	Baxter Healthcare Corp. Columbia, MD 21045
Lamp, Wood's	Wood's Lamp	Burton Div. of Cooper Van Nuys, CA 91406
Lidocaine (1%)	Lidocaine (1%) (HCl Injectable, USP)	Abbott Laboratories North Chicago, IL 60064
Lubricant	Surgilube Sterile Bacteriostatic Surgical Lubricant	E. Fougera and Co. Div. of Altana, Inc. Melville, NY 11747
Lubricant, Ultrasound	Aquasonic 100 Ultrasound Transmission Gel	Parker, Inc. Orange, NJ 07050

Equipment and Supplies Manufacturers *(continued)*

Description	Trade Name	Manufacturer or Supplier
Lubricant, Water Soluble	K-Y Lubricating Jelly	General Medical Corp. Richmond, VA 23261
Lumbar Puncture Set	Lumbar Puncture Tray	American Pharmaseal Co. American Hospital Supply Co. Valencia, CA 91355
Magnifier, Hand Held	Hand Held Magnifier	Bausch and Lomb Optical Co. Rochester, NY 14692
Mask, Face	Face Mask	Hospitak, Inc. Lindenhurst, NY 11757
Mask, Simple Face	Airlife Aerosol Mask, Pediatric	American Pharmaseal Co. Valencia, CA 91355
Mask, Non-rebreathing	Non-rebreathing Oxygen Mask	Hospitak, Inc. Lindenhurst, NY 11757
Mask, Ventilation • Fitted Mask • Circular Infant Mask • Pocket Mask	Non-rebreathing Oxygen Mask	Hospitak, Inc. Lindenhurst, NY 11757
Mask, Venturi	Venturi Air Entrainment Oxygen Mask	Hospitak, Inc. Lindenhurst, NY 11757
Measure, Tape	Tape, Measuring, Cloth Double Scale	Graham-Field, Inc. Hauppauge, NY 11788
Medium, Dermatophyte Test	ACU-DTM	Acuderm, Inc. Fort Lauderdale, FL 33314
Methanol (95%)	Methanol	Fisher Scientific Fair Lawn, NJ 07410
Microlancet	Microlance	Becton-Dickinson and Co. Rutherford, NJ 07070
Mirror, Head	Head Mirror	Storz Instrument Co. St. Louis, MO 63122
Moleskin (Adhesive-backed)	Moleskin, Adhesive, Tinted, 4 inches × 4 yds.	Johnson & Johnson Products, Inc. New Brunswick, NJ 08903
Monitor, Cardiac	Hemodynamic Monitor	Hewlett-Packard Rockville, MD 20850
Monitor, Oscillometric Vital Signs	Dinamap Vital Signs Monitor	Critikon Sub. of Johnson & Johnson Tampa, FL 33614
Mouthpiece, Plastic	Capillary Pipette	Becton-Dickinson and Co. Rutherford, NJ 07070
Mouthpiece, T-tube attachment	T-tube connector	Hospitak, Inc. Lindenhurst, NY 11757
Nebulizer	Pulmosonic	The DeVilbiss Co. Somerset, PA 15501
Needle	Monoject Hypodermic Needle	Monoject Div. of Sherwood Medical St. Louis, MO 63103

Equipment and Supplies Manufacturers *(continued)*

Description	Trade Name	Manufacturer or Supplier
Needle, Bone Biopsy	Jamshidi Bone Marrow Biopsy Needle	American-Pharmaseal Co. Div. of American Hospital Supply Corp. Valencia, CA 91355
Needle, Bone Marrow	Osgood Bone Marrow Needle	Owens and Minor, Inc. Richmond, VA 23230
Needle, Butterfly	Butterfly Infusion Set	Abbott Laboratories Inc. North Chicago, IL 60064
Needle, Butterfly Heparin Lock Plastic Cap	Intermittent Infusion Set	Abbott Laboratories Inc. North Chicago, IL 60064
Needle Holder	Crile Wood Needle Holder	Hu-Friedy Manufacturing Chicago, IL 60618
Needle, 23- or 24-gauge Intercath	IV Catheter Placement Unit	Critikon Sub. of Johnson & Johnson Tampa, FL 33614
Needle, Spinal	Spinal Needle	Becton-Dickinson and Co. Rutherford, NJ 07070
Nitrate, Pilocarpine	0.5% Pilo-Gel Discs	Wescor, Inc. Logan, UT 84321
Nitrate, Sodium	Sodium Nitrate	Advanced Instruments, Inc. Needham Heights, MA 02194
Nitrogen, Liquid	Liquid Nitrogen	Air and Chemical Products, Inc. Bladensburg, MD 20710
Occluder	Occluder	R.O. Golden Elkins Park, PA 19117
Oil, Immersion	Immersion Oil	Image Systems, Inc. Columbia, MD 21044
Oil, Mineral	Muri-Lube Mineral Oil	Lymphomed, Inc. Rosemont, IL 60018
Ointment, Antibacterial	Triple Antibiotic Ointment	NMC Laboratories, Inc. Glendale, NY 11385
Ointment, Bland	Vaseline Petroleum Jelly	Chesebrough-Ponds, Inc. Greenwich, CT 06830
Ointment, Povidone-Iodine	Operand Povidone-Iodine Ointment	Redi-Products Prichard, WV 25555
Ointment, Zinc Oxide	Zinc Oxide	Pharmaderm Melville, NY 11747
Otoscope • Diagnostic Head • Operating Head	Halogen Diagnostic Otoscope Halogen Operating Otoscope	Welch Allyn Skaneateles Falls, NY 13153
Oximeter	Pulse Oximeter	Blue Ridge Anesthesia and Critical Care, Inc. Lynchburg, VA 24502
Pad, Gauze, 2 × 2 inches	2 × 2 inches, 8-Ply Gauze Sponge	Johnson & Johnson Products, Inc. New Brunswick, NJ 08903

Equipment and Supplies Manufacturers *(continued)*

Description	Trade Name	Manufacturer or Supplier
Pad, Gauze, 4 × 4 inches	4 × 4 inches, 12-Ply Gauze Sponge	Johnson & Johnson Products, Inc. New Brunswick, NJ 08903
Pad, Isopropyl Alcohol	Medi-Pak Disposable Absorbent Prep Pad	General Medical Corp. Richmond, VA 23228
Pad, Oval Eye Sterile	Oval Eye Pad	Johnson & Johnson Products, Inc. New Brunswick, NJ 08903
Pad, Povidone-Iodine	Betadine Solution Swab Aid	Purdue-Frederick Co. Norwalk, CT 06856
Pad, Rubber (Crutch Handgrips)	Pads, Rubber Handgrips	Guardian Products, Inc. Sun Valley, CA 91352
Pad, Rubber (Crutch Tops)	Pads, Rubber Underarm Cushions	Guardian Products, Inc. Sun Valley, CA 91352
Pad, Waterproof, Disposable	Durasorb Underpads	Professional Medical Products, Inc. Greenwood, SC 29646
Padding, Cotton	Sof-rol Orthopaedic Padding, 4 in. × 4 yd.	Johnson & Johnson Products, Inc. New Brunswick, NJ 08903
Paddle, Defibrillator	Defibrillator Paddles, 4.5 cm/8 cm	Biomedical Specialties Crofton, MD 21114
Paper, Filter	Filter Paper	Curtin Matheson Scientific, Inc. Beltsville, MD 20705
Paper, pH	pH Test Paper	Baxter Healthcare Corp. Columbia, MD 21045
Paper, pH (Broad Range)	pHydrion Instant-Chek 0-13	Micro Essential Laboratory Brooklyn, NY 11210
Paper, Scale	Advent Baby Scale Protector	Baxter Hospital Supply Div. McGaw Park, IL 60085
Patch, Flesh Colored, Adhesive Backed	Opticlude	3M Personal Care Products St. Paul, MN 55144
Pen, Surgical Marking	Securline	Precision Dynamics Corp. Bath, PA 18104
Petrolatum	Petrolatum	E. Fougera and Co. Melville, NY 11747
Phenylephrine Hydrochloride (¼%)	AK-Dilate	Akorn, Inc. Abita Springs, LA 70420
Pins, Safety (Large)	Safety Pins, Large	Owens and Minor, Inc. Richmond, VA 23230
Podophyllin in Tincture of Benzoin	Podoban	Pharmaceutical Manufacturers Maurry Biological Co. Los Angeles, CA 90047
Polymyxin B-bacitracin	Polysporin	Burroughs Wellcome Co. Research Triangle Park, NC 27709
PPD	Tubersol Tuberculin Purified Protein Derivative (Mantoux) (PPD)	Connaught Laboratories, Inc. Swift Water, PA 18370
Probe	Probe	General Medical Corp. Richmond, VA 23228

Equipment and Supplies Manufacturers *(continued)*

Description	Trade Name	Manufacturer or Supplier
Proparacaine HCl	Alcaine	Alcon, Inc. Humacao, PR 00701
Restraints, Ankle	Vel-Cro Restraints, Posey Limb Holders	J.T. Posey Corp. Arcadia, CA 91006
Restraints, Elbow	"No-No" Arm-Elbow Restraints	H & H Research Birmingham, MI 48009
Restraints, Wrist	"Lamb's Wool" Restraints (buckle)	Skill-Care Corp. Yonkers, NY 10701
Roll, Elastic Bandage	Ace Wrap	Kendall Healthcare Mansfield, MA 02048
Scale, Basket or Pan	Olympic Smart Scale	Olympic Medical Seattle, WA 98108
Scale, Platform Manual	Detecto Pediatric Scale	Baxter Hospital Supply Div. Baxter Healthcare Corp. McGaw Park, IL 60085
Scale, Platform Electronic	Acme Infant Scale	Baxter Hospital Supply Div. Baxter Healthcare Corp. McGaw Park, IL 60085
Scarifier, Metal	Sterile Metal Scarifier	Johnson & Johnson Co. Sommerville, NJ 08876
Scarifier, Plastic	Disposable Plastic Scarifier	Greer Laboratory Lenior, NC 28645
Scissors, Bandage	Bandage Scissors, 5.5 inch	McCoy Surgical Supplies Maryland Heights, MO 63043
Scissors, Iris	Straight Iris Scissors, 4.5 inch	McCoy Surgical Supplies Maryland Heights, MO 63043
Scissors, Metzenbaum	Metzenbaum Scissors, Standard Pattern	Henry Schein, Inc. Port Washington, NY 11050
Scissors, Small	Straight Iris Scissors	McCoy Surgical Supplies Maryland Heights, MO 63043
Scissors, Straight	Straight Scissors	Baxter Healthcare Corp. V. Mueller Div. McGaw Park, IL 60085
Scissors, Surgical	Surgical Scissors, 5.5 inch	McCoy Surgical Supplies Maryland Heights, MO 63043
Scissors, Suture	Kelly Curved Tissue Scissors	Hu-Friedy Manufacturing Chicago, IL 60618
Scissors, Universal	Universal Scissors	DuPuy Warsaw, IN 47801
Scraper	Fingernail File	Jonel Div. of Barristos, Ltd. Chicago, IL 60611
Sealer, Clay	Critoseal	Monoject Div. of Sherwood Medical St. Louis, MO 63122

Equipment and Supplies Manufacturers *(continued)*

Description	Trade Name	Manufacturer or Supplier
Shield, Fox	Storz E-5691 A50	Storz Ophthalmic Instrument Co. St. Louis, MO 63122
Sigmoidoscope, Flexible	Flexible Sigmoidoscope	Olympus Corp. Columbia, MD 21045
Sigmoidoscope, Rigid	Rigid Sigmoidoscope	Welch Allyn Skaneateles Falls, NY 13153
Slides, Glass Microscope	Microscope Slides	General Scientific Richmond, VA 23228
Slide, Occult Blood Detection	Hemoccult Slide	SmithKline Diagnostics, Inc. A SmithKline Beckman Co. Sunnyvale, CA 94088
Sling (Commercial)	Standard Arm Sling	Orthomedic Jefferson City, TN 37760
Solution, Buffered Saline	Diluent	Hollister-Stier Div. of Miles Labs, Inc. Spokane, WA 99220
Solution, Buffered Saline with Phenol	Buffered Saline with Phenol	Hollister-Stier Div. of Miles Labs, Inc. Spokane, WA 99220
Solution, Formalin (10%)	10% Neutral Buffered Formalin	Richard-Allan Medical Industries Richland, MI 49083
Solution, Heparin	Heparin Sodium Injection USP	Elkins-Sinn, Inc. Cherry Hill, NJ 08034
Solution, Histamine Acid Phosphate	Histamine Acid Phosphate	Center Laboratories Port Washington, NY 11050
Solution, Hydrogen Peroxide	Hydrogen Peroxide	Whittaker General Medical Richmond, VA 23228
Solution, Lactated Ringer's	Intravenous Injection Solution	Travenol Laboratories, Inc. Deerfield, IL 60015
Solution, Ophthalmic Irrigating	Dacriose	Iolab Pharmaceuticals Div. of Iolab Corp. A Johnson & Johnson Co. Claremont, CA 91711
Solution, Potassium Hydroxide (10%)	KOH	J.T. Baker Chemical Co. Phillipsburg, NJ 08865
Solution, Povidone-Iodine	Povadyne	Acme/Chaston Dayville, CT 06241
Solution, Povidone-Iodine Scrub	Povidone-Iodine Scrub Solution	Purdue-Frederick Norwalk, CT 06850
Solution, Saline Irrigation	0.9% Sodium Chloride Irrigation USP	Travenol Laboratories, Inc. Deerfield, IL 60015
Solution, Saline Non-Bacteriostatic	Non-Bacteriostatic 0.9% Sodium Chloride, Injectable	Lymphomed, Inc. Rosemont, IL 60018
Solution, Saline Sterile	Sterile Saline	Travenol Laboratories, Inc. Deerfield, IL 60015

Equipment and Supplies Manufacturers *(continued)*

Description	Trade Name	Manufacturer or Supplier
Spacer	Aerochamber	Forrest Pharmaceuticals, Inc. St. Louis, MO 63043
Spacer	Inhalaid or InspirEase	Key Pharmaceuticals, Inc. Miami, FL 33269
Spatula, Cytology, Wooden	Cytology Scraper	Baxter Healthcare Corp. Scientific Products Div. McGaw Park, IL 60085
Spatula, Platinum	No. E-1091	Storz Ophthalmic Instrument Co. St. Louis, MO 63122
Specula, Veterinary Otoscope	Veterinary Otoscope Speculars (4, 5, 7, 9 inches)	Welch Allyn Skaneateles Falls, NY 13153
Speculum, Bivalved Nasal	Guillord-Wright Speculum	Storz Instrument Co. St. Louis, MO 63122
Speculum, Nasal	Vienna Speculum	Storz Instrument Co. St. Louis, MO 63122
Speculum, Vaginal • Child Size	Pedersen Vaginal Specula Small ½ × 3 inches	Miltex Owens and Minor, Inc. Richmond, VA 23230
• Pederson	Pederson Vaginal Specula Small, ½ × 3 inches Medium, ⅞ × 4 inches Large, 1 × 4¾ inches	Miltex Owens and Minor, Inc. Richmond, VA 23230
• Graves	Graves Vaginal Specula Small, ¾ × 3 inches Medium, 1⅜ × 4 inches Large, 1½ × 4½ inches	Miltex Owens and Minor, Inc. Richmond, VA 23230
• Huffman	Huffman Vaginal Specula	Baxter Healthcare Corp. V. Mueller Div. McGaw Park, IL 60085
Sphygmomanometer	Baumanomet Blood Pressure Standard	W.A. Baum Co., Inc. Copiague, NY 11726
Spirometer	Breon 2400	Spirometrics, Inc. Andover, MA 01810
Spirometer	Vitalograph	Vitalograph Lenexa, KS 66215
Splints, Aluminum	Alumafoam Finger Splint, 9 × ½ inches	Conco Medical Co. Bridgeport, CT 06610
Splints, Bandage (2, 3, 4, or 6 inches)	Elastoplast, Elastic Adhesive Bandage	Belersdorf, Inc. Norwalk, CT 06854
Splints, Canvas and Felt	Padded Splint with Link Adj.	Zimmer-USA Warsaw, IN 46580
Splints, Inflatable	Pressure Splints	J.A. Preston Corp. Clifton, NJ 07012
Splints, Metal	Metal, Finger Splint Strips, 9 × ½ inches	Conco Medical Co. Bridgeport, CT 06610

Equipment and Supplies Manufacturers *(continued)*

Description	Trade Name	Manufacturer or Supplier
Splints, Plaster	Specialist Plaster Bandage, Fast-setting, 3 in. × 3 yd.	Johnson & Johnson Products, Inc. New Brunswick, NJ 08903
Sponge, Absorbable Gelatin	Gelfoam	Upjohn Co. Washington, DC 20013
Spray, Ethyl Chloride	Ethyl Chloride	Gebauer Chemical Co. Cleveland, OH 44104
Spray, Topical Anesthetic	Hurricaine	Beutlich, Inc. Pharmaceuticals Chicago, IL 60645
Spud	Storz E-0840	Storz Ophthalmic Instrument Co. St. Louis, MO 63122
Sticks, Silver Nitrate Cautery	Silver Nitrate Applicators	Graham-Field, Inc. Hauppauge, NY 11788
Stick, Wooden Applicator	Wood Applicator Stick	Solon Manufacturing Co. Solon, ME 04979
Stockinette (3- or 4-inch tube)	Orthopaedic Stockinet	Johnson & Johnson Products, Inc. New Brunswick, NJ 08903
Stockinette, Cotton Tube	Orthopaedic Stockinet, Cotton Tubular, 2 in. × 2.5 yd.	Johnson & Johnson Products, Inc. New Brunswick, NJ 08903
Strips, Fluorescein	Flu-Glo Fluorescein Sodium Ophthalmic Strip, 0.6 mg	Barnes-Hind Pharmaceuticals, Inc. Sunnyvale, CA 94086
Strips, Skin Closure	Steri-Strip Skin Closures	3M Co. 3M Center St. Paul, MN 55101
Strips, Sterile Adhesive Bandage	Curad Plastic Strip Curity (Ouchless)	Colgate-Palmolive Co. New York, NY 10022
Stylet	Stylet, Plastic Disposable, Infant and Adult	Baxter Healthcare Corp. American Hospital Div. Virginia Beach, VA. 23452
Suction Machine, Portable, Electric	Medi-pump Model 5711-130	Schuco New York, NY 10011
Suture, Non-absorbable Material	3-0/4-0 Non-absorbable Suture Material	Owens and Minor, Inc. Richmond, VA 23230
Suture Material	Sutures	Ethicon, Inc. Div. of Johnson & Johnson Summerville, NJ 08876
Suture, Chromic Material	Chromic Gut Suture	Davis-Geck, Inc. Manati, PR 00701
Swab, Calcium Alginate	Calgiswab	Spectrum Diagnostics, Inc. Glenwood, IL 60425
Swab, Cotton-tipped	Medi-Pak Sterile Cotton Tipped Applicator	Whittaker General Medical Richmond, VA 23228
Swab, Cotton-tipped Culture	Q-tips Single Tipped Applicator	Chesebrough-Ponds, Inc. Hospital Products Div. Greenwich, CT 06830

Equipment and Supplies Manufacturers *(continued)*

Description	Trade Name	Manufacturer or Supplier
Swab, Fiber-tipped Applicator	Cotton-tipped Applicator	Whittaker General Medical Richmond, VA 23228
Swab, Fiber-tipped Dual	Culturette	Marion Scientific Kansas, MO 64114
Swab, Povidone-Iodine	Betadine Solution Swab Aid	Purdue-Frederick Co. Norwalk, CT 06856
Swab, Sterile	Calgiswab (Type I)	Spectrum Diagnostics, Inc. Glenwood, IL 60425
Swathe	Shoulder Immobilizer, Velpeau Dressing	Zimmer-USA Warsaw, IN 46580
Syringe	Monoject Luer Lock Syringe	Monoject Div. of Sherwood Medical St. Louis, MO 63103
Syringe, Bulb	Daval Irrigation Syringe	Bard Medsystems North Reading, MA 01864
Syringe, Dental, Blunt Tip	Monoject 412 Syringe	Monoject Div. of Sherwood Medical St. Louis, MO 63103
Syringe, Ear (Irrigating)	All Rubber Ear Syringe	Southeastern Hospital Supply Richmond, VA 23228
Syringe, Tuberculin	Monoject Tuberculin	Monoject Div. of Sherwood Medical St. Louis, MO 63103
Tape, Adhesive	Orthaletic Porous Tape	Professional Medical Products, Inc. Greenwood, SC 29646
Tape, Adhesive Clear	Scotch Magic Tape	3M Co. Commercial Office Supply St. Paul, MN 55144
Tape, Measuring Non-stretchable	Inser-Tape Ross Insertion Tape	Ross Laboratories Columbus, OH 43216
Tape, Non-Allergenic	Blenderm	3M Co. Medical Products Div. St. Paul, MN 55101
Tape, 1-Inch Silk or Cloth	Dermiform Hypoallergenic Knitted Tape	Johnson & Johnson Patient Care, Inc. New Brunswick, NJ 08903
Tape, Paper	Micropore	3M Co. Medical Products Div. St. Paul, MN 55144
Tape, Tracheostomy Twill	Tracheostomy Twill Cloth Tape	Owens and Minor, Inc. Richmond, VA 23230
Tent, Oxygen	Oxygen Tent	Ohmeda Medical Madison, WI 53707
Test, Tine	Tuberculin Tine Test	Lederle Laboratories Div. American Cyanamid Co. Pearl River, NY 10965

Equipment and Supplies Manufacturers *(continued)*

Description	Trade Name	Manufacturer or Supplier
Tetracaine 2%	Pontocaine	Winthrop-Breon Div. of Sterling Drug, Inc. New York, NY 10016
Thermometer, Electronic	Diatek 600 Thermometer System	Diatek Inc. San Diego, CA 92121
Thermometer, Mercury	Thermometer (Fahrenheit or Centigrade Scales)	Becton-Dickinson and Co. Rutherford, NJ 07070
Tips, Metal Suction	House-Baron Suction Tube	Storz Instrument Co. St. Louis, MO 63122
Tips, Rubber (Crutch Bottoms)	Tips, Rubber Crutch Floor Grips	Guardian Products, Inc. Sun Valley, CA 91352
Tourniquets • Small Drainage Tubing	Penrose Drain Tube	Southeastern Hospital Supply Richmond, VA 23228
• 1-Inch Flat Rubber Strips	Hygienic Tourniquet Straps	Hygienic Corp. Akron, OH 44310
Transilluminator, Cranial	Neoscan	Sylvan Corp. Irwin, PA 15642
Transilluminator, Sinus	Halogen Transilluminator	Welch Allyn Skaneateles Falls, NY 13153
Trap, Collection	Juhn Tym-Tap Middle Ear Fluid Aspirator/Collector	Xomed, Inc. Jacksonville, FL 32216
Tube, Collection (Hematocrit/Capillary)	Heparinized Capillary Tube	Columbia Diagnostics, Inc. Springfield, VA 22153
Tube, Collection (Milliliter)	Microtainer Tube	Becton-Dickinson, Inc. Rutherford, NJ 07070
Tube, Culture	Culture Tube, Plastic, Sterile, Screwtop, Black	Becton-Dickinson, Inc. Rochelle Park, NJ 07662
Tube, Endotracheal	Endotracheal Tube	Portex, Inc. Wilmington, MA 01887
Tube, Feeding	Feeding Tube Number 5	Argyle, Div. of Sherwood Medical St. Louis, MO 63103
Tube, Nasogastric	Stomach Tube	Argyle, Div. of Sherwood Medical St. Louis, MO 63103
Tube, Orogastric Lavage	Orotracheal Lavage Tube	Ohmeda Medical Madison, WI 53707
Tube, Orotracheal Uncuffed	Orotracheal Uncuffed Tube	Ohmeda Medical Madison, WI 53707
Tube, Polyvinyl Chloride, Silastic or Polyurethane	Enteral Intubation Tube (Endotracheal Tube)	Portex, Inc. Wilmington, MA 01887
T-tube	T-tube Connector	Hospitak, Inc. Lindenhurst, NY 11757

Equipment and Supplies Manufacturers *(continued)*

Description	Trade Name	Manufacturer or Supplier
Tube, Test	Test Tube	Corning R & D Fisher Scientific Columbia, MD 21046
Tubing, Intravenous Connector	Intravenous Connector Tubing (*without* Secure Lock)	Abbott Laboratories Inc. North Chicago, IL 60064
Tubing, Oxygen Administration	Airlife Crush Resistant Oxygen Tubing	American Pharmaseal Co. Div. of American Hospital Supply Co. Valencia, CA 91355
Tubing, Suction	Argyle Non-conductive Connective Tubing	Argyle, Div. of Sherwood Medical St. Louis, MO 63103
Tweezers	Forceps, Thumb Plain, 4.5 inches	SMS Products Owens and Minor, Inc. Richmond, VA 23230
Unit, Air Compressor, Portable	Maxi-Mist Compressor	Mead Johnson Laboratories Evansville, IN 47721
Unit, Air Compressor, Portable	Pulmo-Aide	The DeVilbiss Co. Somerset, PA 15501
Wick, Otic	Oto-Wick (Ear Wick)	Xomed, Inc. Jacksonville, FL 32216
Wire, Stiffening	Keofeed Tube 7.3	Chesebrough-Ponds, Inc. Greenwich, CT 06830
Wrap, Clear Plastic	Saran Wrap	Dow Brands Inc. Indianapolis, IN 46268

Index

Page numbers followed by t or f indicates tables or figures, respectively.

ISBN 0-397-50897-2

90000

9 780397 508976